Atlas of General Thoracic Surgery

MARK M. RAVITCH, M.D.
Professor of Surgery
University of Pittsburgh
Surgeon-in-Chief Emeritus
Montefiore Hospital
Pittsburgh, Pennsylvania

FELICIEN M. STEICHEN, M.D.
Professor of Surgery
New York Medical College
Valhalla, New York

Illustrator
LEON SCHLOSSBERG
Associate Professor of
Art As Applied To Medicine
The Johns Hopkins Medical School
Baltimore, Maryland

1988
W. B. SAUNDERS COMPANY
Harcourt Brace Jovanovich, Inc.

Philadelphia • London • Toronto
Montreal • Sydney • Tokyo

W. B. SAUNDERS COMPANY
Harcourt Brace Jovanovich, Inc.

West Washington Square
Philadelphia, PA 19105

Library of Congress Cataloging-in-Publication Data

Ravitch, Mark M., 1910–

Atlas of general thoracic surgery.

1. Chest—Surgery—Atlases.   I. Steichen, Felicien M.,
    1926–   II. Title.   [DNLM: 1. Thoracic
    Surgery—atlases. WF 17 R256a]

RD536.R38 1988   617′.54   87–4946

ISBN 0–7216–7474–7

Editor: Dean Manke
Designer: W. B. Saunders Staff
Production Manager: Carolyn Naylor
Manuscript Editor: Linda Mills
Illustration Coordinator: Walt Verbitski
Page Layout Artist: W. B. Saunders Staff
Indexer: Ann Cassar

Atlas of General Thoracic Surgery   ISBN 0–7216–7474–7

Last digit is the print number: 9   8   7   6   5   4   3   2   1

PREFACE

already in existence drawings made by Mr. Schlossberg for colleagues now or formerly at Johns Hopkins. It seemed appropriate to use these rather than to make new drawings of the same procedures by the same artist. We are grateful to the original publishers and to our colleagues for their permission and for supplying the original drawings—in one instance removed for the purpose from its place of honor, framed and hanging on the wall of a surgeon's study. The specific attributions are in each case to be found in the accompanying legends.

Selected references to the literature, not always a routine matter in atlases, we have chosen to include for a number of reasons—to cite the historic early papers, the classical later papers, or the particularly clear or lucid papers of whatever period, or because the papers were presented at meetings at which the discussion threw light on the state of the art at the time, and the arguments about a procedure or technique.

ACKNOWLEDGMENTS

This book has been in work since October 1977 and we are grateful to Mr. Robert B. Rowan, then Executive Vice President of W. B. Saunders Company, for the original encouragement and his decision to accept a work of this scope and size and complexity of production. Subsequently, Mr. Carroll C. Cann, then Executive Editor, patiently and wisely counseled us and continued the warm support we have always found at W. B. Saunders. Mr. Dean J. Manke, Medical Editor of Saunders, continued in the understanding, tolerance, and cooperativeness of his predecessors and saw the work to its completion. Linda Mills did a superb and understanding job of copy editing and Karen O'Keefe was imaginative, efficient, and accommodating in the design of the book. Mr. Walter Verbitski's efforts with Mr. Schlossberg's superb illustrations are particularly appreciated. We are indebted to Miss Carolyn Naylor for her care and splendid supervision of the overall production of the book.

Ruth Jacobson, an Editorial Assistant without peer, and Mary Beth Madalinsky have tirelessly typed and retyped, tracked down the literature, corrected references, uncomplainingly accepted revisions and reorganization, and kept flawless track of the many illustrations, protecting them from harm over the years. We are enormously grateful to them both.

CONTENTS

CONTENTS

THE TRACHEA

293

Dr. Hermes Grillo

Anatomy

Anatomy

RIGHT ANTERIOR OBLIQUE VIEW OF TORSO

A. Superficial view of the musculature. The pectoral muscles often approach the midline more closely than shown, particularly superiorly. The gap between the sternal and clavicular heads of the sternocleidomastoid is variable and frequently not as pronounced as shown. The width and shape of the costal arch, the angle of the arch made by the 10th cartilage in the nipple line, and the manner in which the 8th, 9th, or 10th cartilages attach to each other and to the sternum are subject to great variation.

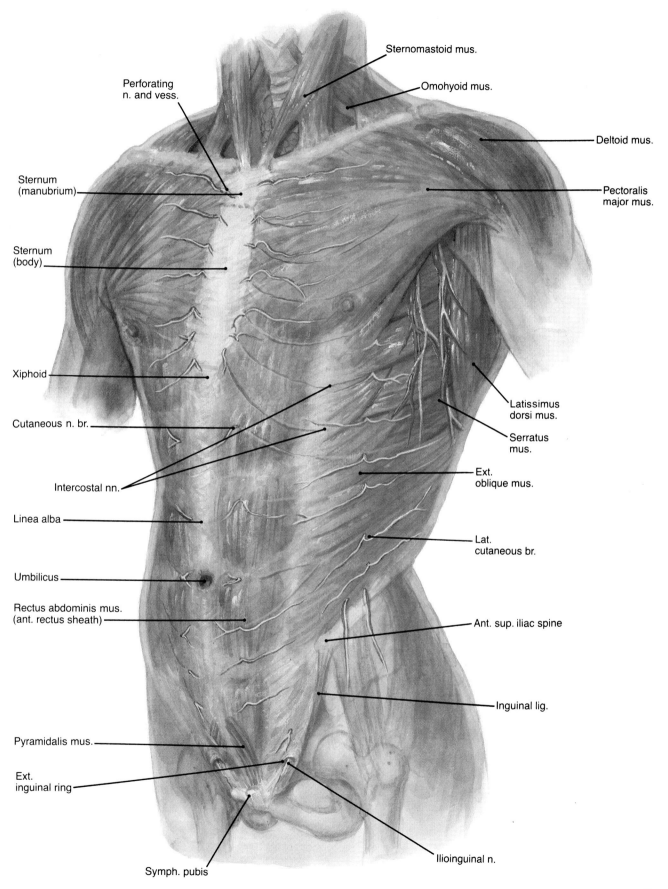

Sternomastoid mus.

Omohyoid mus.

Perforating
n. and vess.

Deltoid mus.

Sternum
(manubrium)

Pectoralis
major mus.

Sternum
(body)

Xiphoid

Latissimus
dorsi mus.

Cutaneous n. br.

Serratus
mus.

Intercostal nn.

Ext.
oblique mus.

Linea alba

Lat.
cutaneous br.

Umbilicus

Rectus abdominis mus.
(ant. rectus sheath)

Ant. sup. iliac spine

Inguinal lig.

Pyramidalis mus.

Ext.
inguinal ring

Ilioinguinal n.

Symph. pubis

3

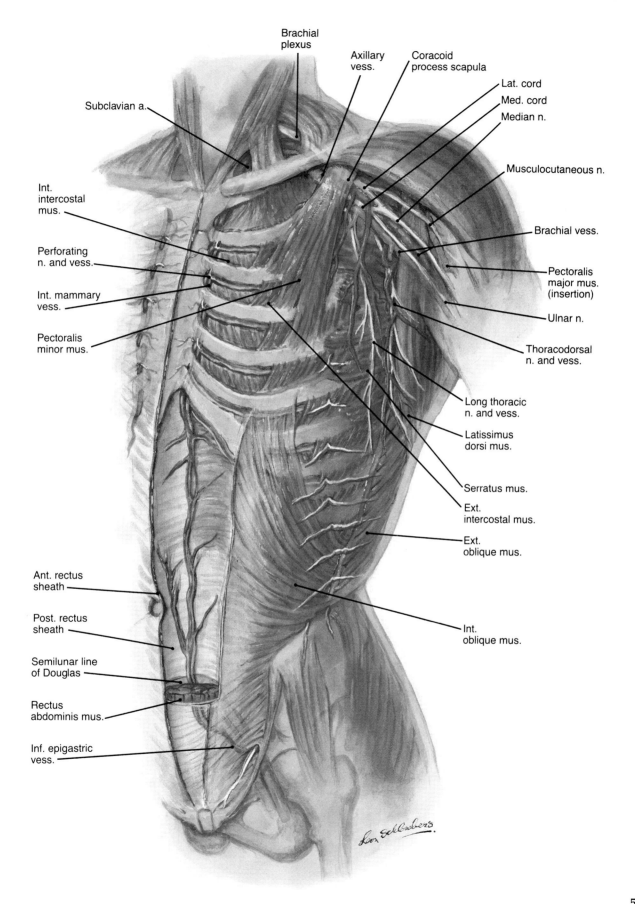

Brachial plexus

Axillary vess.

Coracoid process scapula

Lat. cord

Med. cord

Median n.

Musculocutaneous n.

Subclavian a.

Int. intercostal mus.

Perforating n. and vess.

Int. mammary vess.

Pectoralis minor mus.

Brachial vess.

Pectoralis major mus. (insertion)

Ulnar n.

Thoracodorsal n. and vess.

Long thoracic n. and vess.

Latissimus dorsi mus.

Serratus mus.

Ext. intercostal mus.

Ext. oblique mus.

Ant. rectus sheath

Post. rectus sheath

Semilunar line of Douglas

Rectus abdominis mus.

Inf. epigastric vess.

Int. oblique mus.

POSTERIOR ANATOMICAL VIEW

The right shoulder is elevated, rotating and elevating the scapula. Portions of the latissimus dorsi and the trapezius have been removed. The rhomboids are shown on stretch but not divided. Sections of four ribs have been removed together with the overlying spinal muscles to show the intercostal nerves, the spinal ganglia, the sympathetic rami, the sympathetic trunk, and the greater splanchnic nerve.

Incisions (See also *Thoracic Incisions,* pages 110–155)

Note that a median sternotomy involves no muscle division and that an anterior thoracotomy must necessarily divide and split fibers of the pectoralis major and minor, unless one chooses to divide their costal attachments and reflect them upward. The formal posterolateral thoracotomy, in its anterior extent, usually comes below the pectoralis major. Posteriorly, it necessarily transects a portion of the trapezius and of the rhomboids and the whole of the latissimus dorsi, denervating the portion distal to the level at which the thoracodorsal nerve is transected, and divides the distal portion of the long thoracic, denervating the lower portions of the serratus.

In connection with operation for congenital deformities of the chest wall, note particularly that cephalad the anterior sheath of the rectus fuses with the pectoralis major fascia and the sternum and 5th costal cartilage, the superior belly of the rectus being attached usually to cartilages V, VI, and VII.

The lateral (axillary) thoracotomy is made in the interval between pectoralis major and latissimus dorsi. It can be extended anteriorly and posteriorly under those muscles. The latissimus dorsi may be incised a short distance to permit wide distraction of the ribs. The nerves are retracted and spared.

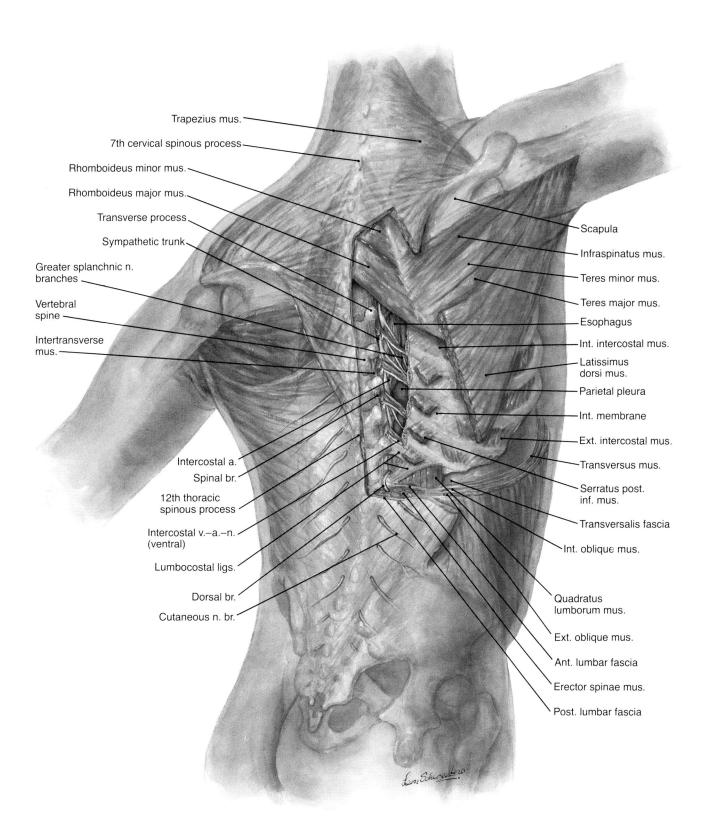

Trapezius mus.

7th cervical spinous process

Rhomboideus minor mus.

Rhomboideus major mus.

Transverse process

Sympathetic trunk

Greater splanchnic n. branches

Vertebral spine

Intertransverse mus.

Intercostal a.

Spinal br.

12th thoracic spinous process

Intercostal v.–a.–n. (ventral)

Lumbocostal ligs.

Dorsal br.

Cutaneous n. br.

Scapula

Infraspinatus mus.

Teres minor mus.

Teres major mus.

Esophagus

Int. intercostal mus.

Latissimus dorsi mus.

Parietal pleura

Int. membrane

Ext. intercostal mus.

Transversus mus.

Serratus post. inf. mus.

Transversalis fascia

Int. oblique mus.

Quadratus lumborum mus.

Ext. oblique mus.

Ant. lumbar fascia

Erector spinae mus.

Post. lumbar fascia

Congenital Deformities

CORRECTION OF PECTUS EXCAVATUM

A. Ordinarily a midline incision is employed, since it is quicker, drier, and does not require mobilization of such large flaps as are necessary for a transverse incision. (In small girls, the submammary incision is employed, slightly arched in the midline, and with the development of the breasts it becomes an essentially concealed incision.) The incision is carried down to the sternum, and with the fine needle–tipped electrocautery, flaps of skin, fat, and pectoralis major are reflected as one. The perforating branches of the internal mammary artery can be seen, clamped, and coagulated. There is essentially no bleeding, and the entire dissection is performed with the electrocautery.

B. The pectoral muscles have been laid back to expose the deformed cartilages for the entire extent of the deformity. The two lowermost cartilages will generally be exposed by making an oblique incision (not shown) through the rectus muscle, which is not detached. The cartilages are excised subperichondrially, after the perichondrium has been incised longitudinally for the full extent of the deformity, and transversely at either end of the longitudinal incision so that rectangular perichondrial flaps can be elevated. If the edges of these flaps are seized with a number of fine hemostats, and traction made upon these, the cartilage can be freed with a delicate elevator such as a Freer.

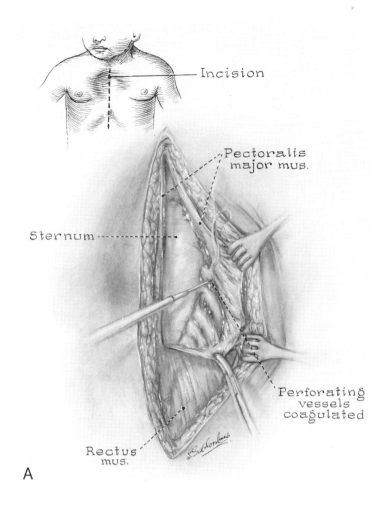

Incision

Pectoralis
major mus.

Sternum

Perforating
vessels
coagulated

Rectus
mus.

A

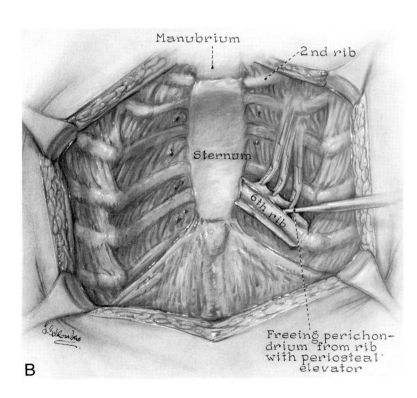

Manubrium

2nd rib

Sternum

6th rib

Freeing perichon-
drium from rib
with periosteal
elevator

B

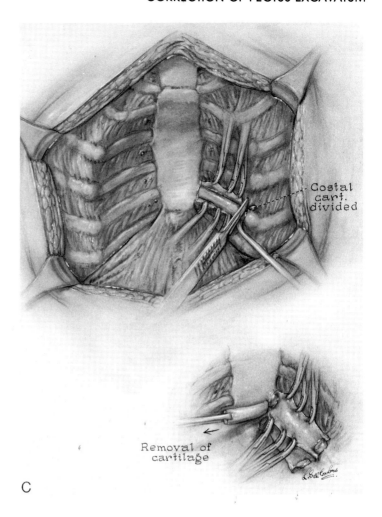

Costal
cart.
divided

Removal of
cartilage

C

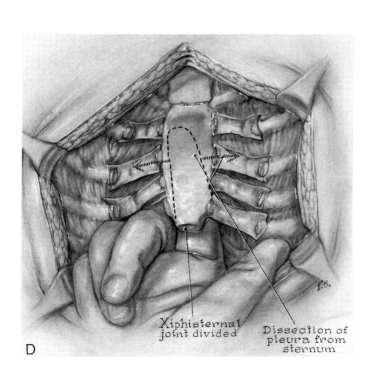

Xiphisternal
joint divided

Dissection of
pleura from
sternum

D

13

CORRECTION OF PECTUS EXCAVATUM *(Continued)*

E. The sternum is elevated with a bone hook, and the intercostal bundles are divided from the sternum by cutting between the internal mammary vessels and the sternal border. A wedge of rib bone (shown) is taken for placement in the sternal osteotomy. Perforating vessels from the internal mammary may bleed and require coagulation.

F. If the sternal osteotomy is performed just above the highest abnormal cartilage, it will be found that the sternal osteotomy will, in fact, be in a portion of the sternum in which the declivity has already begun, and the correction will not be optimal. For this reason, the sternal osteotomy should be performed one interspace higher, and the lowest normal cartilage, sometimes the 3rd, often the 2nd, is divided obliquely, from the front medially to laterally and behind. The intercostal vessels at this level must be secured and the intercostal muscles divided into the upper interspace in order to provide free access to the border of the sternum.

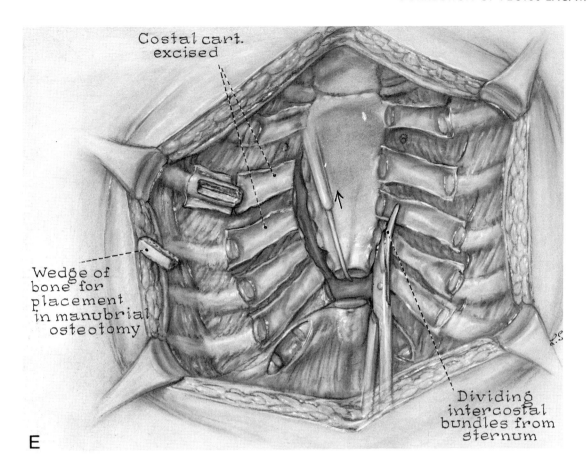

Costal cart. excised

Wedge of bone for placement in manubrial osteotomy

Dividing intercostal bundles from sternum

E

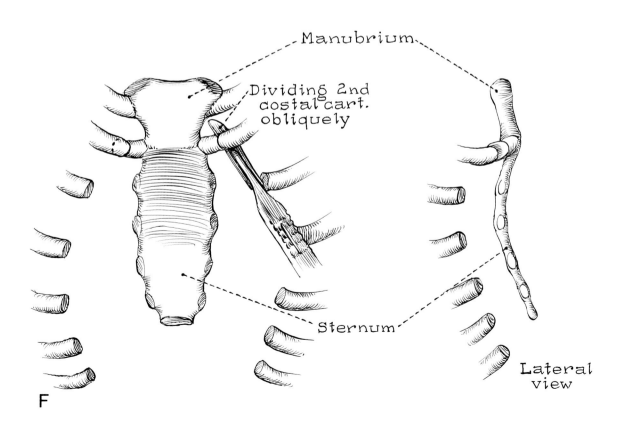

Manubrium

Dividing 2nd costal cart. obliquely

Sternum

Lateral view

F

G. While the sternum is held forward, the posterior cortex is deeply scored in an accurately transverse line in the intercostal space above the obliquely divided cartilage. This brings the new osteotomy site well above the original takeoff of the downward sternal curve. The sternum is now elevated, and the anterior cortical lamella is fractured. The fragment of rib bone, shown removed in E, is transfixed with sutures carried through the anterior sternal cortex and periosteum, and the wedge is firmly secured in place as a chock block. For infants and small children, we remain quite happy with using our original technique of an anterior transverse cuneiform sternal osteotomy closed with heavy sutures through the sternum and additional sutures through the periosteum. With such an anterior sternal osteotomy in older children and in adults, we have noted a tendency of the sternum distal to the osteotomy to slip back after such a procedure, producing a stepdown deformity, probably because the posterior periosteum had been significantly loosened in the operative manipulation.

H. When the sternum is remarkably scaphoid, so that the distal end begins to point anteriorly, the overcorrection resulting from the sternal osteotomy would leave the distal end of the sternum tilted forward undesirably. In such instances, a more distal anterior transverse osteotomy is performed, and another wedge of bone is packed into this to hold it open, correcting the anterior angulation of the distal sternal segment. Additional sutures of heavy silk are placed through-and-through the sternum across the osteotomy site and around the bone block. As the sternum is lifted forward, the sternal ends of the obliquely divided 2nd or 3rd cartilage come to lie upon the lateral ends. Fixation of the sternum is by heavy sutures through the sternum across the osteotomy (one of them passed around the bone block), by sutures in the sternal periosteum, and by sutures through the overlapping cartilage ends on either side. This provides a three-point fixation of the sternal repair—costal cartilage, sternum, costal cartilage. In smaller children, sutures may be forced through the sternum with a heavy needle. In older children and adults, one may need to use an awl or a twist drill to pass a suture (0 silk or equivalent synthetic). To pass the suture through the rib fragment–bone block, we use a Keith needle as a drill, rolled between thumb and finger.

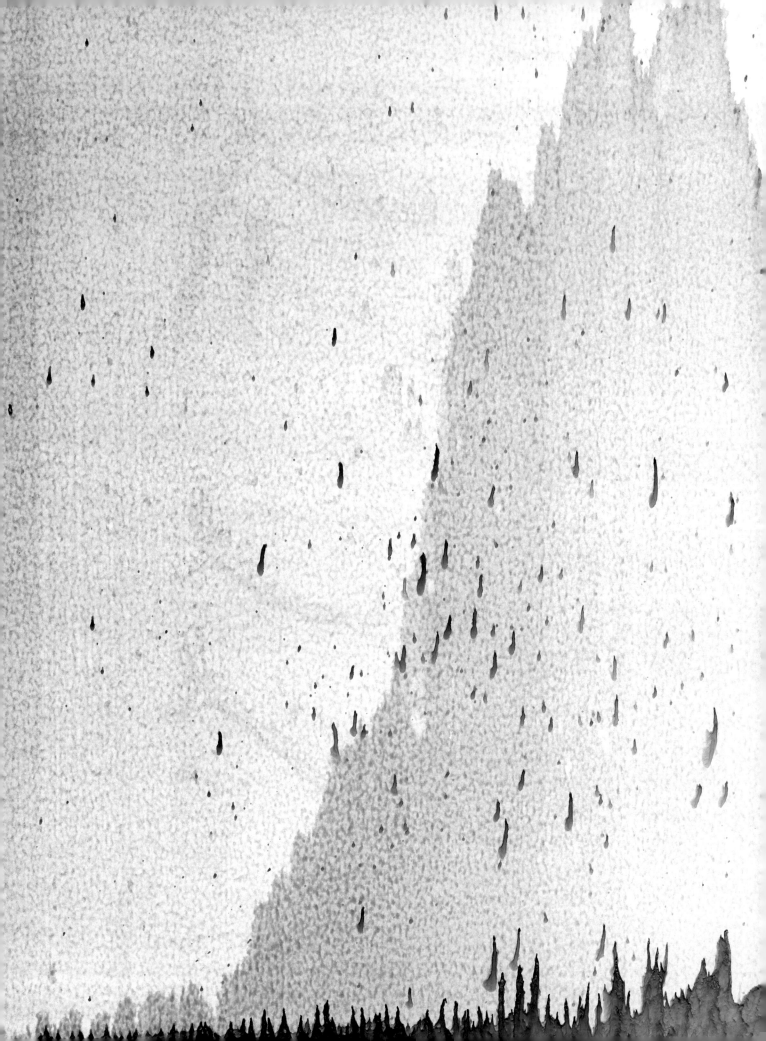

CORRECTION OF PECTUS EXCAVATUM *(Continued)*

I. Although we generally find the repair described in these illustrations all that is required, we do employ internal wire fixation in some special instances: (1) In extremely broad deformities in which unusually long segments of ribs have been resected, and in patients with other cardiac or respiratory problems—this fixation eliminates the paradox seen in the first few days after operation. (2) In adults and large teenagers in whom the length of the sternum would impose excessive leverage on the repair. (3) In recurrences requiring a major reconstruction. The technique pictured is simple and effective. A Kirschner wire or Steinmann pin of caliber appropriate to the subject is drilled through the sternum and cut to proper length; the ends, lying on the chest wall under the pectorals, are closed in loops. Two or three heavy sutures through or around the rib hold the wire in place at each end. The wire may be bent to arch it slightly forward. Occasionally we employ two wires. The wires need not be removed unless they migrate to project against the skin. Then, through a small incision and with the patient under local anesthesia, one loop is cut off and the wire pulled out the other side through another incision.

J. The pectoral muscles are sutured to each other and to the sternal periosteum, and the fat and skin are closed in two or three layers. Closure of the pectoral muscles helps to hold the sternum forward and cushions the midline scar.

In small children, no drain at all is required and any fluid that accumulates may be aspirated percutaneously. With larger operations, we frequently employ a percutaneous mediastinal suction catheter, and in large adolescents and in adults with a large dissection, we deliberately open the right pleura and drain the chest with an intercostal tube.

From Ravitch, M.M.: *Congenital Deformities of the Chest Wall and Their Operative Correction.* Philadelphia, W.B. Saunders Company, 1977, with permission.
Full description of alternative operations and exhaustive bibliography.

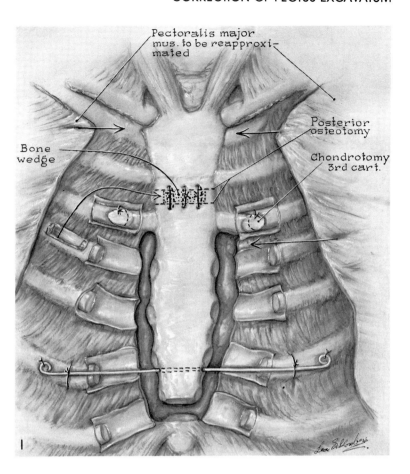

Pectoralis major mus. to be reapproximated

Posterior osteotomy

Chondrotomy 3rd cart.

Bone wedge

I

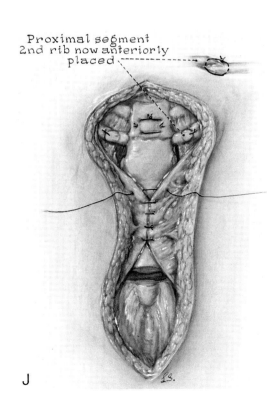

Proximal segment 2nd rib now anteriorly placed

J

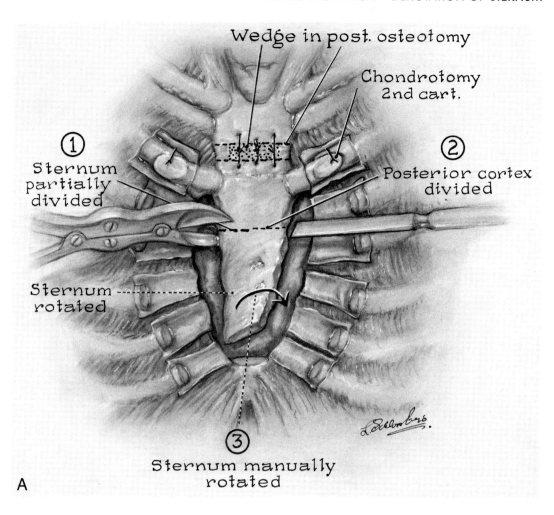

A

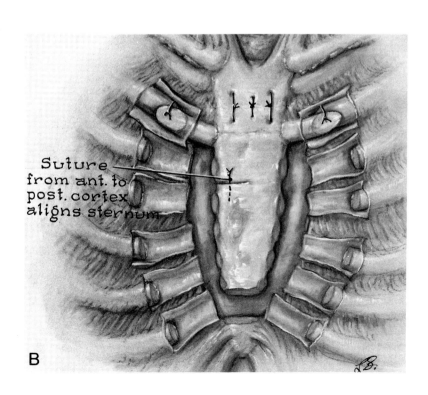

B

TURNOVER PROCEDURE FOR PECTUS EXCAVATUM

One has misgivings about the massive free graft that is produced in the turnover operation, but in point of fact our conventional operation for pectus excavatum, shown on the preceding pages, leaves only the anterior periosteum intact and the sternum otherwise totally devascularized, and only once in over 500 such repairs have we had reason to suspect that there had been interference with the growth of the sternum. On the other hand, the turnover graft procedure creates devascularized intercostal muscles and costal cartilages, which is not the case in our standard operation. The turnover operation is in a sense simpler and more straightforward and does produce immediate stability of the chest wall. Since 1960 on very special indications, we have occasionally performed the turnover operation, usually for an extremely broad and long defect in which we have been particularly concerned about the stability of the repair.

A. The pectorals have already been reflected widely to either side. The xiphoid has been divided from the gladiolus, the underside of the sternum is dissected from the pericardium, and the pleural envelopes are stripped back. Starting from below and proceeding upward, the costal cartilages or ribs are serially divided at the lateral margin of the deformity and the intercostal vessels are taken serially as the plastron is elevated. The internal mammary vessels are left, as shown. The manubrium is transected with a saw or osteotome.

B. The sternum with attached costal cartilages is rotated 180°.

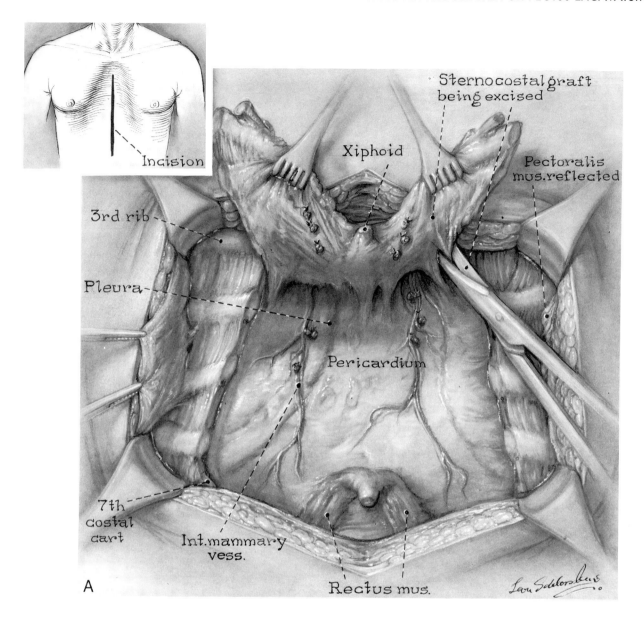

Incision

Sternocostal graft
being excised

Xiphoid

Pectoralis
mus. reflected

3rd rib

Pleura

Pericardium

7th
costal
cart

Int. mammary
vess.

Rectus mus.

A

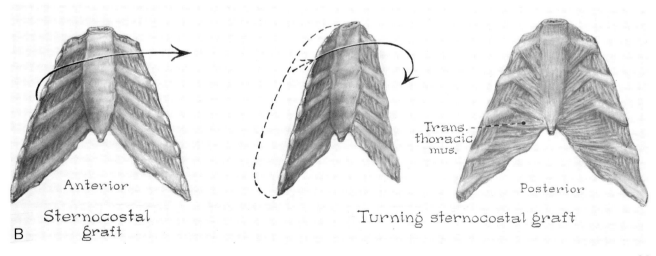

Anterior

Sternocostal
graft

Trans.
thoracic
mus.

Posterior

Turning sternocostal graft

B

TURNOVER PROCEDURE FOR PECTUS EXCAVATUM
(Continued)

C. The sternum is fitted and then reattached with heavy nonabsorbable sutures to bone, cartilage, and muscle, as shown. With a wound of this size, a considerable accumulation of fluid can be expected after operation, and we usually use both a percutaneous mediastinal catheter and a right intercostal tube, deliberately incising the right pleura if it has not already been opened. The pectoral muscles are sutured back to each other and to the sternal midline with a row of closely spaced nonabsorbable sutures as in the usual operation for pectus excavatum.

D. The final fit is variable. We have usually preferred to have the sternal ends superiorly abut directly against each other, but the graft may overlap as shown. Laterally, the plastron tends to overlap the edges of the defect. The rib ends do not usually correspond as nicely as shown in the drawing, and heavy sutures must be placed at angles. The immediate effect is one of very strong stabilization.

Some operators excise the intercostal muscles; others pull the perichondrium from the cartilages before the elevation and turnover.

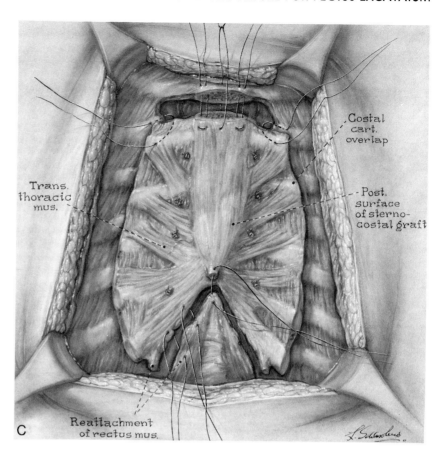

Trans. thoracic mus.

Costal cart. overlap

Post. surface of sterno-costal graft

Reattachment of rectus mus.

C

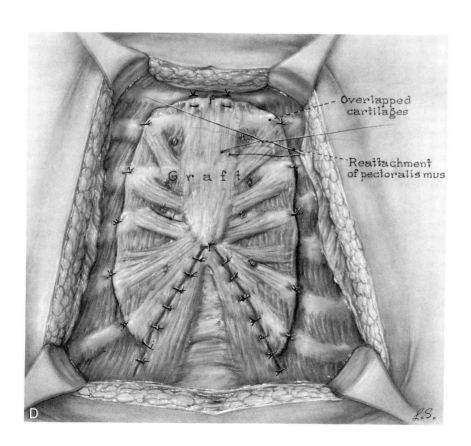

Overlapped cartilages

Reattachment of pectoralis mus

Graft

D

25

TURNOVER PROCEDURE FOR PECTUS EXCAVATUM
(Continued)

E. We have performed the turnover operation infrequently, perhaps 10 times in the 25 years since we first undertook it. In the last two patients, we have experimented with one of the several techniques (Scheer) described for leaving the sternum attached to the recti and leaving attached to the sternum the internal mammary vessels, which are divided above. The internal mammary vein in this preparation continues to fill, and the tissues appear to bleed oxygenated blood. The operation is substantially more difficult, since one must secure the intercostals and divide the cartilages or ribs on either side while the sternum is held down by its attachments to the recti. It is easiest to divide the ribs or cartilages on the right from below up, transect the manubrium, and then elevate the plastron and divide the costal elements on the left. Any loose tags of muscle are trimmed away from the underside of the sternum. The sternum is then rotated 180° on its attachment to the recti, and the costal cartilages on each side preferably are allowed to overlap. The fixation of the sternum after its reversal, and the drainage, are as noted previously.

After the turnover procedure by either method, the chest wall is at once solid and remains solid. Since we have employed the procedure almost exclusively in broad, flat, symmetrical defects, the reversed sternum has not presented an unpleasing appearance. Others, apparently applying the turnover for deep central defects, have noted the resulting prominent boss of the distal sternum, which they have corrected by a variety of osteoplastic procedures.

Figures A through D from Ravitch, M.M.: *Congenital Deformities of the Chest Wall and Their Operative Correction.* Philadelphia, W.B. Saunders Company, 1977, with permission.

REFERENCES

1. Judet, J., and Judet, R.: Thorax en entonnoir. Un procédé opératoire. Revue D'Orthopedie 40:248–257, 1954
2. Scheer, R.: Über eine neue Methode der chirurgischen Behandlung der Trichterbrust. Die "gestielte Umwendungsplastik." Der Chirurg. 28:312–314, 1957
3. Wada, J.: Surgical correction of the funnel chest "Sternoturnover." West. J. Surg., Obst. & Gynec. 69:358–361, 1961
4. Ravitch, M.M.: *Congenital Deformities of the Chest Wall and Their Operative Correction.* Philadelphia, W.B. Saunders Company, 1977

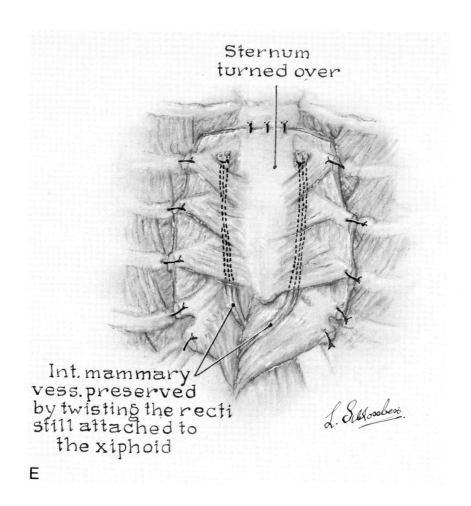

Sternum turned over

Int. mammary vess. preserved by twisting the recti still attached to the xiphoid

E

UNILATERAL DEPRESSION OF THE ANTERIOR CHEST WALL

A. We have seen this condition only on the right side. All of the cartilages, even to some degree the first, are depressed well out to beyond the costochondral junctions. The sternum, as shown, may be sharply rotated to the right, but it is not depressed or scaphoid. The chest wall is exposed as in the operation for pectus excavatum, the xiphoid divided from the sternum, and the posterior surface of the sternum freed. All of the involved costal elements on the right are treated by a very short parasternal resection, an osteotomy in the depth of the depression, and another just beyond the junction with normal rib laterally. On the uninvolved left side, a small wedge chondrotomy is performed in each cartilage so that when the sternum is lifted up and its position corrected, the chondrotomy will be closed.

B. The resection of the costal cartilage on the right may be a very short one, and the wedge chondrotomy on the left can be closer to the sternum than shown.

C. To correct the rotation of the manubrium, the right half of the sternum is cut through with the bone shears *(left)* and the anterior cortex on the left divided, so the sternum can be derotated by traction with a bone hook as shown *(right)*.

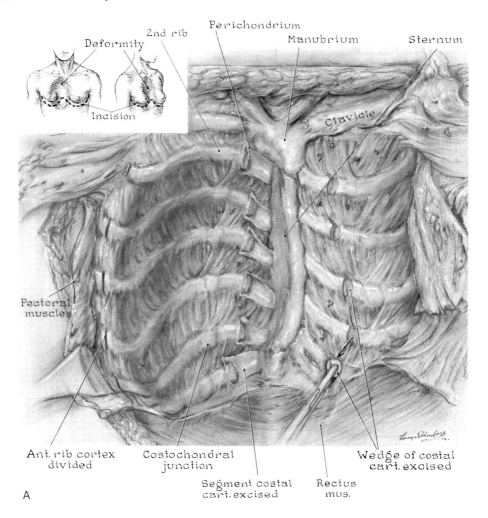

A

28

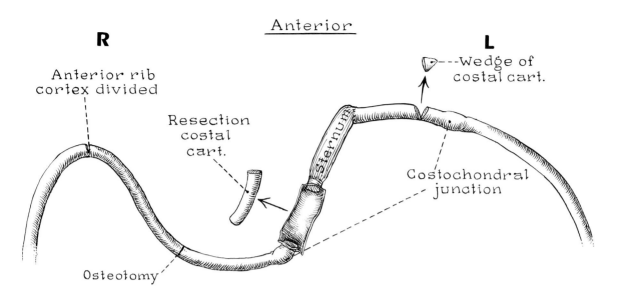

Anterior

R

L

Anterior rib cortex divided

Resection costal cart.

Wedge of costal cart.

sternum

Costochondral junction

Osteotomy

Transverse section at level of fourth ribs —

B

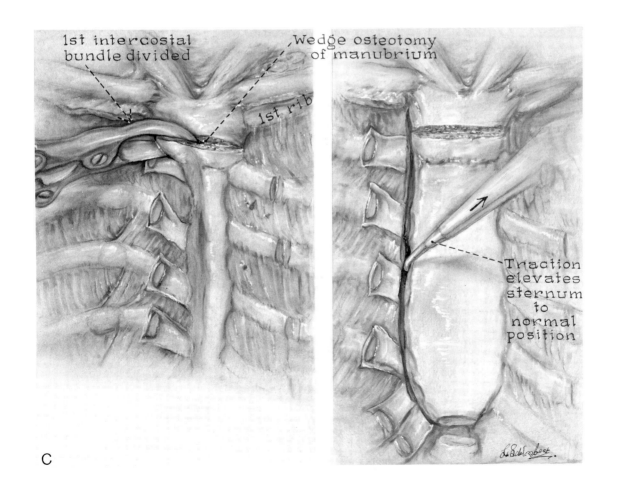

1st intercostal bundle divided

Wedge osteotomy of manubrium

1st rib

Traction elevates sternum to normal position

C

UNILATERAL DEPRESSION OF THE ANTERIOR CHEST
WALL *(Continued)*

D. An extensive reconstruction of this kind requires skeletal support. In the instance shown, two Kirschner wires are placed through the sternum and under the medial chest wall on the right, emerging lateral to the costal osteotomies. The mobilized segments of the right chondrocostal elements are elevated forward and fixed to the Kirschner wires in the manner shown in the drawing and the diagram. Superiorly, it has usually proved easier to employ a Rehbein splint. The small end at the right is driven through a perforation of the anterior cortex and into the marrow of the rib beyond the osteotomy. The remainder of the splint is actually arched and acts as a spring, so that when the costal elements and the sternum are sutured to it and the medial end is anchored to the solid chest wall on the left, the splint tends to lift

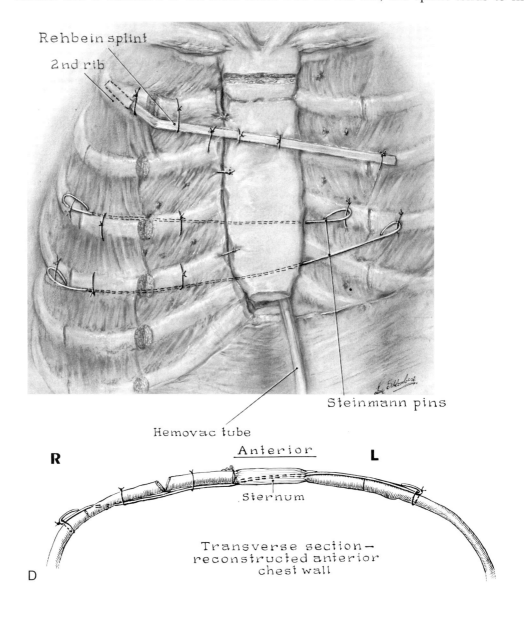

Rehbein splint

2nd rib

Steinmann pins

Hemovac tube

Anterior

R   L

Sternum

Transverse section—
reconstructed anterior
chest wall

D

forward the reconstructed chest wall. The metallic devices need not be removed. Heavy sutures still must be placed across the sternal osteotomy to maintain the derotation.

E. The pectoral muscles are sutured to each other and to the sternal midline, a percutaneous drain is placed in the mediastinum, and another is placed into the right pleural cavity after the right pleura has been widely opened. The xiphoid is not reattached to the sternum lest it create unacceptable tension.

From Ravitch, M.M.: Asymmetric congenital deformity of the ribs. Ann. Surg. 191:534–538, 1980, with permission.

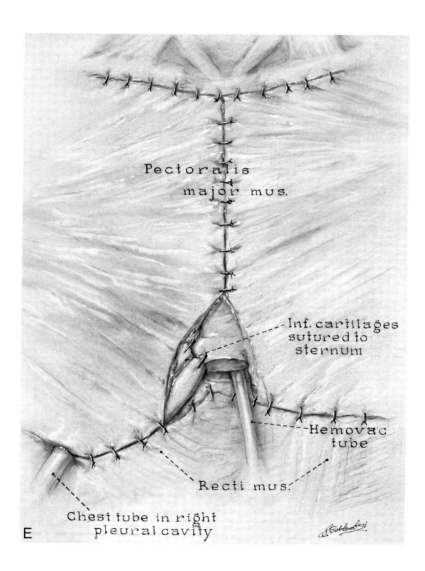

CORRECTION OF PECTUS CARINATUM

A. These very wide defects are best repaired through a transverse submammary incision arched upward in the midline. Flaps of skin and subcutaneous tissue are raised in both directions and the pectoral muscles are separately elevated and dissected free, in the manner illustrated in the dissection for pectus excavatum. Whereas in pectus excavatum the lower cartilages are conveniently exposed by oblique incisions in the recti, for pectus carinatum we find it necessary to dissect the recti free from the cartilages, sternum, and xiphoid, and laterally to free also the upper attachments of the abdominal muscles. The deformities are frequently asymmetrical. Any bosses at the chondrosternal junctions are shaved away, and occasionally one or several humped cartilages along the edge of the sternum and superior to those involved in the concavity are resected. Almost never need anything be done to the sternum.

B. The involved cartilages, with any involved bony rib, are resected subperichondrially and subperiosteally for the full extent of the deformity. As each element is resected, that portion of the chest wall lifts forward with respiration in a manner that was not before possible, and it is obvious that the perichondrial beds are now redundant. Reefing sutures of nonabsorbable material are placed to take up the slack in the perichondrial beds, providing them with a straight run from the lateral border of the defect to the sternum. The perichondrium is made as taut as possible. The anterior prominence of the sternum is not attacked in any way, because (1) it is often more apparent than real, being exaggerated by the lateral depressions in the costal cartilages, and (2) the tension of the reconstruction and, perhaps in growing children, the elimination of the need for compensatory expansion of the chest anteriorly usually result in what is essentially a restitution to a normal contour.

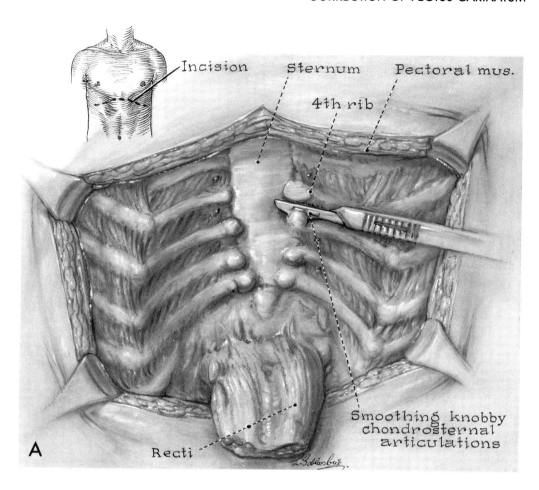

Incision   Sternum   Pectoral mus.

4th rib

Smoothing knobby
chondrosternal
articulations

Recti

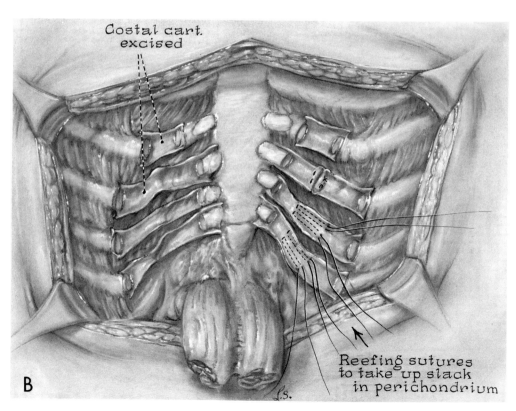

Costal cart.
excised

Reefing sutures
to take up slack
in perichondrium

C. The pectoral muscles are sutured to each other and to the sternal midline.

D. At the time of elevating the muscles, we usually mark by sutures the lower medial corners of the pectorals and the points at which the recti and obliques will be attached to the pectorals, for guidance at this point in the closure. These wounds are usually quite dry. For the most part we employ no drains, and the wounds usually require no subsequent aspiration.

Occasionally, the xiphoid and a bit of the distal sternum point straight backward. In such cases, we perform an anterior transverse cuneiform osteotomy. Closing the osteotomy with heavy nonabsorbable sutures elevates the tip of the sternum and makes it level with the rest of the bone; this contributes remarkably to a restoration of a normal appearance.

From Ravitch, M.M.: *Congenital Deformities of the Chest Wall and Their Operative Correction.* Philadelphia, W.B. Saunders Company, 1977, with permission.

REFERENCES

1. Ravitch, M.M.: The operative correction of pectus carinatum (pigeon breast). Ann. Surg. 151:705–714, 1960
2. Ravitch, M.M.: *Congenital Deformities of the Chest Wall and Their Operative Correction.* Philadelphia, W.B. Saunders Company, 1977

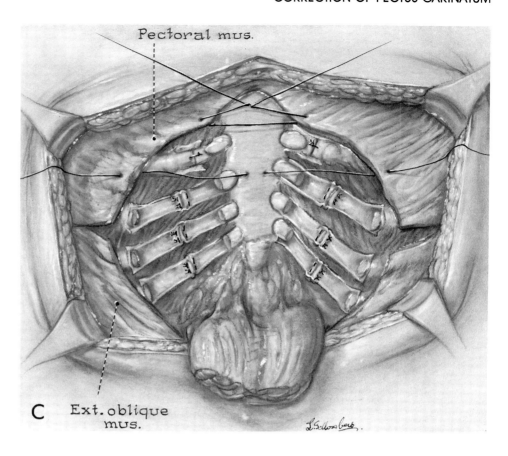

Pectoral mus.

C   Ext. oblique
        mus.

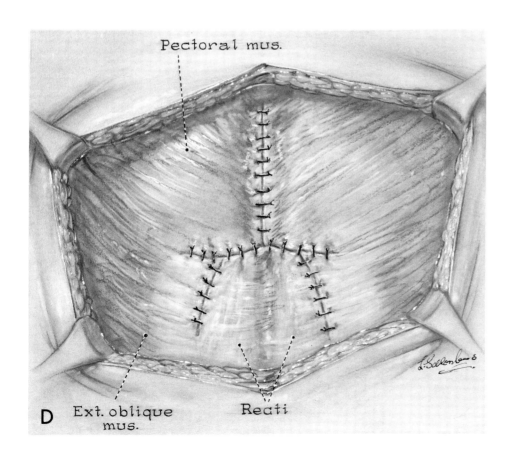

Pectoral mus.

D   Ext. oblique   Recti
        mus.

PECTUS CARINATUM—POUTER PIGEON TYPE

In this deformity, there is usually a double curve of the sternum: the upper portion of the manubrium may slope sharply forward, distal to that is a backward curve to the middle of the manubrium, and then there is a sharp anterior curve. The sternum is unusually broad and frequently has a double xiphoid. The sternebrae are usually prematurely fused. The deformity is readily corrected, actually by a modification of the operation for pectus excavatum.

A. Through a midline incision, the usual flaps of skin, fat, and pectoralis major are elevated; the short, depressed segments of the costal cartilages are excised subperichondrially; the xiphoid is divided from the sternum; and the pleural envelopes are reflected to both sides with the finger, as in the operation for pectus excavatum.

B. Because of the Z-shaped configuration of the sternum, seen in the lateral view, if a wedge osteotomy alone is performed at the superior angulation, the result is to bring the distal sternum far forward. Therefore, the fragments of bone removed from the superior wedge osteotomy are now fixed in a distal anterior osteotomy, producing a very satisfactory correction.

From Ravitch, M.M.: Unusual sternal deformity with cardiac symptoms—operative correction. J. Thorac. Surg. 23:138–144, 1952, with permission.

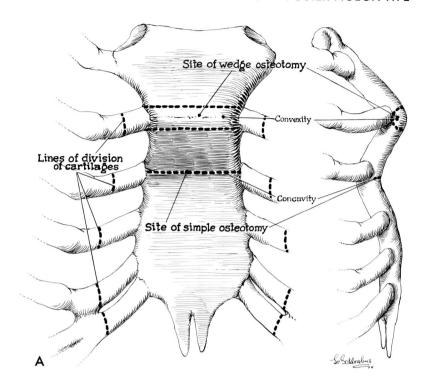

Site of wedge osteotomy

Convexity

Lines of division of cartilages

Concavity

Site of simple osteotomy

A

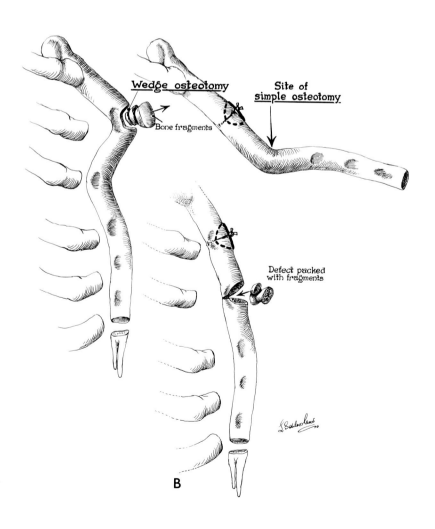

Wedge osteotomy

Site of simple osteotomy

Bone fragments

Defect packed with fragments

B

STERNAL CLEFTS*

Repair of Sternal Cleft in Early Infancy

In infants within the first weeks of life, a cleft, whether a broad U or a narrower V, can usually be completely closed by direct approximation of the sternal halves.

A. As shown, it may be necessary to resect a V from the distal portion of the sternum, to avoid buckling when the sternal halves are brought together.

B. Short cuts in the sternal bars tend to permit the concave inner borders to straighten out when the sternal halves are brought together by several heavy peristernal sutures. Some sutures may be placed through the sternum. A series of finer sutures is taken through periosteum and bone. It is not difficult to dissect the mediastinal tissues away from the undersurface of the sternal bar without entering the pleura. Not shown is the incision of the fascioperiosteal covering over the medial edges of the two sternal bars so that firm bony union can be achieved. With particularly broad defects, and hence expected tension, narrow Teflon bands instead of sutures may be employed for the heavy peristernal approximating mechanism.

---

*NOTE: In all of the sternal cleft drawings, we have, for simplicity, not shown the pectorals and the recti. To a greater or lesser degree, reflection of the pectorals will be necessary for exposure. In any case, the resuture of the muscles in the midline, over the operative closure of the sternum, is an important part of the repair.

From Ravitch, M.M.: *Congenital Deformities of the Chest Wall and Their Operative Correction.* Philadelphia, W.B. Saunders Company, 1977, with permission.

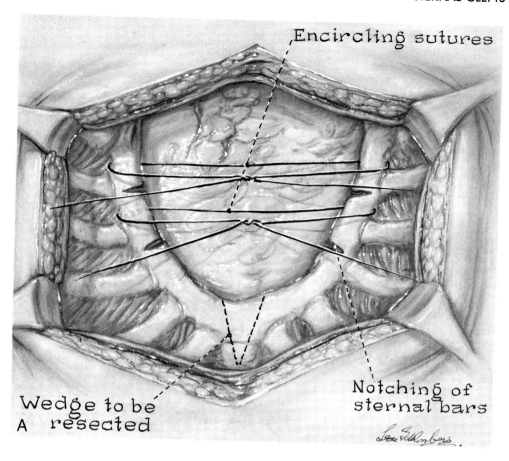

Encircling sutures

Wedge to be
A resected

Notching of
sternal bars

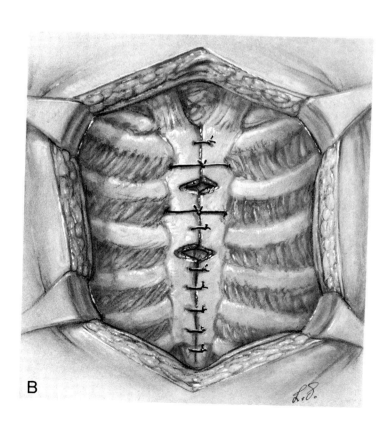

B

Repair of Sternal Cleft in Childhood

By the time children are three or four years of age, and sometimes even earlier, direct approximation of the sternal halves without releasing the cartilages is no longer feasible.

A. Once more, it may be necessary to perform a V-resection in the distal, fused portion of the sternum.

B. Oblique chondrotomies are performed on the several cartilages attached to the sternal bars, most particularly the upper cartilages. The intercostal vessels are more readily avoided if the chondrotomies are done after a subperichondrial dissection has been completed. By pulling the sternal halves together with the encircling suture (carefully placed medial to the internal mammary vessels, as shown), one can determine whether or not it is necessary to divide the posterior perichondrium to allow for full approximation of the sternum.

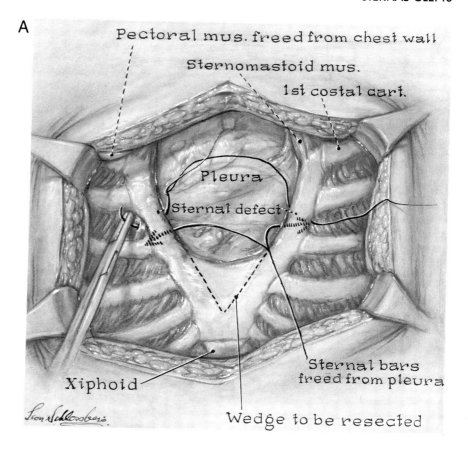

A

Pectoral mus. freed from chest wall

Sternomastoid mus.

1st costal cart.

Pleura

Sternal defect

Sternal bars freed from pleura

Xiphoid

Wedge to be resected

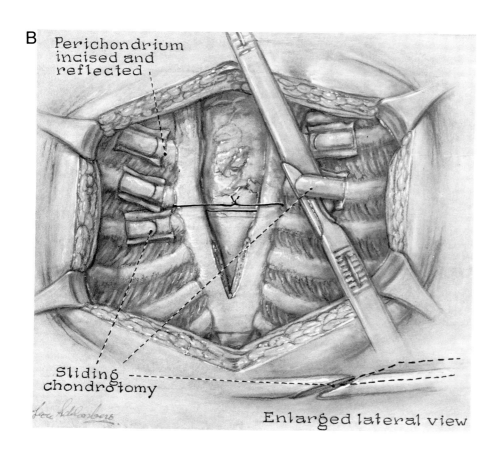

B

Perichondrium incised and reflected

Sliding chondrotomy

Enlarged lateral view

Repair of Sternal Cleft in Childhood *(Continued)*

C. The sternal edges are dissected free to promote bony union of the approximated sternal bars.

D. The sternal halves are tightly approximated by the peristernal sutures, and the sternal periosteum is carefully sutured with multiple 2–0 silk sutures. The drawing shows the degree to which the sliding chondrotomies have relaxed the chest wall. The pectoral muscles are now resutured to each other and to the sternal periosteum in the midline. The attachments of the sternal heads of the sternocleidomastoids and the ribbon muscles are often much more widely separated than shown and require to be approximated, or slid over and approximated, to prevent an area of paradox in the suprasternal notch.

From Ravitch, M.M.: *Congenital Deformities of the Chest Wall and Their Operative Correction.* Philadelphia, W.B. Saunders Company, 1977, with permission.

REFERENCES

1. Sabiston, D.C., Jr.: The surgical management of congenital bifid sternum with partial ectopia cordis. J. Thorac. Surg. 35:118–122, 1958
2. Asp, K., and Sulamaa, M.: Ectopia cordis. Acta Chir. Scand. 283:52–56, 1961
3. Daum, R., and Hecker W. Ch.: Zur operativen Korrektur der totalen Sternumspalte. Thoraxchirurgie Vaskuläre Chirurgie 12:333–339, 1964

C

Periosteal flaps

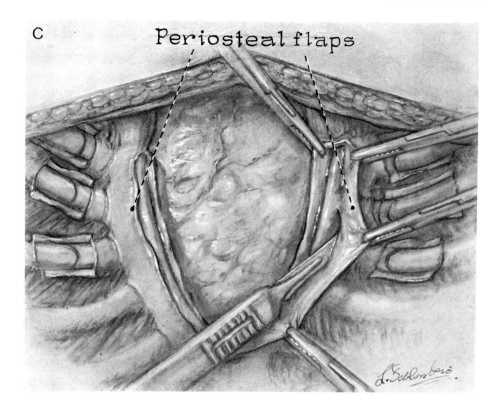

D

Sliding
chondrotomies
open

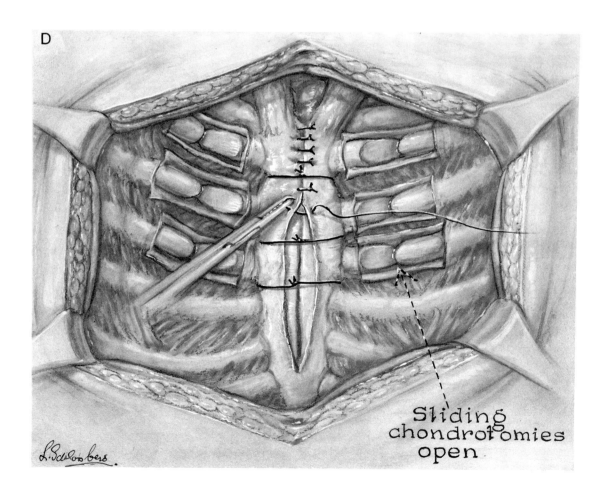

Repair of Sternal Cleft in Adolescence

A. By the time of adolescence, it is no longer possible to approximate the sternal edges.
B. If the two sternal bars are divided at their inferior ends and chondrotomies performed on all of the involved cartilages, when the sternal halves are brought together, as shown in the diagram, the circumference of the chest is significantly reduced, and the decreased anteroposterior diameter results in compression of the heart, marked by bradycardia and hypotension.
C. In such cases, prosthetic support is necessary and no chondrotomies are performed. A synthetic fabric as shown, or fascia lata, will soon tend to sag and must be supported by rib grafts for a defect of any width. Teflon felt is somewhat thicker but may still require a rib graft in order to construct and demarcate the upper margin of the new manubrium. A compound prosthesis of Marlex and acrylic, with the acrylic providing rigidity and the edges of the Marlex sheets beyond the acrylic permitting ingrowth of fibrous tissue from the chest wall, is probably best for wide clefts, just as it is for sternal resections (see pages 84–85, *Sternal Resection*).

From Ravitch, M.M.: *Congenital Deformities of the Chest Wall and Their Operative Correction*. Philadelphia, W.B. Saunders Company, 1977, with permission.

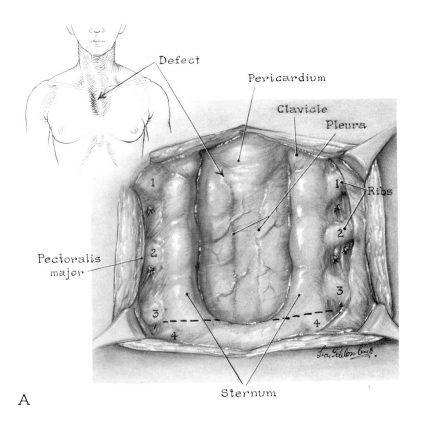

A

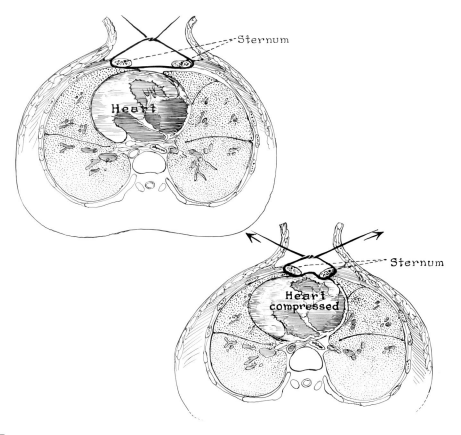

Sternum

Heart

Sternum

Heart
compressed

B

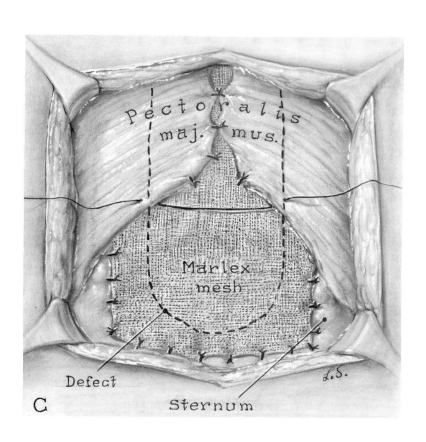

Pectoralis
maj. mus.

Marlex
mesh

Defect

Sternum

C

CORRECTION OF CHEST WALL DEFECT IN POLAND SYNDROME

In Poland syndrome—which consists of brachysyndactyly or even ectromelia, hypoplasia or absence of either breast or nipple or both, hypoplasia of subcutaneous tissue, axillary hypotrichosis, absence of the costosternal portion of the pectoralis major, absence of the pectoralis minor, absence of the costal cartilages or ribs II, III, and IV or III, IV, and V—there is a wide variation in the degree of expression and in the combination of the elements of the malformation. The operation shown is undertaken when there is a substantial chondral or costochondral defect.

A. A curved incision is placed so that it falls well outside the defect. A thin fascia, all that remains of the costosternal portion of the pectoralis major, lies directly upon the pleura. In the involved area there are no intercostal muscles. Cartilages III, IV, and V have variable segments missing, as shown. Abortive stubs represent the medial ends of III and IV. At either end, a bed is prepared for the rib graft. Laterally, the stump of the cartilage or rib is freshened. Medially, with a hemostat pressed into the sternum, as shown, a recess is created into which the pointed medial end of the rib graft will be inserted.

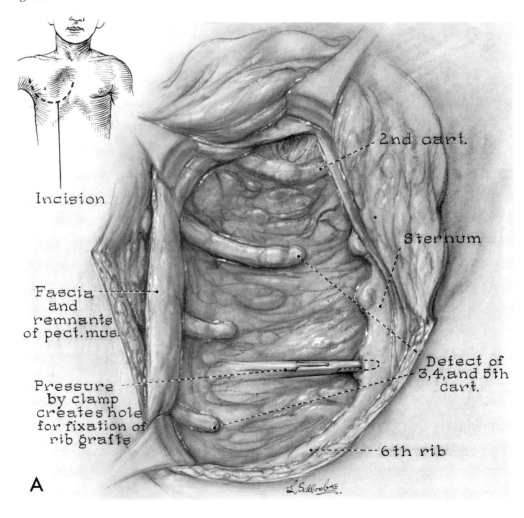

Incision

Fascia and remnants of pect. mus.

Pressure by clamp creates hole for fixation of rib grafts

2nd cart.

Sternum

Defect of 3, 4, and 5th cart.

6th rib

A

L. Schlossberg.

B. Rib grafts from the contralateral side are taken subperiosteally and split with an oscillating saw. The rib graft is pointed in order to press into the sternum medially and is notched as shown to hold the encircling ligatures, since it is usually too small for passage of a suture through it.

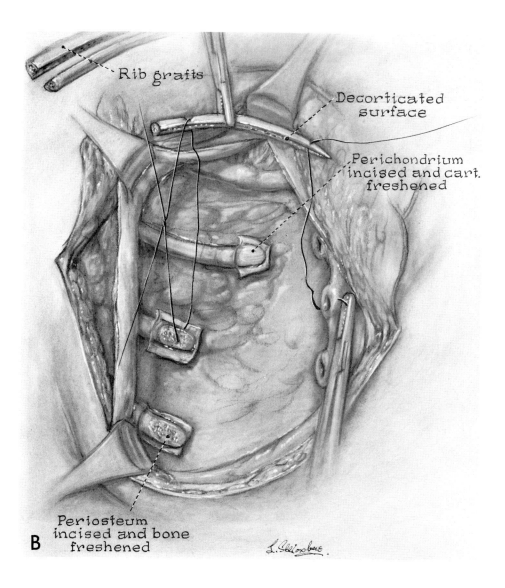

C   and D. A sheet of prosthetic material (we have preferred Teflon felt because it adds some thickness to the chest wall) is sutured to each of the grafts and to the surrounding tissue; it is drawn tautly over the defect. A subcutaneous drain is required.

In some patients with Poland syndrome, there is an associated sternal deformity, generally a tilting of the sternum, which will require additional steps that may possibly require metallic support as shown on page 30 *(Unilateral Depression of the Anterior Chest Wall)* to stabilize the repositioned sternum as an anchor for the rib struts.

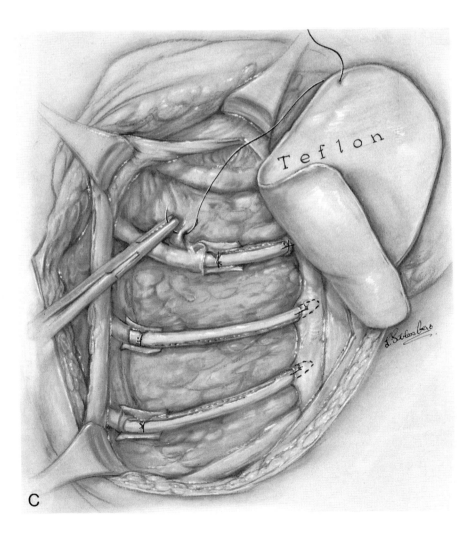

C

A number of surgeons have reported use of a latissimus dorsi muscle flap appropriately designed to fill out the depression caused by absence of breast, subcutaneous tissue, and pectoralis major, whether there is a costal defect or not. This seems to us a rather large operation merely to provide thickness and texture. It requires several incisions and may not obviate the need for rib struts or prosthesis. In males, the added thickness is not important. In females, the mammary prosthesis that is usually required will largely obscure the effect of the muscle graft.

From Ravitch, M.M.: *Congenital Deformities of the Chest Wall and Their Operative Correction*. Philadelphia, W.B. Saunders Company, 1977, with permission.

REFERENCES

1. Ravitch, M.M.: *Congenital Deformities of the Chest Wall and Their Operative Correction*. Philadelphia, W.B. Saunders Company, 1977
2. Ravitch, M.M.: Poland's syndrome—a study of an eponym. Plast. Reconstr. Surg. 59:508–512, 1977
3. Haller, J.A., Jr., Colombani, P.M., Miller, D., and Manson, P.: Early reconstruction of Poland's syndrome using autologous rib grafts combined with a latissimus muscle flap. J. Pediatr. Surg. 19:423–429, 1984.

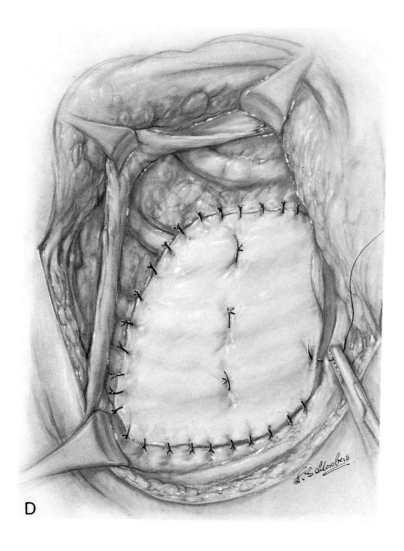

D

Resection of Chest Wall for Tumors of Ribs and Sternum

THE PRINCIPLES OF RESECTION OF THE CHEST WALL FOR TUMOR

The diagram shows the shape and relative size of the skin incision, which is planned to be well outside the area of chest wall resection so that the line of incision lies over solid chest wall and not over the reconstructed defect. Clearly, if a preliminary biopsy had been made, it would necessarily be through the center of this flap, which would then become unusable because possible tumor seeding from the biopsy would require wider excision of the biopsy site, jeopardizing the circulation of the flap. Malignant tumors of the chest wall are so much more common than benign ones, and frozen section sufficiently unreliable, that unless there are very strong reasons for suspecting a benign lesion, we proceed directly to resection. If biopsy with frozen section is felt to be required before resection, it should be performed after the flap has been raised, and the wound should be carefully protected from contamination. The principle of the resection indicated here involves removal of long lengths of the involved ribs and substantial lengths of the first apparently uninvolved ribs above and below the tumor; the resection is through the full thickness of chest wall, including the pleura. If the tumor lies deep to an area where, for example, the pectoralis major, rhomboid muscles, latissimus dorsi is not applied to the chest wall, the muscle tissue may properly be spared. As is the case for the area under the scapula, this sparing may obviate the need for reconstitution of the rigid thoracic wall.

After the skin flap is raised, an intercostal incision is made in the interspace below what is thought to be the lowest uninvolved rib to be resected, in this case the 5th rib, and a finger is inserted into the pleural cavity to determine whether the incision avoids the tumor adequately and to ascertain whether the lung is free or whether a portion must be resected with the chest wall. If the sternum is approached by the tumor, or actually involved, a similarly generous resection of the sternum is undertaken. If the ribs are divided from below, upward, the intercostal vessels can be secured below each rib before it is divided, thereby reducing blood loss to a minimum.

After Eijgelaar, A., and van der Haide, J.N.H.: Ergebnisse der radikalen Brustwandresection. Thoraxchirurgie 20:404–407, 1972.

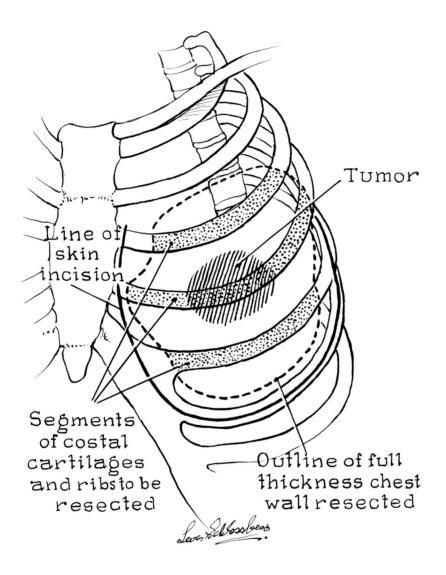

Tumor

Line of skin incision

Segments of costal cartilages and ribs to be resected

Outline of full thickness chest wall resected

RESECTION OF COSTAL TUMOR, RECONSTRUCTION WITH RIB GRAFT AND MARLEX

On the basis of informed clinical suspicion that a chest wall tumor is malignant, we proceed to definitive operation.

A. The curved incision, concave upward, is planned so that it will fall on solid chest wall however large the chest wall resection may turn out to be. If biopsy is insisted upon, it is preferable to perform it at the stage in the operation (the first illustration in the series) at which one has reached the muscle that would have to be resected with the malignant tumor—in this example, the pectoralis major. A biopsy at this point would not risk contamination of tissue that is not to be resected and would not jeopardize the skin flap. On the other hand, frozen section is frequently unreliable for assessing bone and cartilage tumors and, if one merely takes a biopsy of the tumor at this point, closes the wound, and waits for the results from the permanent sections, the subsequent report that the tumor is malignant would require an enormous resection of contaminated chest wall, skin, and fat.

B. The entire dissection is performed with the fine needle–tipped electrocautery. In this case, since the tumor is medial and close to the sternum, the incision goes well past the midline of the sternum. The soft tissues are incised down to bony chest wall with the electrocautery.

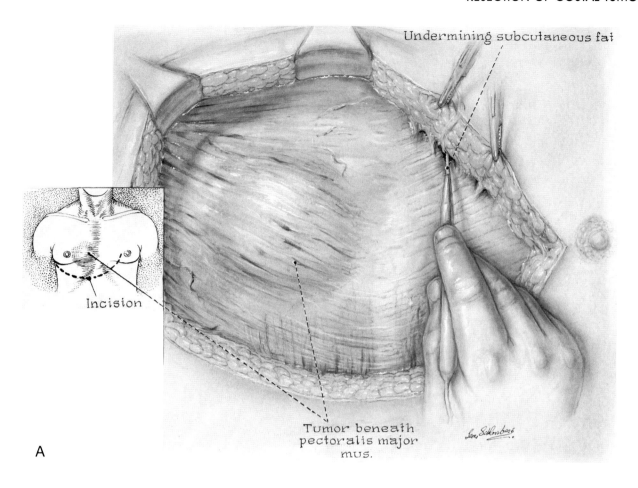

Undermining subcutaneous fat

Incision

Tumor beneath pectoralis major mus.

A

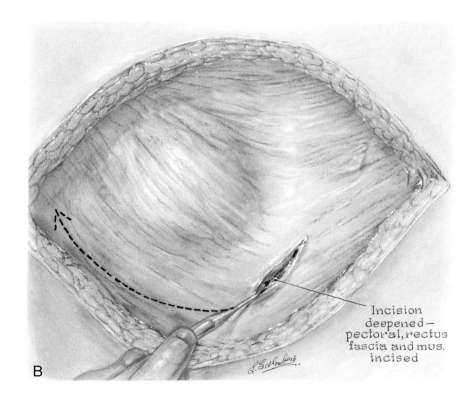

Incision deepened — pectoral, rectus fascia and mus. incised

B

C. Because the 7th rib appears to be uninvolved, the incision is made in the 7th interspace, a finger is inserted, the margin is judged to be adequate, and the lung is found unattached. On the patient's right, the intercostal vessels are sequentially suture-ligated, and the ribs, intercostal muscles, and pleura are divided until one comes superiorly to the interspace above the uninvolved rib to be taken. From above and below, then, the midline is approached; the internal mammary vessels are identified, ligated, and divided; and the sternum is cut along the predetermined path with saw or bone shears.

D. If an autogenous rib graft is to be used, it is removed subperiosteally, exposed either by elevating the wound edges and dissecting beneath them or through a linear extension of the incision (as in this case). The Doyen elevator is shown elevating the periosteum laterally. One measures the defect and measures the rib graft before dividing it. The configuration of the chest and the size of the patient will determine the length of the most useful rib graft obtainable without excessive curvature.

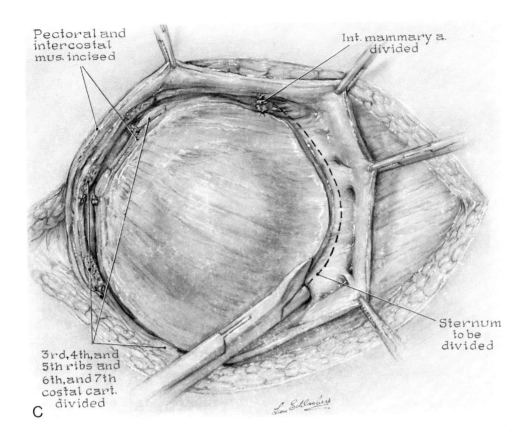

Pectoral and intercostal mus. incised

Int. mammary a. divided

Sternum to be divided

3rd, 4th, and 5th ribs and 6th, and 7th costal cart. divided

C

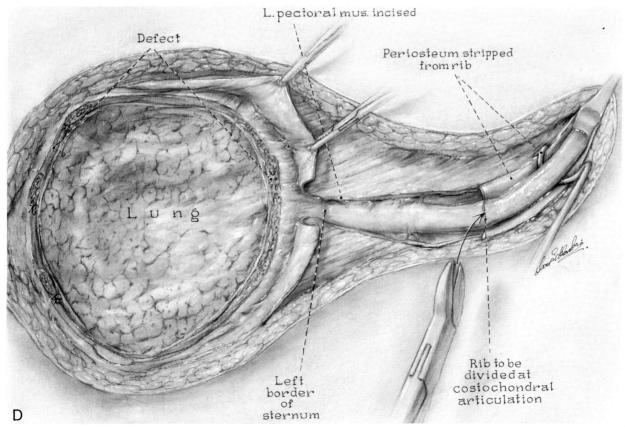

Defect

L. pectoral mus. incised

Periosteum stripped from rib

Lung

Left border of sternum

Rib to be divided at costochondral articulation

D

55

E. The posterior cortical surfaces of the two ends of the graft are resected (not shown), and the graft is laid on bared sternum to the right and in the periosteal bed on the left. It is sutured there by heavy through-and-through, nonabsorbable sutures.

F and G. A Marlex sheet, cut of appropriate size, is sutured over the bony defect, with sutures placed a centimeter or so in from the edge of the Marlex.

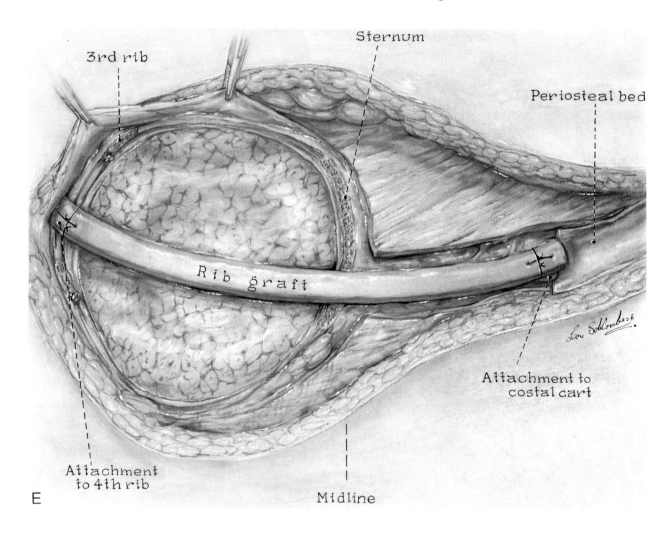

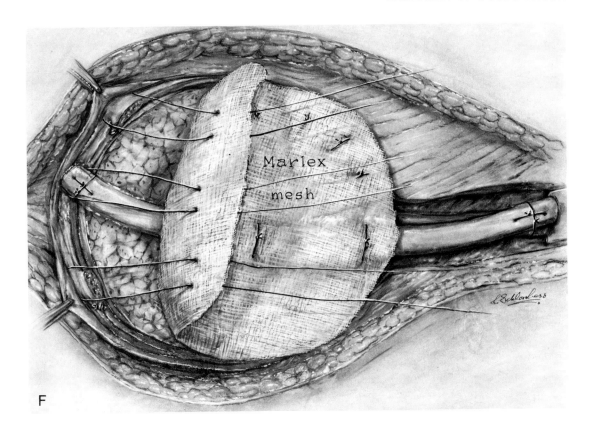

F

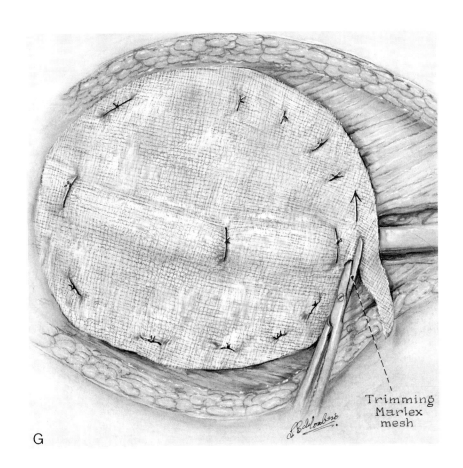

G

Trimming
Marlex
mesh

H. The edge of the muscle is now sutured down over the feathered edge of the prosthesis, and one or two heavy sutures are placed through the Marlex and around the rib graft.
I. Large suction wound drains are employed subcutaneously. An intercostal drainage tube may be used as well. The skin flap is then sutured down.

A modest defect of a size requiring only a single rib graft does not require a rigid prosthesis.

Figures *A, C, D,* and *F* from Yap, S., Ravitch, M.M., and Pataki, K.I.: En bloc chest wall resection for candidal costochondritis in a drug addict. Ann. Thorac. Surg. 31:182–187, 1981, with permission.

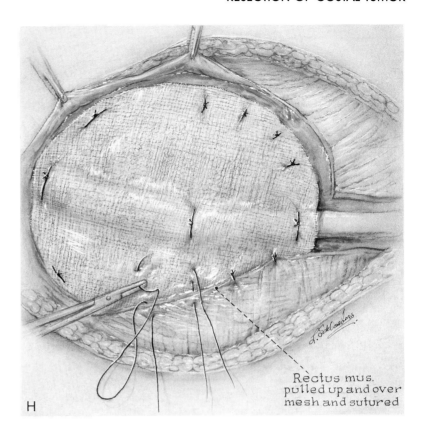

Rectus mus.
pulled up and over
mesh and sutured

H

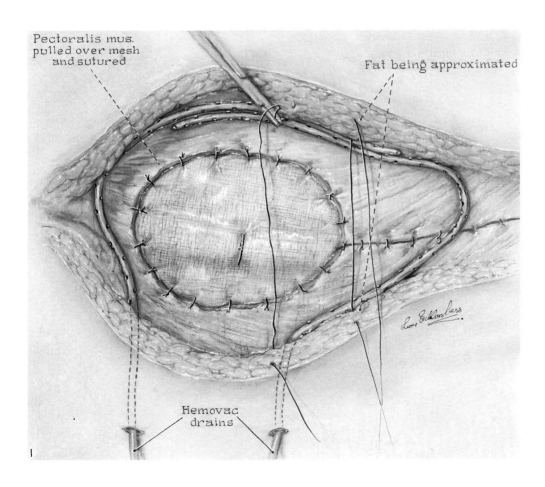

Pectoralis mus.
pulled over mesh
and sutured

Fat being approximated

Hemovac
drains

I

RIB GRAFT STABILIZATION (SECONDARY) OF LARGE POSTOPERATIVE CHEST WALL DEFECT

This patient was referred after a wide chest wall resection in two operations; extensive seeding from the biopsy wound forced the sacrifice of a large area of skin. The thoracic wall had been reconstructed with unreinforced Marlex. The result was a large, soft, depressed area, under which medially the heart beat and laterally an obvious respiratory paradox was apparent.

A. A large transverse incision and reflection of the right pectoralis major (for technique, see pages 10–11, *Correction of Pectus Excavatum*) provide exposure. Long sections of the 6th and 7th ribs from the sound side are removed subperiosteally.

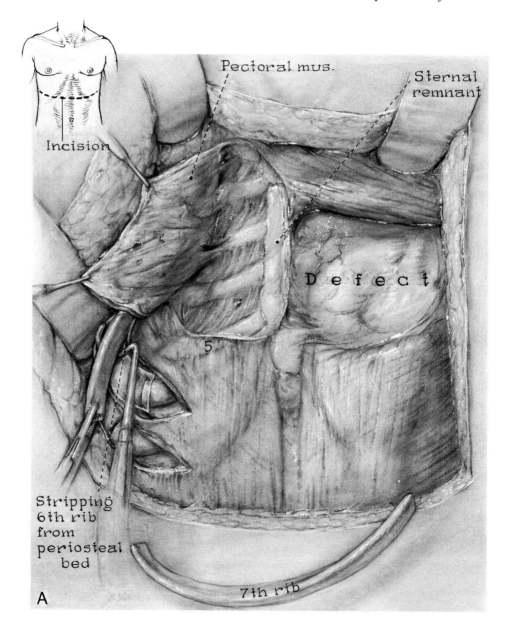

B. Appropriate beds in the sternum are prepared for the medial ends of the grafts by cutting away the anterior sternal cortex with an osteotome. Laterally, the anterior cortex of the matching ribs is cut away with rongeurs. The rib graft is similarly prepared.

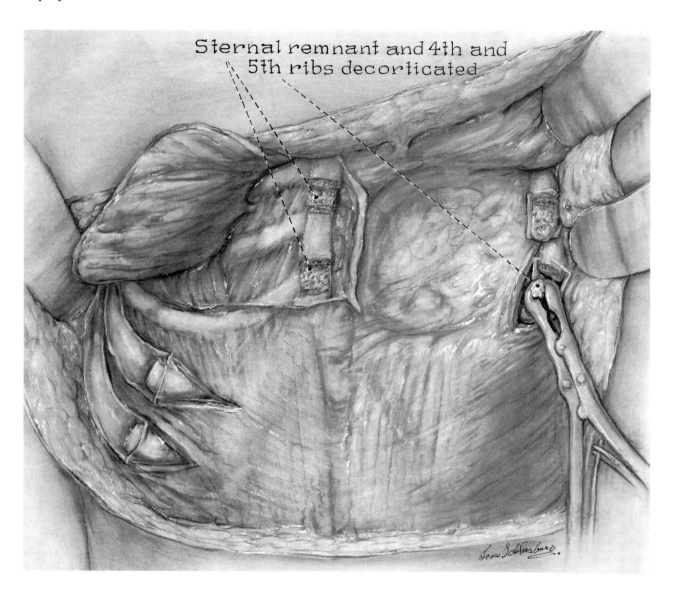

Sternal remnant and 4th and 5th ribs decorticated

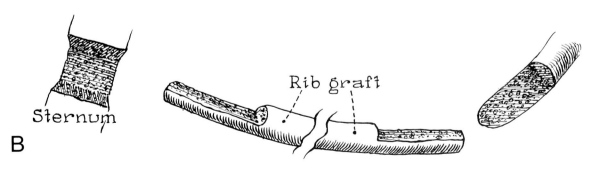

Sternum

Rib graft

B

C and D. Tunnels are created by blunt dissection under the floppy Marlex, and the
grafts are slid into the two tunnels and stoutly sutured to the rib ends, to the sternum,
and to the Marlex. The hardness of the cortices of sternum and ribs varies from
patient to patient. At times, a steady pressure with a strong needle will suffice to
bring sutures through; at others, it is necessary to use an awl or a twist drill.

E. The right pectoral muscle is now sutured to the sternum, to the portion of the left
pectoral remaining, and to the scar over the rectus sheath. Ample experience has
convinced us that, in general, for thoracic wall defects flexible prostheses, whether
of fascia lata, Marlex, or Teflon felt, do not provide sufficient stability or protection
without rigid support.

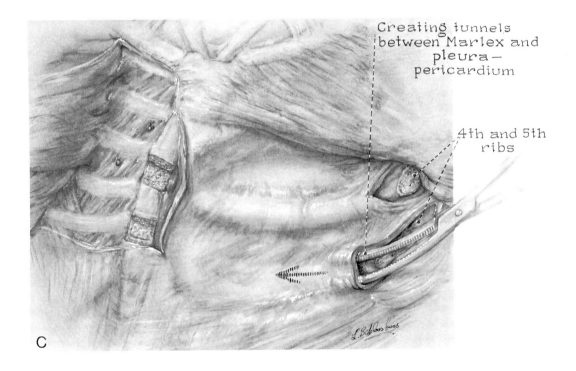

C

Rib graft being placed in tunnel

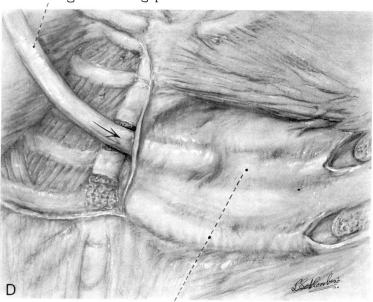

D

Tunnels beneath Marlex

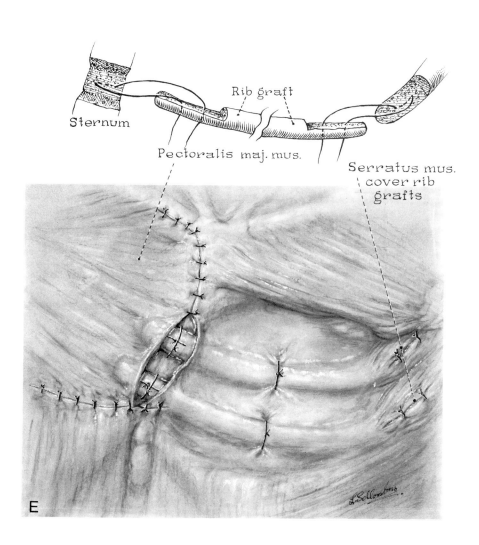

Sternum

Rib graft

Pectoralis maj. mus.

Serratus mus. cover rib grafts

E

Muscle Flaps

PECTORALIS MAJOR MUSCLE FLAPS

A. **Blood Supply.** The rich circulation of the pectoralis major provides a series of options in mobilizing the muscle.

   The principal arterial supply, with parallel venous drainage, is (1) from the subclavian artery via the internal mammary and its perforating branches, reaching the underside of the muscle, and (2) from the axillary artery, via the highest thoracic artery and the thoracoacromial artery, which descend and fan out between the pectoralis major and pectoralis minor muscles and intercommunicate with each other, medially with the internal mammary, and laterally with the lateral thoracic artery, a more distal branch of the axillary artery.

   Depending on the manner in which the muscle is to be moved, one of these two major sources of blood supply may be sacrificed, the remainder sufficing to nourish the transposed muscle and a properly designed island of skin attached to it.

B. **Pectoralis Major Turnover Flap—Unilateral.** For a modest sternal dehiscence *(top)*, if débridement and direct closure are decided against or if the wound is old, the pectoralis major is divided in the anterior axillary line, at least the lateral portion of the superior neurovascular pedicle is divided, and the muscle flap is turned medially *(bottom)* either bridging across the sternotomy (or defect created by a resection) or dipping down into it. The lateral portion of the pectoralis major is sutured to the chest wall. In a narrow defect of this kind, direct skin closure is usually possible.

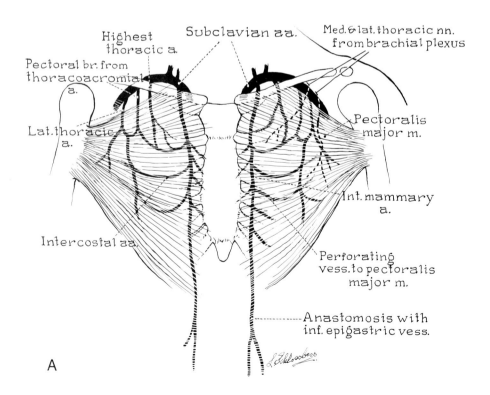

A

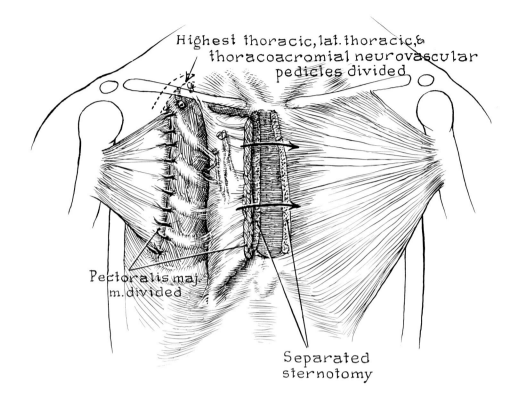

Highest thoracic, lat. thoracic, &
thoracoacromial neurovascular
pedicles divided

Pectoralis maj
m. divided

Separated
sternotomy

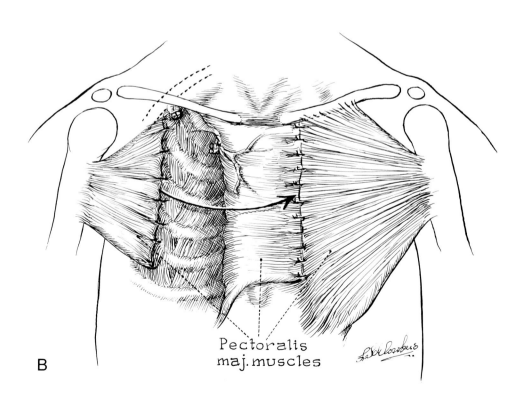

B

Pectoralis
maj. muscles

PECTORALIS MAJOR MUSCLE FLAPS *(Continued)*

C. Pectoralis Major Turnover Flap—Bilateral. With a wider dehiscence and extensive skin loss or larger defect after resection of skin and sternum, the defect may be closed by turning over bilateral flaps of pectoral muscle sutured to each other and turning any excess into the defect. The muscle can accept an immediate split-thickness graft.

D. Sliding Pectoralis Major Graft—Bilateral. The pectoralis major muscle on either side is divided at its origin from the humerus. Skin flaps are elevated to allow the muscle to slide freely, and the muscles are elevated from the chest wall. The carefully preserved neurovascular pedicles coming down from above suffice to nourish the muscle, which is otherwise entirely free. One muscle or both, or only a portion of one, can be moved as the situation requires, and a paddle of skin may be moved on the muscle (see also pages 85–87). It is remarkable how far the pectoralis major muscle, freed in this way, may slide. For large defects we usually provide rigidity of the chest wall by using rib grafts or a prosthetic composite prosthesis of Marlex and acrylic under the muscle flap (see pages 73–75, *Massive Chest Wall Resection for Recurrent Breast Carcinoma*, and pages 85–87, *Chondrosarcoma of the Sternum*).

E. Pectoral Flap Treatment of Dehiscence of the Sternum. If a single pectoral flap is employed, it is simply tucked down into the cleft and sutured to the edges. If bilateral flaps are employed, the second flap is brought over the dehiscence and sutured to the first one in the manner shown. The pectoral muscle in the anterior mediastinum not only fills a good deal of the space, but it also brings in a circulatory base for the vigorous granulation tissue needed to complete healing.

REFERENCES

1. Arnold, P.G., and Pairolero, P.C.: Use of *pectoralis major* muscle flaps to repair defects of anterior chest wall. Plast. Reconstr. Surg. 63:205–213, 1979
2. Jurkiewicz, M.J., Bostwick, J., III, Hester, T.R., Bishop, J.B., and Craver, J.: Infected median sternotomy wound: Successful treatment by muscle flaps. Ann. Surg. 191:738–744, 1980
3. Freeman, J.L., Walker, E.P., Wilson, J.S.P., and Shaw, H.J.: The vascular anatomy of the pectoralis major myocutaneous flap. Br. J. Plast. Surg. 34:3–10, 1981
4. Nahai, F., Morales, L., Jr., Bone, D.K., and Bostwick, J., III: Pectoralis major muscle turnover flaps for closure of the infected sternotomy wound with preservation of form and function. Plast. Reconstr. Surg. 70:471–474, 1982

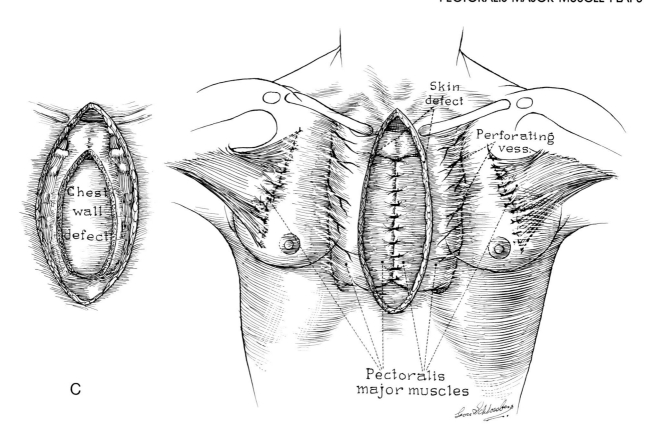

C

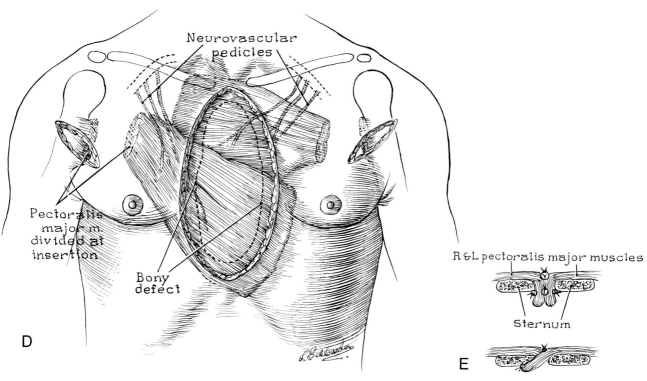

D

E

RECTUS ABDOMINIS FLAP FOR DISTAL STERNAL DEFECT

This is applicable to the relatively common distal sternal dehiscence (and infection) of a median sternotomy. It is, of course, applicable only if the internal mammary vessels were spared. It is also possible, by dividing the muscle superiorly and leaving it attached only by the skeletonized pedicle of the superior epigastric artery, to swing the muscle around on its vascular pedicle with an island graft of skin until what was its lower end reaches the region of the manubrium (see reference). To cover defects at the costal margin, the rectus abdominis may be rotated, with attached skin if need be.

REFERENCE

1. Neale, H.W., Kreilein, J.G., Schreiber, J.T., and Gregory, R.O.: Complete sternectomy for chronic osteomyelitis with reconstruction using a rectus abdominis myocutaneous island flap. Ann. Plast. Surg. 6(4):305–314, 1981

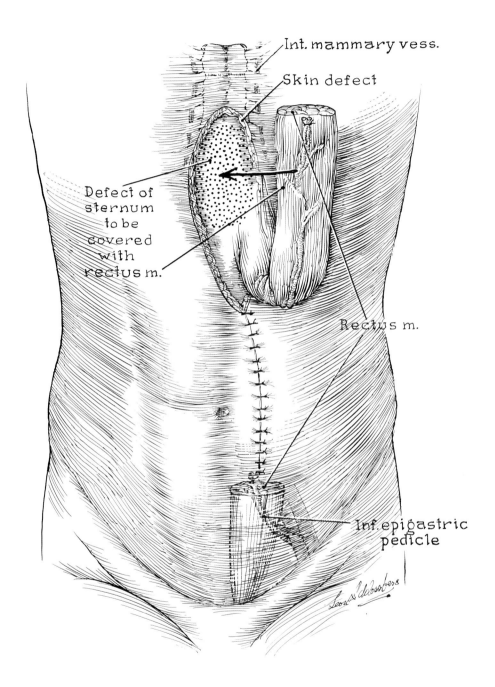

Int. mammary vess.

Skin defect

Defect of
sternum
to be
covered
with
rectus m.

Rectus m.

Inf. epigastric
pedicle

MASSIVE CHEST WALL RESECTION FOR RECURRENT BREAST CARCINOMA, MARLEX-ACRYLIC PROSTHESIS AND LATISSIMUS DORSI MYOCUTANEOUS FLAP

The problem created by a patient with a large area of skin involved by carcinoma and heavy irradiation, and with a dirty ulcer, are exemplified by the patient whose operation is shown.

A. After the usual skin preparation, at the posterior midline, an iodophor-soaked gauze sponge is sutured to the chest wall well beyond the diseased tissue, and the skin is prepared once more and draped. The initial scalpel incision completely around the area of suspected involvement is carried down to the bony chest wall with the electrocautery.

B. An intercostal incision at the lower border of the planned resection has permitted the insertion of a finger in order to determine that the incision is well beyond the lesion and to feel the firm attachment of the lung to the underside of the chest wall in the area of the ulcer. The intercostal vessels laterally have been serially ligated and the ribs sectioned in sequence until elevation of the lower border of the segment of chest wall to be resected has disclosed the attached lung. The lung is divided on a TA 90 stapler, which is applied twice at a comfortable distance from the pleura for two discrete areas of adhesion.

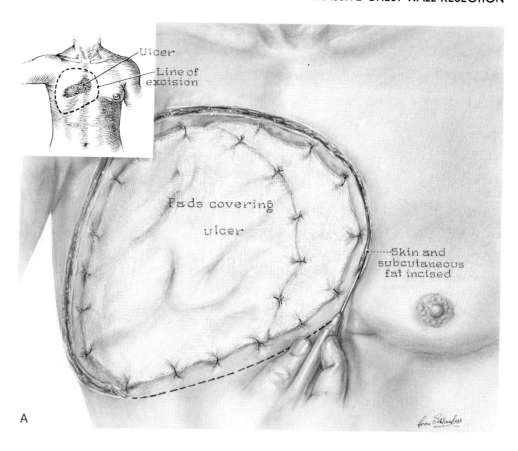

Ulcer

Line of excision

Pads covering ulcer

Skin and subcutaneous fat incised

A

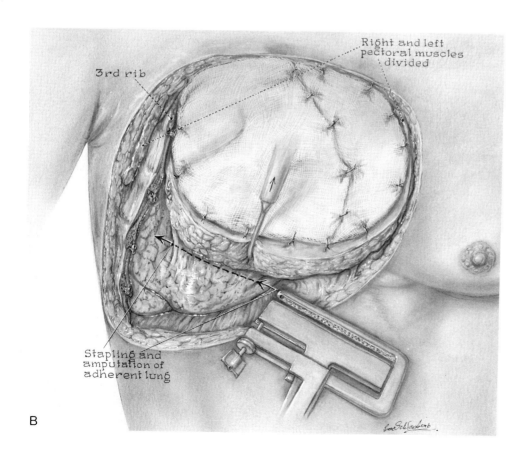

Right and left pectoral muscles divided

3rd rib

Stapling and amputation of adherent lung

B

C. The two staple lines are clearly visible when the specimen has been resected. Superiorly, the specimen has been freed by incision along the first interspace. Above and below, the internal mammary vessels have been exposed and doubly ligated and divided. A good two thirds of most of the length of the sternum has been resected.

D. A "sandwich" composed of two layers of Marlex with acrylic as the filling is shown being applied. The acrylic powder and the plasticizer are stirred until quite thick, then pasted on the surface of one sheet of the Marlex, marked out for appropriate shape and size so as to overlap the defect; then the second layer of Marlex is applied. The border of Marlex, for 1 to 1.5 cm, is kept free of acrylic. The requisite curvature of the prosthesis is obtained by pressing the prosthesis on the side of an overturned stainless steel basin of appropriate size until the acrylic has hardened.

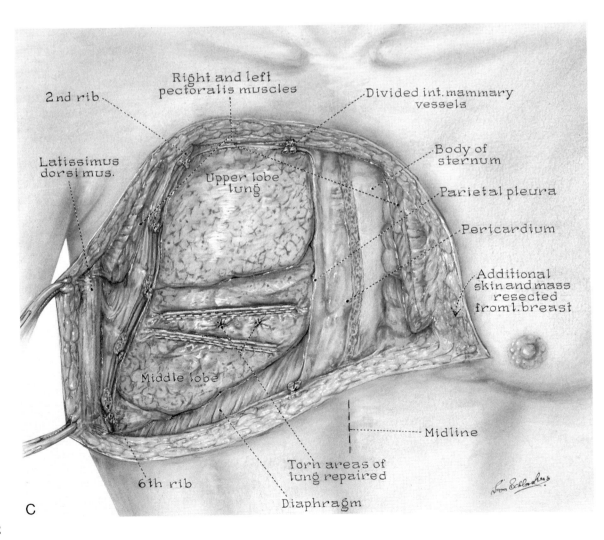

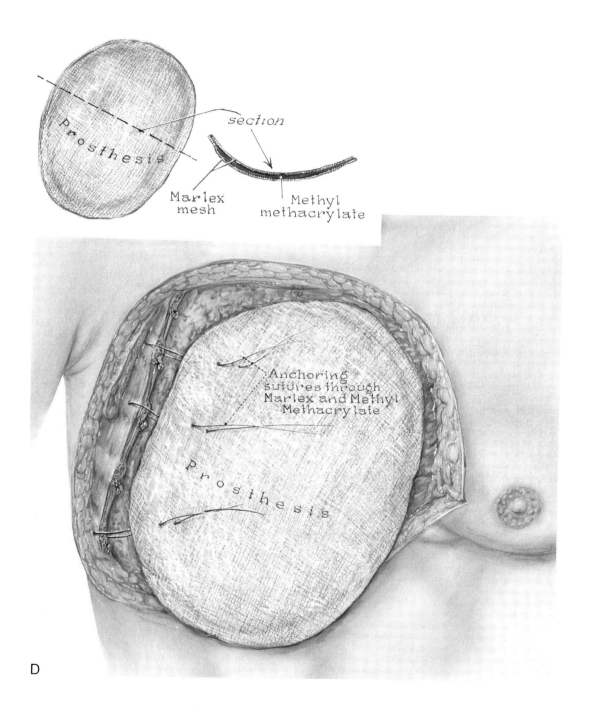

D

E. Several sutures are taken between the acrylic prosthesis and the bone on all sides. The hard acrylic prosthesis must be drilled through in order for the needle to be passed. This firmly seats the prosthesis, the feathered Marlex edge of which is sutured to the muscle and soft tissues beyond the borders of the bony defect.

F. *Top:* The island skin flap, depicted by a dotted line in the illustrations of the torso, had been outlined before the operation and included in the area draped out. *Bottom:* A circular incision is made along the dotted line down to the muscle. The large flap in this patient involves almost the entire latissimus dorsi, so the muscle is divided from the spine posteriorly and from the iliac crest inferiorly, and the attachments of the upper anterior border are dissected free. The upper and anterior border of the skin island outlined is continuous with the cutaneous operative defect. When the entire myocutaneous flap is elevated and rotated, as shown by the arrow, the island flap with its heavy base of full thickness of latissimus dorsi carrying the blood supply of the skin island comfortably overlies the Marlex-acrylic prosthesis and fills the cutaneous defect. Particularly with smaller islands of skin, it is advisable to secure the island to the underlying muscle with a continuous suture to decrease the likelihood that the vessels providing nutrition to the island of skin might be injured in the manipulation.

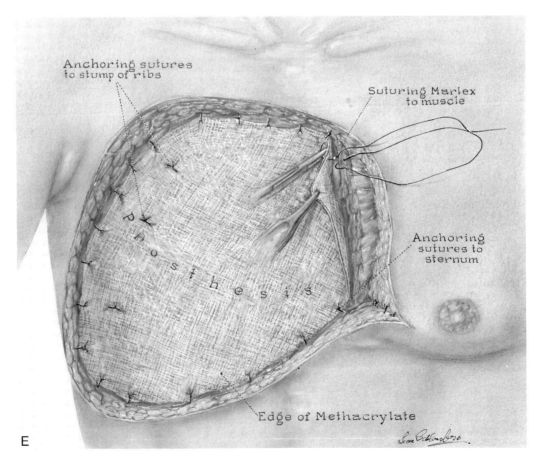

E

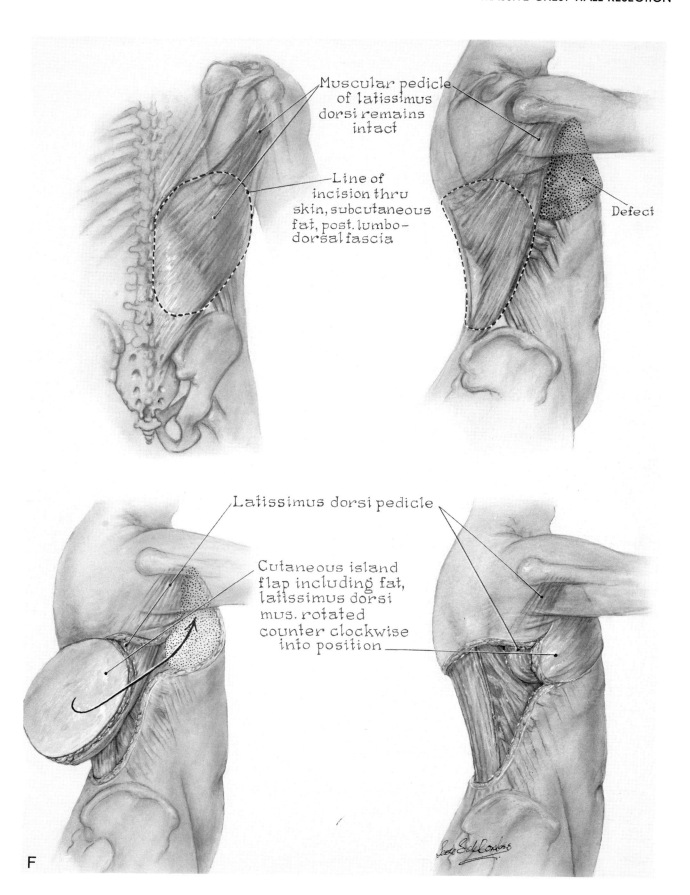

Muscular pedicle of latissimus dorsi remains intact

Line of incision thru skin, subcutaneous fat, post. lumbo-dorsal fascia

Defect

Latissimus dorsi pedicle

Cutaneous island flap including fat, latissimus dorsi mus. rotated counter clockwise into position

F

G. The final illustration shows the flap sutured in place. With a dissection of this size, a chest tube is employed. The very large donor site is closed by split-thickness grafts, either at the time or after a 24- to 48-hour delay.

From Ravitch, M.M., Hurwitz, D., and Wolmark, N.: Chest wall resection. Surgical Rounds, August 1980, pp. 15–24, with permission.

REFERENCES

1. Tansini, I.: Sopra il mio nuovo processo di amputazione della mammella. La Riforma Medica XXII:757–759, 1906
2. Campbell, D.A.: Reconstruction of the anterior thoracic wall. J. Thorac. Surg. 19:456–461, 1950
3. LeRoux, B.T.: Maintenance of chest wall stability. Thorax 19:397–405, 1964
4. Eschapasse, H., Gaillard, J., Fournial, G., Berthomieu, F., Henry, E., Hornus, E., and Hassani, M.: Utilisation de prothèses en résine acrylique pour la réparation des vastes pertes de substance de la paroi thoracique. Acta Chir. Belg. 76:281–285, 1977
5. Mathes, S.J., and Nahai, F.: *Clinical Applications for Muscles and Musculocutaneous Flaps.* St. Louis, C.V. Mosby Company, 1982

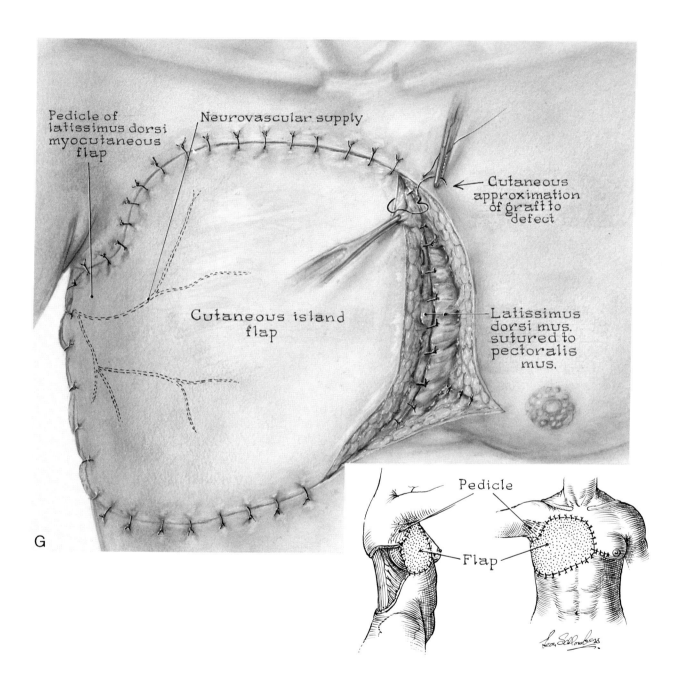

Pedicle of latissimus dorsi myocutaneous flap

Neurovascular supply

Cutaneous approximation of graft to defect

Cutaneous island flap

Latissimus dorsi mus. sutured to pectoralis mus.

G

Pedicle

Flap

CHONDROSARCOMA OF THE STERNUM, PREVIOUSLY BIOPSIED

MARLEX-ACRYLIC PROSTHESIS AND PECTORALIS MAJOR MYOCUTANEOUS GRAFT

A. The latissimus dorsi myocutaneous flap, in the case illustrated, was made necessary by both the obvious contamination of the biopsy wound with tumor and the jeopardy posed to the skin flap usually employed, by a fresh incision within it. The same reconstruction would be required for a tumor invading the skin or for recurrent tumor. The sagittal section shows the substantial inward projection of the tumor. One can be confident, at least at a primary operation, that such a tumor will not invade the intrathoracic structures. It is planned to excise the involved skin together with the chest wall. The only involvement of the skin is expected to be in the immediate vicinity of the biopsy wound, so that the incision comes fairly close to the swelling of the tumor.

B. The lower flap, composed of skin fat and pectoralis major, is elevated.

C. The internal mammary vessels are transfixed, ligated, and divided in the 2nd interspace to the right.

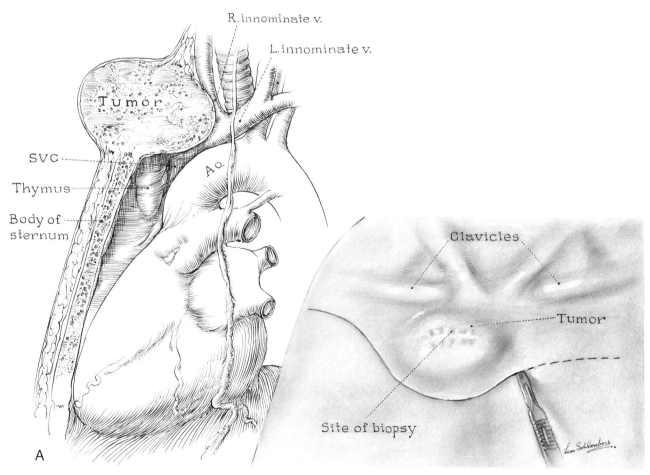

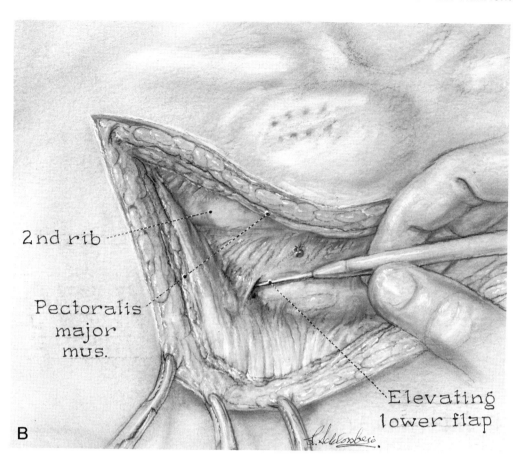

2nd rib

Pectoralis
major
mus.

Elevating
lower flap

B

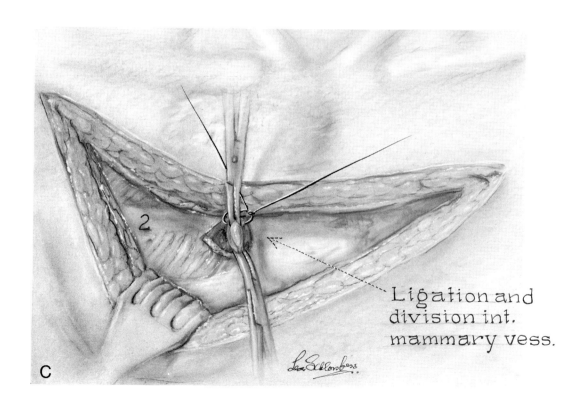

2

Ligation and
division int.
mammary vess.

C

D. The 2nd rib is divided several centimeters lateral to that. The sternum is transected, in this case with the Gigli saw.
E. The 2nd costal cartilage on the left (with the tumor lying more to the right) is divided fairly close to the sternum, and the internal mammary vessels on the left are secured (not shown). The 1st rib on each side is divided as well, and the intercostals secured by suture before the ribs are divided.

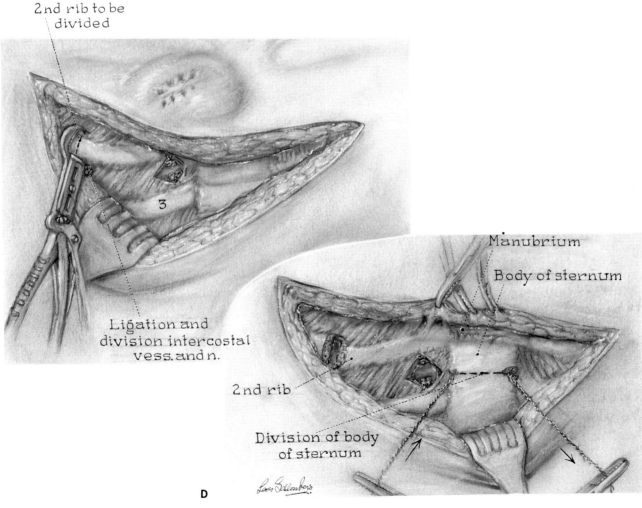

2nd rib to be divided

Ligation and division intercostal vess. and n.

Manubrium

Body of sternum

2nd rib

Division of body of sternum

D

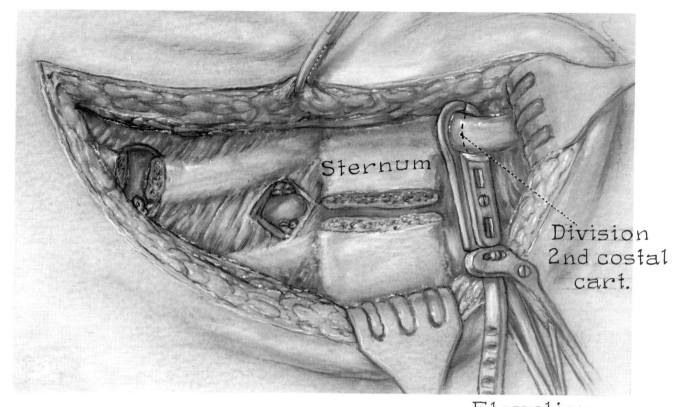

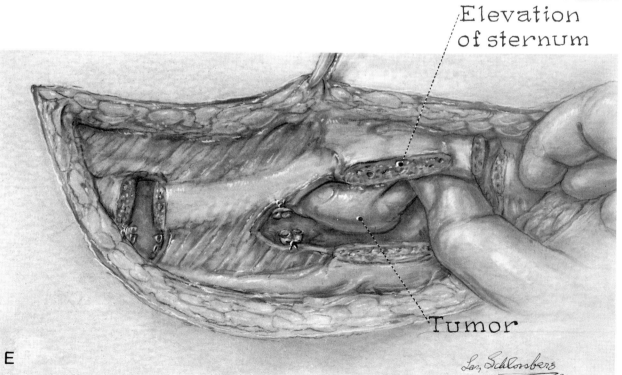

E

F. Elevation of the sternum now exposes the substernal mass and obvious important vascular attachments, so that the decision is made to free the upper border of the chest wall specimen before undertaking the mediastinal dissection.

G. The clavicle is shown divided, with a Gigli saw passed around it first with a clamp, and the subclavius muscle is also being divided. Superiorly, the right sternocleido-mastoid muscle, the ribbon muscles, and a portion of the left sternocleidomastoid are separated from the sternum, and (not shown) the sternoclavicular joint on the left is divided with bone cutters.

H. The specimen, now free but for its mediastinal attachments, is elevated, and the large tributary veins are readily secured.

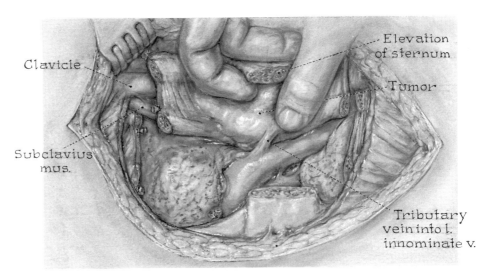

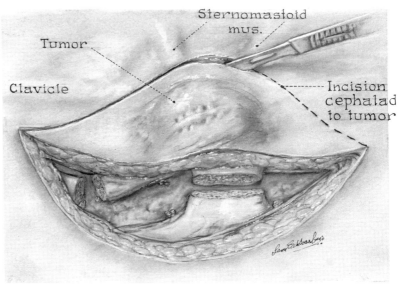

F

82

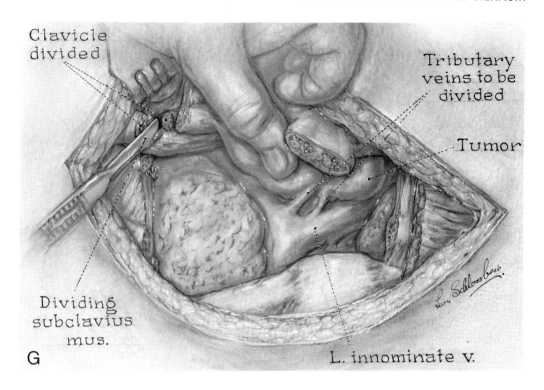

Clavicle divided

Tributary veins to be divided

Tumor

Dividing subclavius mus.

L. innominate v.

G

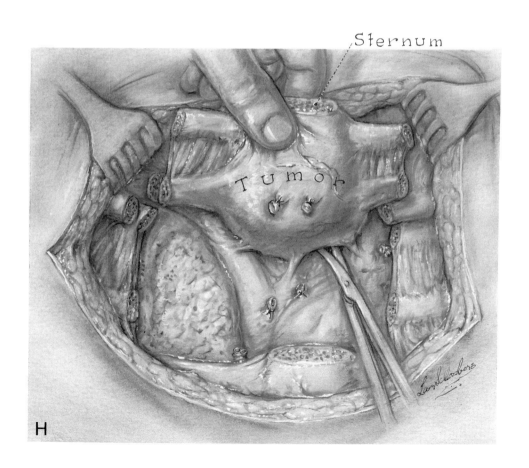

Sternum

Tumor

H

I. The resultant defect shows the innominate veins with the ligated tributaries and the ends of the two clavicles and the divided ribs. A considerable portion of the right pleural cavity is exposed. Drill holes through the clavicles, the ribs, and the methyl methacrylate permit firm seating on the chest wall of the Marlex–methyl methacrylate–Marlex prosthesis. The perforations in the prosthesis permit two-way drainage—there will be both a chest tube and wound suction catheters—and the ingrowth of granulation tissue.

J. The sternocleidomastoid and ribbon muscles superiorly, the pectoralis major laterally, and the rectus fascia inferiorly are sutured over the feathered Marlex edge of the prosthesis.

K. The cutaneous defect is too large to be closed simply by the use of relaxation incisions, and in any case, one would prefer to have more than skin over the acrylic prosthesis. An appropriately sized oval skin flap is elevated together with the underlying pectoralis major muscle and a portion of the sheath of rectus abdominis.

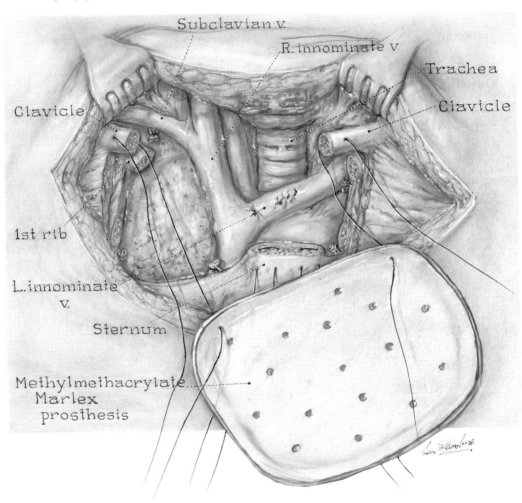

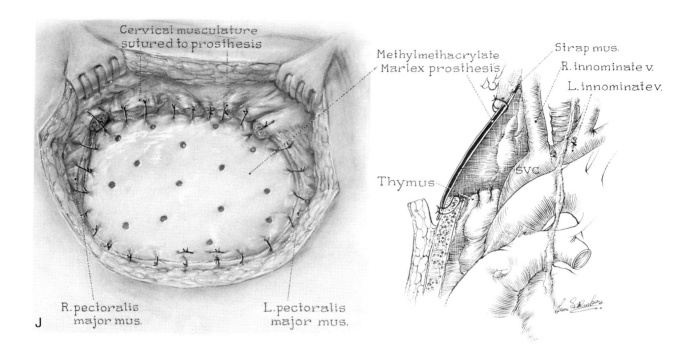

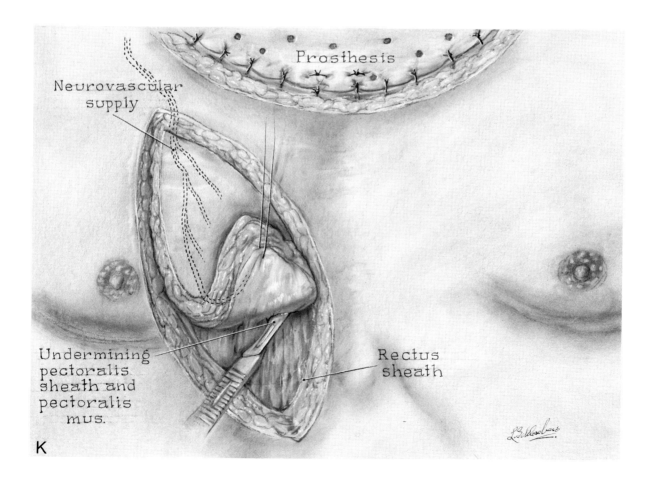

L. The pen-and-ink sketch shows the principle of this type of pectoralis major myocutaneous flap. *Left:* The blood supply nourishing the proposed flap is indicated. *Right:* The flap is elevated and rotated up into the defect by passing it under the bridge of skin and subcutaneous tissue between the defect and the donor site. The margins of the muscle flap are sutured to the muscle edges in the superior wound, and the skin flap is sutured to the surrounding skin. In this instance, the donor wound could be closed by tightly placed sutures. The inset shows the intercostal tube in the pleural cavity below and the wound catheter above, both on suction.

Figures *A, I,* and *L* from Ravitch, M.M.: In: *Gibbon's Surgery of the Chest,* 4th Edition, D.C. Sabiston and F.C. Spencer (Eds.). Philadelphia, W.B. Saunders Company, 1983, with permission.

REFERENCES

1. Brown, R.G., Fleming, W.H., and Jurkiewicz, M.J.: An island flap of the pectoralis major muscle. Br. J. Plast. Surg. 30:161–165, 1977
2. Tobin, G.R., Mavroudis, C., Howe, W.R., and Gray, L.A., Jr.: Reconstruction of complex thoracic defects with myocutaneous and muscle flaps. J. Thorac. Cardiovasc. Surg. 85:219–228, 1983
3. Arnold, P.G., and Pairolero, P.C.: Chest wall reconstruction: Experience with 100 consecutive patients. Ann. Surg. 199:725–732, 1984
4. Pairolero, P.C., and Arnold, P.G.: Chest wall tumors: Experience with 100 consecutive patients. J. Thorac. Cardiovasc. Surg. 90:367–372, 1985

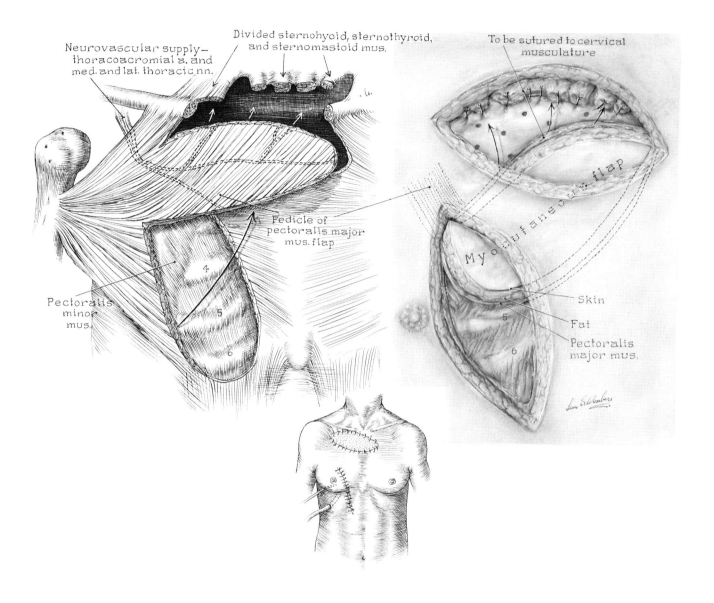

Neurovascular supply—
thoracoacromial a. and
med. and lat. thoracic nn.

Divided sternohyoid, sternothyroid,
and sternomastoid mus.

To be sutured to cervical
musculature

Pedicle of
pectoralis major
mus. flap

Pectoralis
minor
mus.

Myocutaneous flap

Skin

Fat

Pectoralis
major mus.

Diaphragm

DIAPHRAGM SEEN FROM ABOVE

The attachment of the pericardium and the positions of the perforating structures are shown.

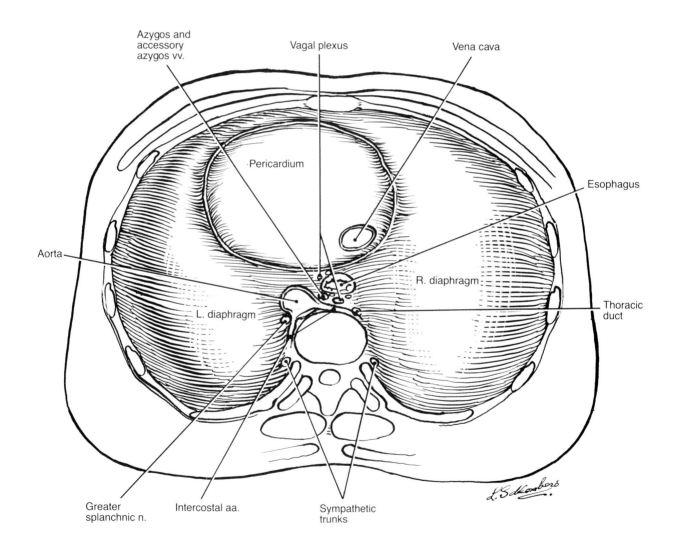

DIAPHRAGM SEEN FROM BELOW

The posterior edge of the diaphragm is applied rather flatly to the posterior wall for some distance, so that the esophageal hiatus, which appears in this drawing to be well anterior to the aorta as well as slightly to its left, is in fact very little anterior to it but emerges through the diaphragm at the more cephalad extent of the diaphragm's posterior fixation.

From Zuidema, G.D. (Ed.) and Schlossberg, L. (Illustrator): *Atlas of Human Functional Anatomy*, 3rd Edition. Baltimore, Johns Hopkins University Press, 1985, with permission.

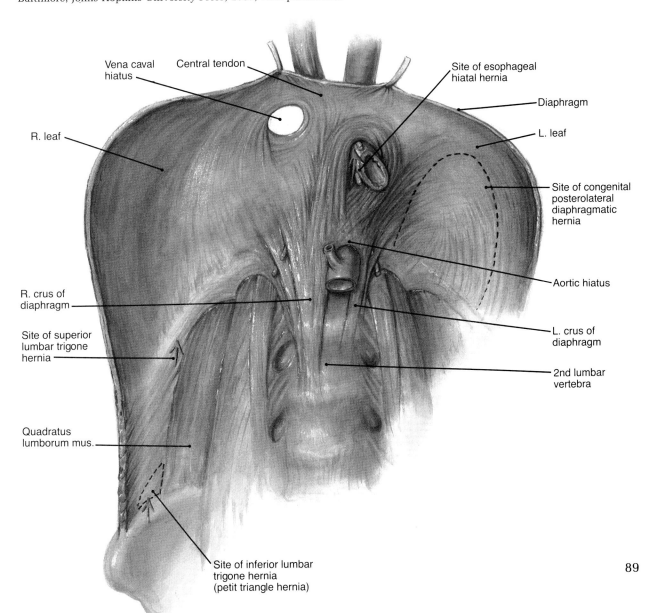

Vena caval hiatus

Central tendon

Site of esophageal hiatal hernia

Diaphragm

R. leaf

L. leaf

Site of congenital posterolateral diaphragmatic hernia

Aortic hiatus

R. crus of diaphragm

L. crus of diaphragm

Site of superior lumbar trigone hernia

2nd lumbar vertebra

Quadratus lumborum mus.

Site of inferior lumbar trigone hernia (petit triangle hernia)

89

Subphrenic Abscess

DRAINAGE OF SUBPHRENIC ABSCESS OR ABSCESS OF LIVER—INTERCOSTAL, TRANSPLEURAL, TRANSDIAPHRAGMATIC

A. The suspected abscess is localized either by direct aspiration on the basis of physical examination or after appropriate imaging. Only enough pus is withdrawn to be certain that the needle is in the cavity, and the needle is left in place (not shown). If for any reason the needle is to be removed, it is worthwhile injecting a small amount (1 to 3 cc) of methylene blue or gentian violet into the cavity, particularly for subphrenic abscesses. This will identify the occasional occurrence that aspiration is of one loculus of the abscess, and drainage of another.

B. A good-sized oval of skin, fat, and muscle is resected down to rib, and 2 or 3 cm of rib is resected with periosteum and intercostal muscles.

C. Incision is made into the pleural cavity, disclosing the pleural surface of the diaphragm. *Left:* The free edges of the pleural opening are rapidly sutured to the diaphragm beneath with a continuous absorbable suture, effectively excluding the pleural cavity from the wound. *Right:* A 4-inch × 4-inch sponge is opened, stretched, twisted, and laid into the wound to protect the soft tissues and reinforce the suture seal.

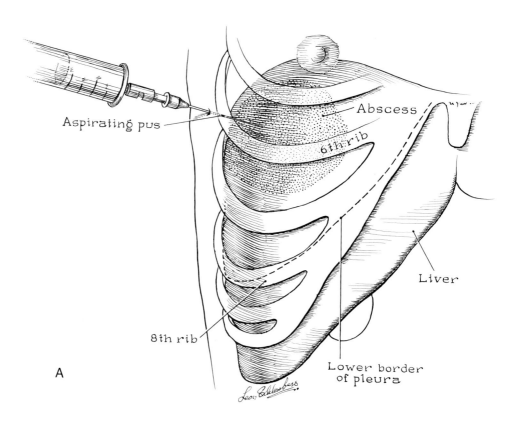

A

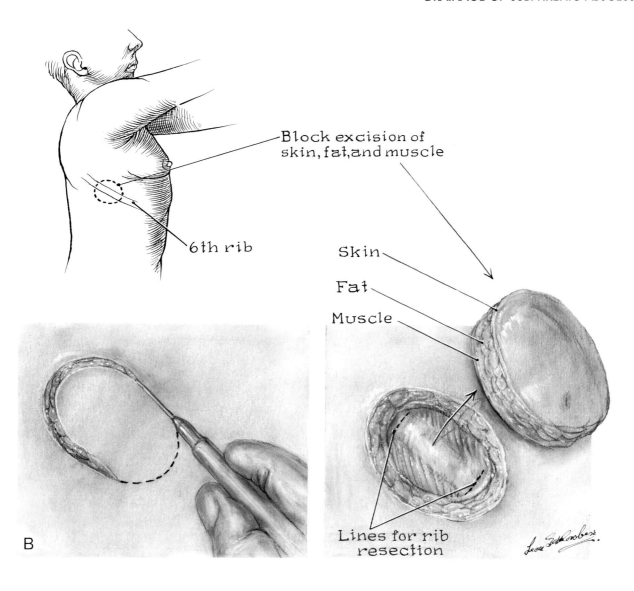

Block excision of
skin, fat, and muscle

6th rib

Skin

Fat

Muscle

Lines for rib
resection

B

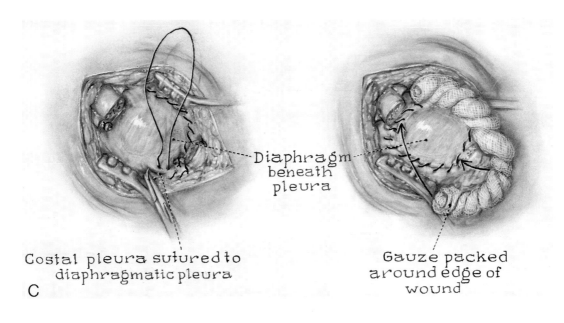

Diaphragm
beneath
pleura

Costal pleura sutured to
diaphragmatic pleura

C

Gauze packed
around edge of
wound

DRAINAGE OF SUBPHRENIC ABSCESS *(Continued)*

D. If the needle is not still in place, the abscess is aspirated and then a clamp is pushed through into the abscess; the opening is enlarged with the finger and then with the knife or cautery.

E. *Top:* With the finger in the cavity, one can now tell whether the abscess is subphrenic, the inner wall of which will be smooth, or an excavation in the liver, the inner wall of which will be ragged. Pus is aspirated and any thick coagulum or necrotic tissue is removed. The amount of recess here shown below the wound edge is permissible. If it were any more, an additional rib below would be removed, bringing the opening of the wound closer to the bottom of the cavity. *Bottom:* Two of the large drainage tubes that we prefer have been placed in the wound and wrapped around with gauze to protect the soft tissues and to promote the adhesion of the pleura to the diaphragm. It is our conviction that the best drainage of a subphrenic abscess is that which ensures dependency and takes the shortest course to the body wall. The same approach is useful for appropriately located liver abscesses. Occasionally in huge abscesses this might, indeed, be by an approach from below the 12th rib or from under the costal margin anteriorly, but not very often. We have used this approach for four decades and have yet to see an empyema, or a pneumothorax amounting to more than a trifling cap of air at the apex. The excision of skin, fat, muscle, and ribs is performed because premature closure of a linear incision, interfering with adequate drainage, is so much more likely than any problem with the healing of a larger wound.

REFERENCES

1. Johnston, G.B.: Symptoms and treatment of hepatic abscess with report of eighteen cases. Transactions of the American Surgical Association XV:225–250, 1897
2. Ochsner, A., and Graves, A.M.: Subphrenic abscess. An analysis of 3,372 collected and personal cases. Transactions of the American Surgical Association LI:349–378, 1933
3. Wooler, G.H.: Subphrenic abscess. Thorax 11:211–222, 1956
4. Boyd, D.P.: The intrathoracic complications of subphrenic abscess. J. Thorac. Cardiovasc. Surg. 38:771–779, 1959

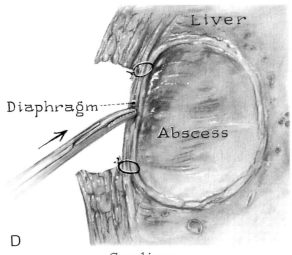

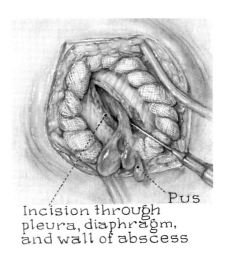

Liver

Diaphragm

Abscess

D

Section

Incision through
pleura, diaphragm,
and wall of abscess

Pus

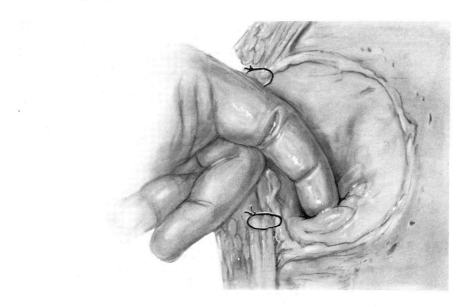

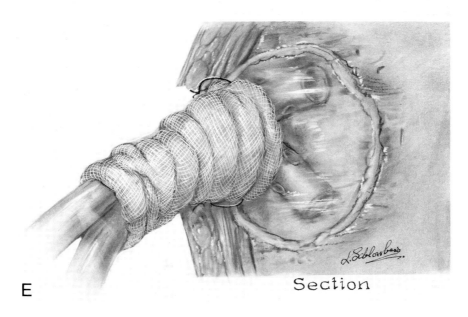

E

Section

DRAINAGE OF SUBPHRENIC ABSCESS OR ABSCESS OF LIVER—INTERCOSTAL, EXTRAPLEURAL, TRANSDIAPHRAGMATIC

A. The drawing shows the abscess centered under the 10th rib, a little behind the posterior axillary line. The dotted outline of the pleural reflections indicates the possibility that the abscess can be approached extrapleurally. After the abscess is appropriately located by physical examination and imaging by CT scan or sonography, the patient is operated upon under local anesthesia. When the patient is on the table and in the lateral position, the location of the abscess is confirmed by aspiration of 1 or 2 cc with a needle; usually the needle is left in place to guide the dissection.

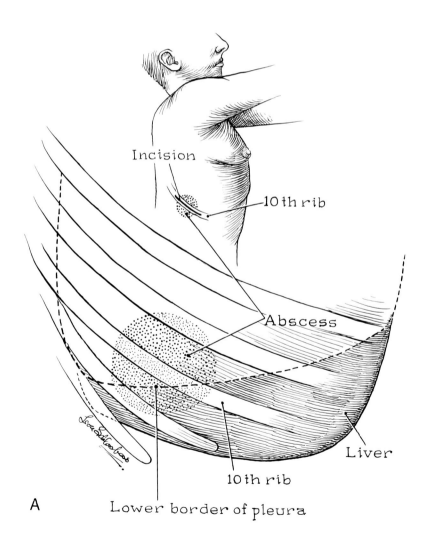

Incision

10th rib

Abscess

Liver

10th rib

A

Lower border of pleura

B. As in the previous illustrations, a generous segment of rib is resected and, if the cavity is at all large, a full thickness of chest wall and a disc of skin are taken. In the present instance it is not expected that prolonged drainage will be required. *Top left:* The reflection of the pleura is identified and stripped upward from the diaphragm, exposing the bare diaphragm below the pleural reflection without ever entering the pleural cavity. *Top right:* If the needle has been withdrawn, the abscess is aspirated directly through the diaphragm, a clamp inserted through the needle hole and spread, and the diaphragm incised with knife or cautery. A finger is inserted to determine the size of the cavity, pus is aspirated, and any large masses of coagulum or necrotic liver are picked out. The finger should probe the abscess cavity to make sure that its lowest limit has been reached. It may at times be necessary to resect another rib, with the intercostal muscles, to eliminate any inferior recess. *Bottom:* We prefer large rubber tubes for drains, with gauze wrapped around them to pack the wound open and prevent its too early closure.

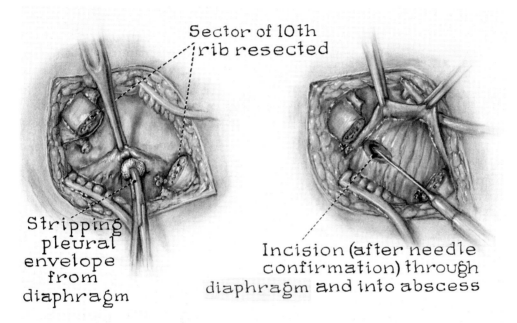

Sector of 10th rib resected

Stripping pleural envelope from diaphragm

Incision (after needle confirmation) through diaphragm and into abscess

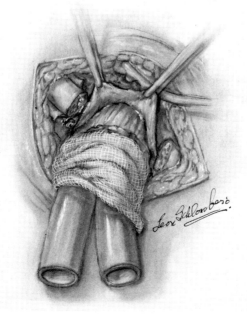

B

Thoracic Outlet Syndrome.
Transaxillary Sympathectomy

THE THORACIC OUTLET

Emphasized are the passage of the subclavian artery over the first rib and between the scaleni as the vein and the artery diverge around the anterior scalenus muscle, the course of the brachial plexus behind and above the artery at the level of the first rib, and the phrenic nerve lying on the belly of the anterior scalenus. Depending upon the configuration of the first rib, its degree of elevation, and the presence or absence of a cervical rib (not shown), scalenotomy alone may or may not relieve the subclavian compression in the thoracic outlet syndrome. Resection of the first rib and of any cervical rib or ligament is the more definitive procedure.

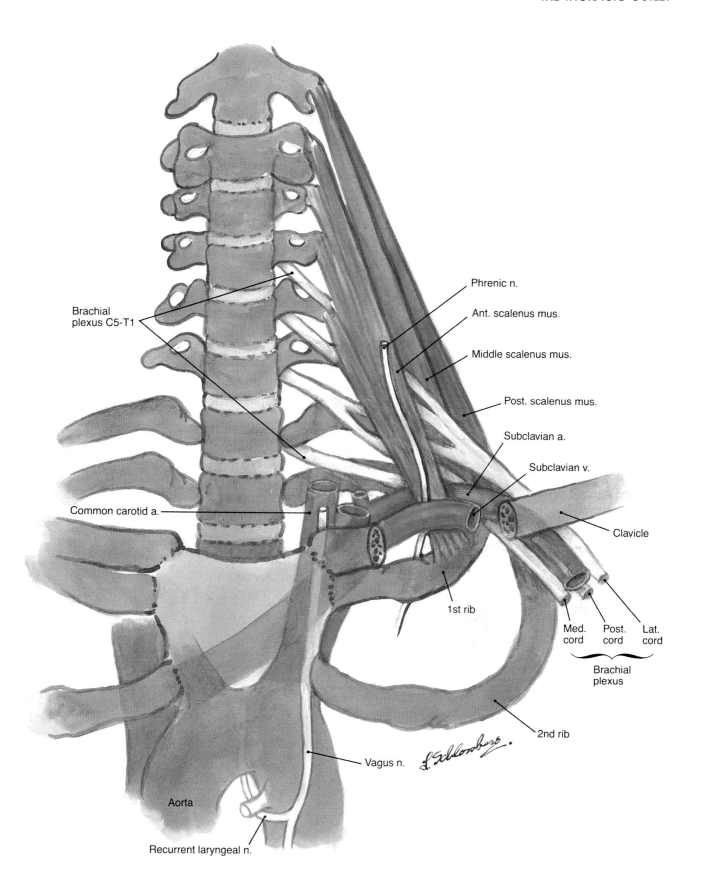

Brachial
plexus C5-T1

Phrenic n.

Ant. scalenus mus.

Middle scalenus mus.

Post. scalenus mus.

Subclavian a.

Subclavian v.

Clavicle

Common carotid a.

1st rib

Med. cord

Post. cord

Lat. cord

Brachial plexus

2nd rib

Vagus n.

Aorta

Recurrent laryngeal n.

TRANSAXILLARY RESECTION OF THE FIRST RIB FOR THORACIC OUTLET SYNDROME

A. The patient is placed in the lateral decubitus position with the involved extremity abducted to 90° by an assistant. Traction on the arm by the assistant can be released intermittently.

A transverse, slightly curved incision, made in the axilla below the hair line, extends between the borders of the pectoralis major anteriorly and the latissimus dorsi posteriorly.

As the incision is deepened to the external thoracic fascia, care is taken to preserve the intercostobrachial cutaneous nerve, which lies in the center of the operative field. The axillary vein emerges between the clavicle and the 1st rib. Note that with the arm elevated, the vessels and nerves ascend vertically into the extremity. Dissecting superiorly, one encounters the anterior scalenus muscle, inserting on the 1st rib, followed by the axillary artery and the elements of the brachial plexus. The most posterior structures are the middle scalenus muscle, inserting on the 1st rib, and the posterior scalenus muscle, inserting on the 2nd rib. The apex of the pleura is behind the artery and vein and the anterior scalenus muscle.

B. The dissection is carried toward the apex of the axilla along the external thoracic fascia up to the 1st rib. With gentle dissection, the axillary vein and artery, the brachial plexus, and the anterior and middle scaleni are delineated clearly. After clear identification of the insertion of the anterior scalenus, the muscle is divided directly upon the upper border of the 1st rib. The periosteum of the rib is then incised with the cautery and the rib dissected out subperiosteally. The insertion of the middle scalenus muscle should be elevated from the rib, rather than transected, in order to avoid injury to the long thoracic nerve, which runs along the posterior margin of the middle scalenus muscle.

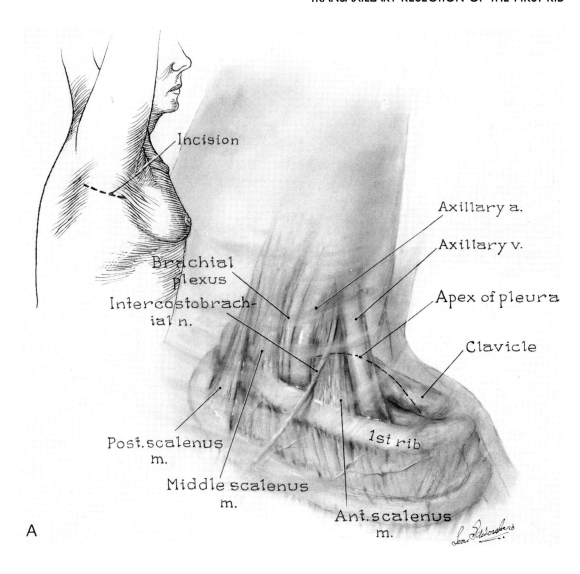

Incision

Brachial plexus

Intercostobrach-
ial n.

Axillary a.

Axillary v.

Apex of pleura

Clavicle

1st rib

Post. scalenus
m.

Middle scalenus
m.

Ant. scalenus
m.

A

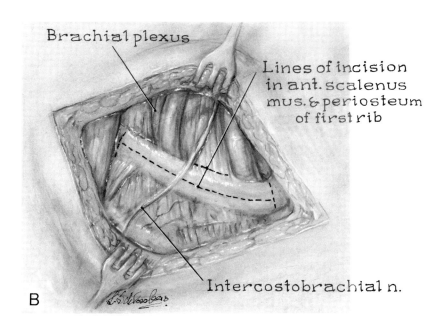

Brachial plexus

Lines of incision
in ant. scalenus
mus. & periosteum
of first rib

Intercostobrachial n.

B

99

TRANSAXILLARY RESECTION OF THE FIRST RIB *(Continued)*

C. The rib is then freed up subperiosteally, thus protecting artery, vein, and brachial plexus. It may well be resected in one piece, with the transections placed posteriorly at the level of the articulation with the transverse process and anteriorly at the costochondral junction. It is often more practical to divide the rib halfway and then to dissect anteriorly and posteriorly, resecting the rib in two segments or even three.

Following complete removal of the neck and head of the 1st rib, the 8th cervical and the 1st thoracic nerve roots are clearly seen. If a cervical rib is present, its anterior portion usually attaches to the 1st rib, and it is resected after the posterior half of the 1st rib has been removed, providing better access to the cervical rib. A suction drain is placed.

REFERENCE

1. Roos, D.B.: Transaxillary approach for first rib resection to relieve thoracic outlet syndrome. Ann. Surg. 163:354–358, 1966

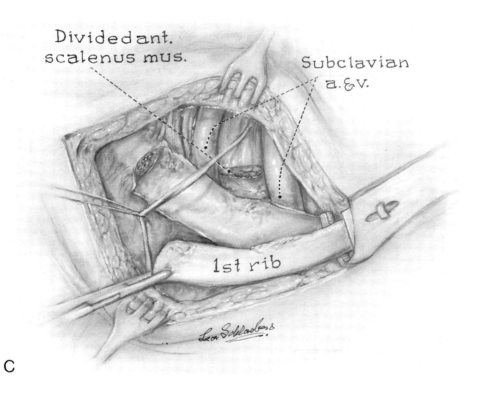

C

CERVICODORSAL SYMPATHECTOMY

Transaxillary, Transpleural Approach*

A. The arm is held at a right angle to the body. The usual transaxillary thoracotomy is made through the periosteal bed of the 3rd rib. The rib need not be removed (see pages 138–144, *Axillary Thoracotomy*).

B. The sympathetic trunk and ganglia can be palpated paravertebrally and exposed by incising the pleura over them. The sympathetic trunk is exposed to the stellate ganglion above and the 3rd or 4th ganglion below.

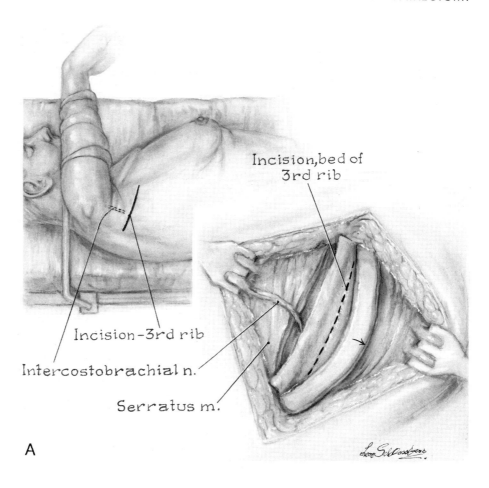

Incision, bed of 3rd rib

Incision-3rd rib

Intercostobrachial n.

Serratus m.

A

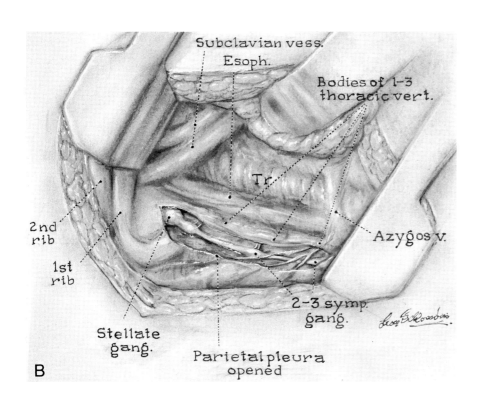

Subclavian vess.

Esoph.

Bodies of 1-3 thoracic vert.

Tr

Azygos v.

2nd rib

1st rib

2-3 symp. gang.

Stellate gang.

Parietal pleura opened

B

CERVICODORSAL SYMPATHECTOMY *(Continued)*

Transaxillary, Transpleural Approach* *(Continued)*

C. The trunk is clipped and divided below the 3rd or 4th dorsal ganglion as the operator chooses, the proximal stump is held up, and the rami communicantes are serially divided, with the trunk elevated until the stellate ganglion is reached. In the usual sympathectomy, the lower half of the stellate ganglion may be taken for a more complete sympathectomy, with some increase in the risk of Horner's syndrome. The metal clips are used in part from tradition and in part so that later roentgenograms can confirm the topographical extent of the resection.

It is scarcely necessary to drain the chest, which is evacuated of air by inflating the lungs and withdrawing a catheter under aspiration as the last suture in the periosteal bed is tied.

REFERENCES

1. Atkins, H.J.B.: Sympathectomy by the axillary approach. Lancet 1:538–539, 1954
   In an earlier "letter to the editor," Lancet December 17, 1949, p. 1152, Atkins said, "When Prof. R.H. Goetz, of Cape Town, visited this country last summer he persuaded me to adopt the periaxillary approach to the stellate and upper thoracic sympathetic ganglia." In the 1954 article Atkins says, "the procedure was devised by W.G. Schulze and Prof. R.H. Goetz, at the Groote Schuur Hospital, Cape Town." A letter from Professor R.P. Hewitson, of the Groote Schuur Hospital in Cape Town, December 20, 1984, says, "Professor Cole Rous, who succeeded Professor Saint when he retired at the end of 1946, was doing sympathectomies through an anterolateral second rib approach. Naturally, this leaves an ugly scar, particularly in females, and so Bill Schulze in 1947 made the approach through the second rib entirely in the axilla. He says that Professor Goetz had no part in this but the latter was, as is well known, very interested in the sympathetic nervous system and its outflow from the chest. Schulze approached Goetz to describe the sympathetic anatomy, with the idea that he [Schulze] would describe his axillary approach in the same article—but Goetz never responded and so Schulze did not get around to publishing. Schulze went over to London for a period (to get his FRCS amongst other things) and demonstrated this approach to Hedley Atkins amongst others. . . ."
2. Little, J.M.: Transaxillary transpleural thoracic sympathectomy. Surgical Techniques Illustrated 2:15–27, 1977
3. Linder, F., Jenal, G., and Assmus, H.: Axillary transpleural sympathectomy: Indication, technique, and results. World J. Surg. 7:437–439, 1983
   See also references after Lateral Thoracotomy without Division of Muscle (Axillary Thoracotomy, page 144).

---

*Note: As for many operative approaches, this one has been discovered and rediscovered by surgeons in various places and at various times.

104

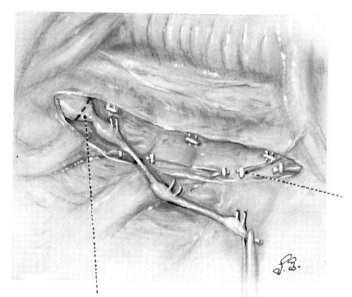

Divided
intercostal
vv.

Excision of
lower portion
of stellate gang. and
1st, 2nd, and
C   3rd symp. gang.

CERVICODORSAL SYMPATHECTOMY *(Continued)*

Supraclavicular Approach

Although the axillary, transthoracic approach shown in the previous plates (pages 102–105) has become particularly popular in recent years, there has been a long and satisfactory experience with the supraclavicular approach, which is direct and straightforward and obviates thoracotomy.

The patient is placed with a roll between the scapulae, with the ipsilateral arm pulled down.

A. The approach is through a short, transverse supraclavicular incision. Making the incision medially tends to avoid annoying venous bleeding from veins commonly found lateral to the muscle. The clavicular head of the sternocleidomastoid is held up by a right-angle clamp passed under it and is divided.

B. Clearing away the fat and areolar tissue behind the muscle exposes the phrenic nerve lying on the anterior scalenus muscle. The nerve is carefully retracted medially together with the carotid sheath, and the scalenus is dissected free, held up by a clamp passed under it, and divided.

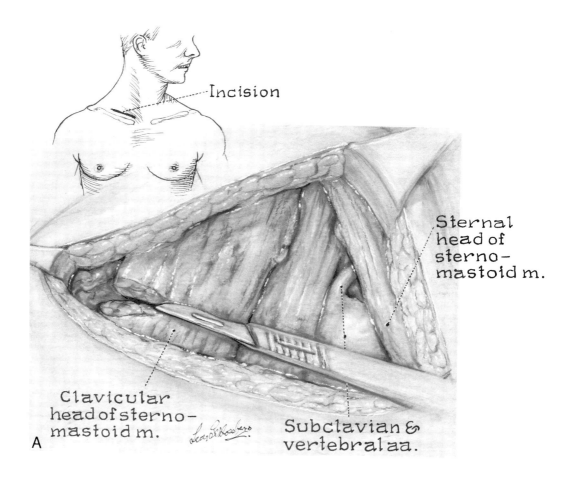

Incision

Sternal
head of
sterno-
mastoid m.

Clavicular
head of sterno-
mastoid m.

Subclavian &
vertebral aa.

A

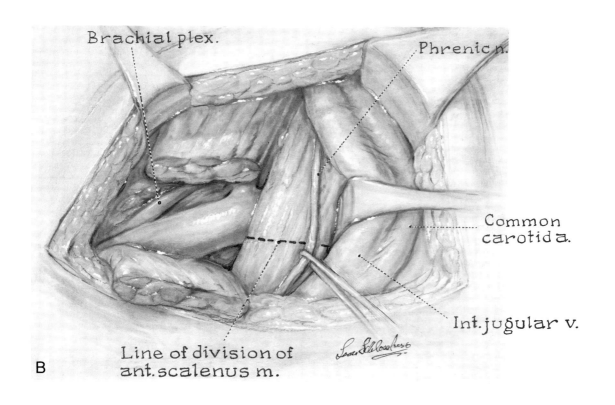

Brachial plex.

Phrenic n.

Common
carotid a.

Int. jugular v.

Line of division of
ant. scalenus m.

B

CERVICODORSAL SYMPATHECTOMY (Continued)

Supraclavicular Approach (Continued)

C. The subclavian artery presents, arching up from beneath the clavicle. When its upper surface is cleared of fat, the thyroid axis and vertebral arteries can be seen. In order to mobilize the subclavian sufficiently to depress it out of the way, the thyroid axis may have to be divided. A space is exposed between the middle scalenus muscle and inner cord of the brachial plexus laterally, the internal jugular vein medially (retracted out of harm's way), and the subclavian artery and the clavicle below. Sibson's fascia, flooring this space, overlies the apex of the pleura. As the fascia is divided, the extrapleural space is entered and the pleura gently dissected back with a gauze dissector and fingers, pressing upon the very junction between the necks of the ribs, or the vertebrae, and the edge of the pleura.

D. Carrying the dissection down to the neck of the 3rd rib provides the exposure shown, confirmed by finger palpation of the stellate ganglion and the sympathetic chain below it. The trunk is usually divided distal to the 3rd or 4th thoracic ganglion, the ganglion grasped and elevated, and the rami divided, freeing the trunk and ganglia upward progressively. The rami of the stellate ganglion are divided, and either the ganglion is entirely spared or the distal portion is resected. The upper and distal limits of resection of the chain are usually marked with silver clips. Elaborate treatment of the cephalad end to prevent regeneration is no longer in vogue.

REFERENCES

1. Nanson, E.M.: The anterior approach to upper dorsal sympathectomy. Surg. Gynecol. Obstet. 104:118–120, 1957
2. Johnson, R.M., and Southwick, W.O.: Surgical approaches to the spine. In: R.H. Rothman and F.A. Simeone (Eds.). *The Spine*, Volume I. Philadelphia, W.B. Saunders Company, 1975, pp. 69–156

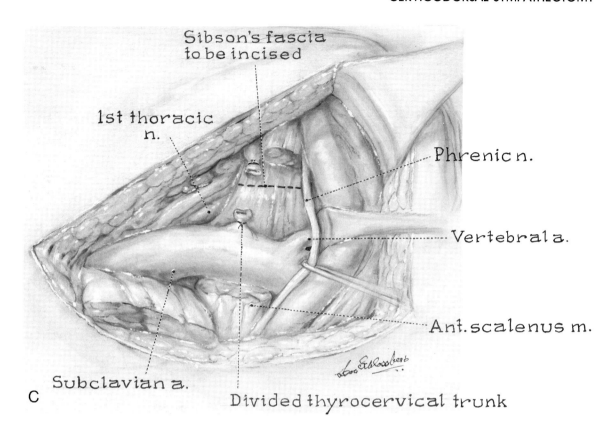

Sibson's fascia
to be incised

1st thoracic
n.

Phrenic n.

Vertebral a.

Ant. scalenus m.

Subclavian a.

C

Divided thyrocervical trunk

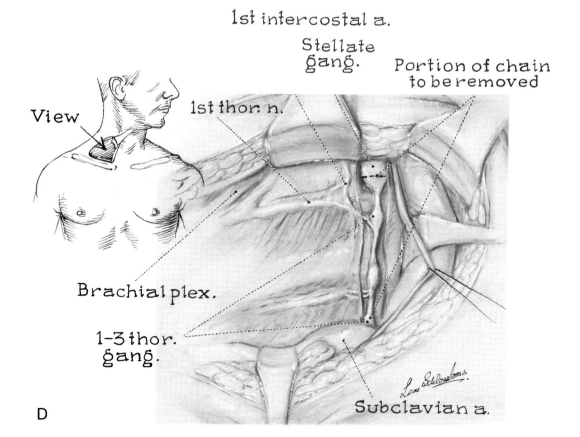

1st intercostal a.

Stellate
gang.

Portion of chain
to be removed

1st thor. n.

View

Brachial plex.

1-3 thor.
gang.

Subclavian a.

D

Thoracic Incisions

Thoracic Incisions

MEDIAN STERNOTOMY

This incision provides the quickest access and best exposure for resection of the thymus and most anterior mediastinal cysts and tumors, as well as for operations upon the heart and great vessels. It can provide good exposure of the lung if there are reasons to avoid anterior or lateral thoracotomy, and it can be used for some bilateral pulmonary operations. The left lower lobe is not easily accessible through a median sternotomy.

A. The less the subcutaneous fat is dissected away from the sternum, the less space there will ultimately be for the accumulation of fluid.

B. It is usually advisable to separate the posterior aspect of the sternum from the mediastinal structures by blunt finger dissection from behind the manubrium downward, and from the xiphoid process upward, to be sure that there is space between the heart and great vessels and the saw. Many operators eschew this step.

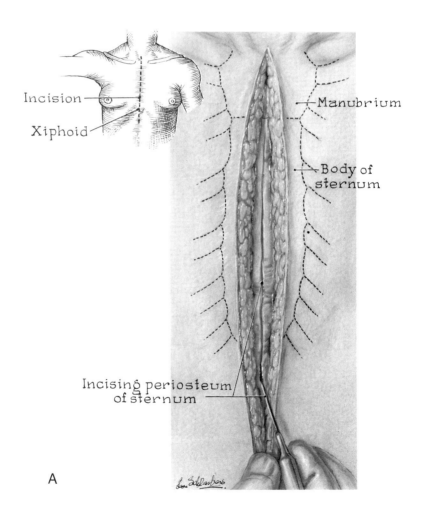

A

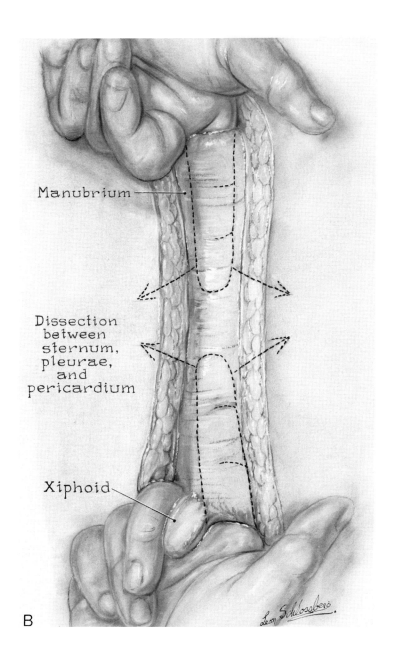

Manubrium

Dissection
between
sternum,
pleurae,
and
pericardium

Xiphoid

B

C. *Left*: A powered saw, preferably with a guide that passes behind the sternum, is employed after incision of the anterior periosteum with the electrocautery to minimize bleeding. The saw cut may be made from above downward as shown, or in the reverse direction. The right ventricle has been known to be incised by an oscillating saw, without a guide, that was pressed down too vigorously as it cut the sternum. *Right*: Bleeding from the bone is controlled with the electrocautery, applied to a fine hemostat on the bleeding points, or with bone wax. The hemostatic scalpel (hot knife) lends itself ideally to control of bleeding from the periosteum and bone.

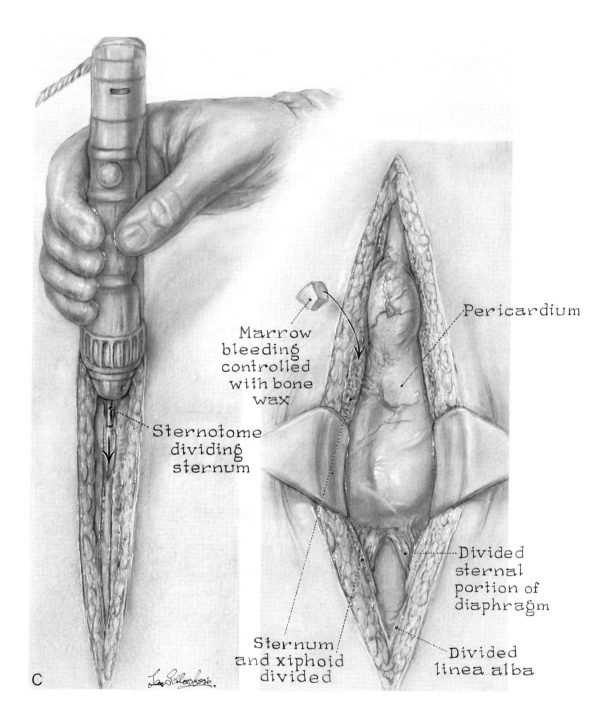

Marrow
bleeding
controlled
with bone
wax

Pericardium

Sternotome
dividing
sternum

Sternum
and xiphoid
divided

Divided
sternal
portion of
diaphragm

Divided
linea alba

C

D. As the sternal spreading retractor is opened gradually, the pleura is stripped back from mediastinum and chest wall, exposing the anterior mediastinum.
E. Closure is with heavy wire or synthetic sutures, passed either *(left)* through perforations in the sternum made with an awl, or in the less sclerotic sternum, with the heavy cutting needle. Alternatively *(right)*, the suture is placed around the sternum. If the sternum tends to buckle forward, it is well to insert special sutures to resist this tendency, in addition to the usual sutures in the periosteum and anterior cortex.

REFERENCES

1. Milton, H.: Mediastinal surgery. Lancet 1:872–875, 1897
   The historic description of median sternotomy by its inventor, who predicted then that it would be useful for surgery of the heart and great vessels.
2. Holman, E., and Willett, F.: The surgical correction of constrictive pericarditis. Surg. Gynecol. Obstet. 89:129–144, 1949
3. Julian, O.C., Lopez-Belio, M., Dye, W.S., et al.: The median sternal incision in intracardiac surgery with extracorporeal circulation: A general evaluation of its use in heart surgery. Surgery 42:753–761, 1957
4. Robicsek, F., Daugherty, H.K., and Cook, J.W.: The prevention and treatment of sternum separation following open-heart surgery. J. Thorac. Cardiovasc. Surg. 73:267–268, 1977
   For the osteoporotic sternum—parasternal wires passed under and over the costal cartilages to prevent the circumsternal wires from cutting through.

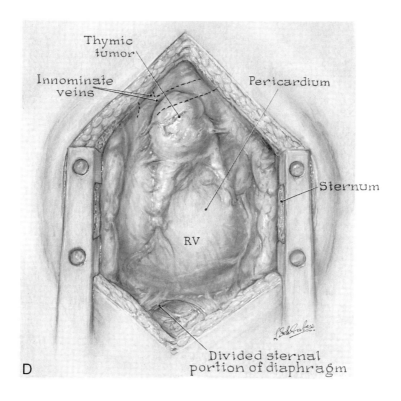

D

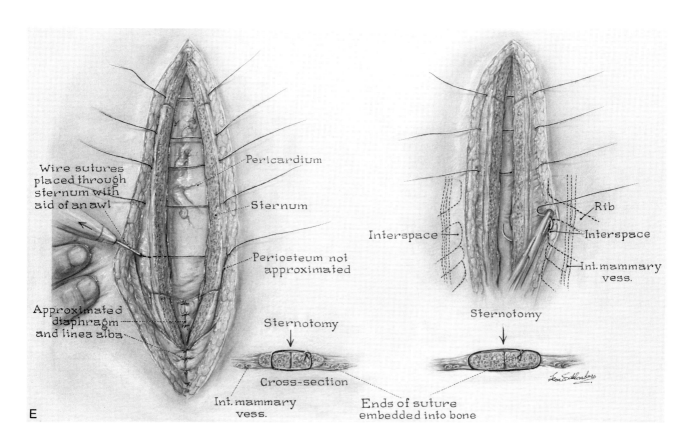

E

Alternative approximations of
the sternum

POSTEROLATERAL THORACOTOMY

The formal posterolateral thoracotomy provides the widest exposure and the safest manipulation of the intrathoracic viscera, but it must be recognized that an incision of this magnitude carries a certain morbidity of its own, apart from the time involved in making and closing it.

A. The patient is lying on the right side, tilted about 15° forward from a straight lateral position, and the left arm is carefully tied with swathed wrappings to a support. The incision begins often as high as the upper border of the scapula, passes down paraspinally, and then swings around anteriorly 2 or 3 cm below the inferior angle of the scapula to beyond the anterior axillary line or farther forward. In many cases, the vertical portion of the incision is not needed and a purely lateral thoracotomy incision is employed—straight line or slightly curved.

B. With scissors and the fingers, the areolar and fibrous tissues are opened in the triangle of auscultation, the space under the latissimus dorsi is exposed, and the latissimus dorsi is held up with the fingers (as shown) and cut with the cutting current of the fine needle–tipped electrocautery. (Obviously, the cold scalpel, and for that matter, the hemostatic scalpel—hot knife—have their uses and their proponents.) Any individual vessels large enough to continue bleeding are seized with a fine hemostat and electrocoagulated as the operation proceeds.

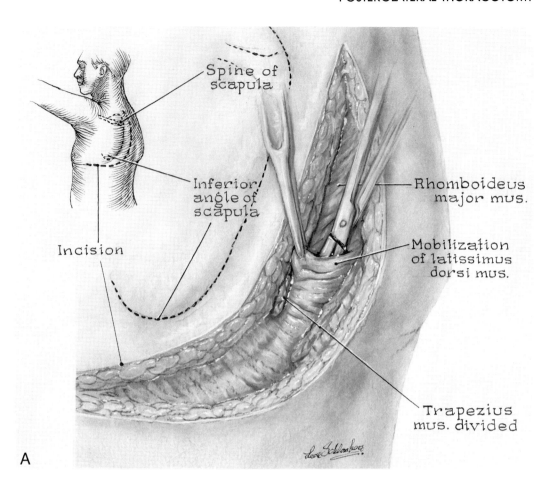

Spine of scapula

Inferior angle of scapula

Incision

Rhomboideus major mus.

Mobilization of latissimus dorsi mus.

Trapezius mus. divided

A

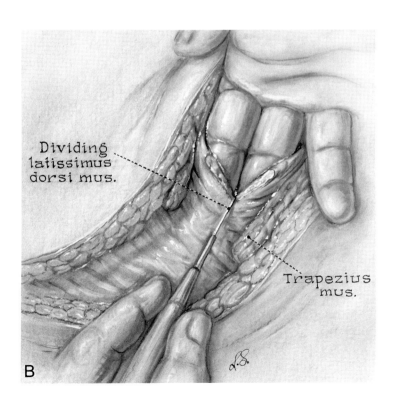

Dividing latissimus dorsi mus.

Trapezius mus.

B

119

C. Posteriorly, one applies the same maneuvers, proceeding upward, to divide the trapezius and the rhomboids. The farther posteriorly the incisions in the latissimus and trapezius are made, the more ligamentous and less heavily muscular is the structure, the less the bleeding, and the more secure the sutured closure. In the lateral (axillary) thoracotomy, the incision does not involve the trapezius and rhomboids (see pages 138–141, *Lateral Thoracotomy without Division of Muscle [Axillary Thoracotomy]*).

D. The standard posterolateral thoracotomy for pneumonectomy or other major thoracic procedure is through the bed of the 5th rib, or the 5th interspace.

For operations involving the lower esophagus or diaphragm, a substantially lower incision can be made, and for lesions involving dissection at the cupola of the hemithorax, an incision at the 3rd or 4th rib or interspace can be made. In rare instances and for special purposes, through the approach shown, two chest wall incisions are made—for example, in the 4th and 8th interspaces.

The scapula is held up by an elevator and a hand is slipped up under it and slid along the chest wall, around and above the posterior scalenus until the first rib is unequivocally identified. The ribs are then counted down from above.

Depending upon the level of access into the chest, the pectoralis major is transected or split. Particularly in children, it may be worthwhile to detach the origins of the pectoralis major from the ribs and reapply them at the conclusion. The fibers of the anterior serratus are usually split or may, like the pectorals, be detached.

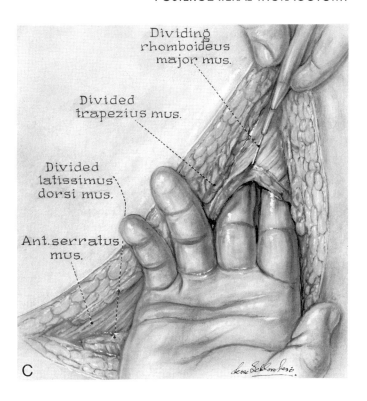

C

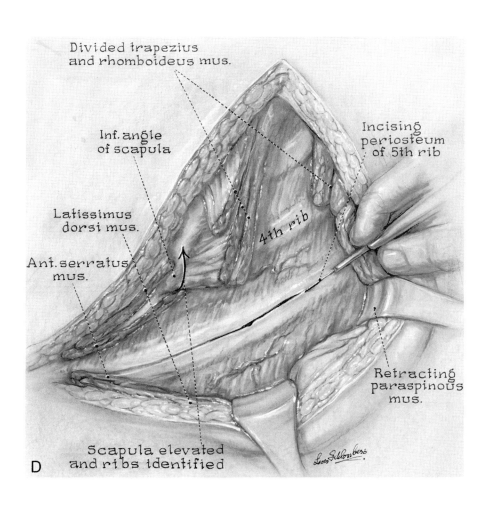

D

E. The periosteum of the 5th rib is incised and reflected, its vessels are sealed with the electrocautery, and it is dissected back from the superior half of the rib. *The exposure yielded by any thoracotomy is largely determined by the length of the parietal incision, not by whether ribs are resected or not. For major exposure, the incision in periosteum and pleura should go from sternum to spine.*

F. The exposure anteriorly or posteriorly can be increased by dividing costal cartilage or excising sections of rib, respectively, so that at the end of the incision, as the spreader is opened, the ribs fold like the splines of a closing fan. To gain exposure of the ribs posteriorly, a longitudinal incision is made along the anterior border of the spinal muscles, which are retracted posteriorly, exposing the ribs and the interspace posterior to the angle. We believe there is less pain if a small portion of the rib is resected, as shown, than if the rib is merely divided.

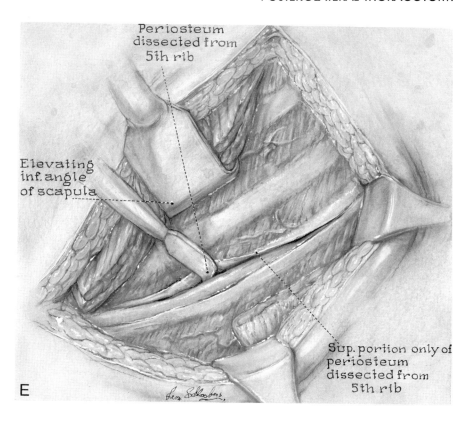

Periosteum
dissected from
5th rib

Elevating
inf. angle
of scapula

Sup. portion only of
periosteum
dissected from
5th rib

E

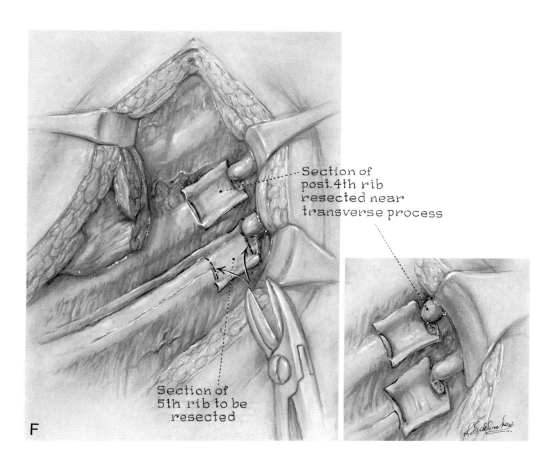

Section of
post. 4th rib
resected near
transverse process

Section of
5th rib to be
resected

F

POSTEROLATERAL THORACOTOMY *(Continued)*

G. With the interspace widened by a Richardson retractor inserted so as to hug the rib and then turned 90° so as to spread the ribs apart, the thorax is entered through the periosteal bed of the 5th rib. This provides rather stronger tissues for closure than does a simple intercostal incision, which is somewhat more quickly made. The resection of the length of a rib for access to the thorax presents essentially no advantage and is seldom performed by us.

H. With the posterior periosteum of the rib and the pleura incised and the Richardson retractor in the interspace rotated so as to wedge the ribs apart, the incision is continued with the scissor as shown. The retractor is advanced and repositioned as necessary to separate the ribs as the incision is completed. This gradual spreading of the ribs also tends to decrease the likelihood of fracturing the ribs, so often the result of immediate insertion and rapid opening of a Finochietto rib spreader.

I. The exposure gained by the formal posterolateral incision through the bed of the 5th rib is viewed from in front, with the lung depressed.

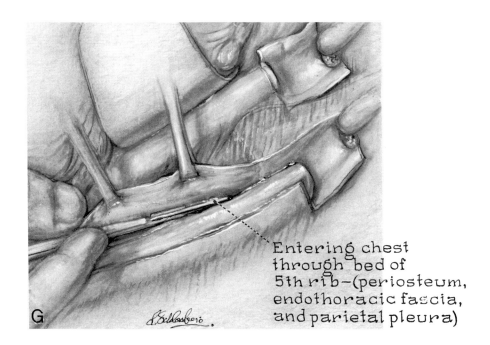

Entering chest through bed of 5th rib—(periosteum, endothoracic fascia, and parietal pleura)

124

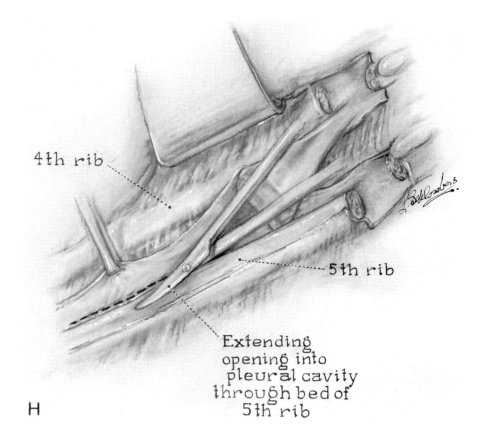

4th rib

5th rib

Extending
opening into
pleural cavity
through bed of
5th rib

H

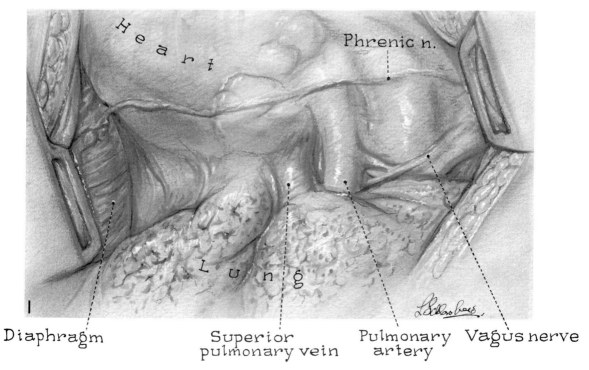

Heart

Phrenic n.

Lung

I

Diaphragm

Superior
pulmonary vein

Pulmonary
artery

Vagus nerve

POSTEROLATERAL THORACOTOMY *(Continued)*

J. The posterior exposure gained by the formal posterolateral thoracotomy through the bed of the 5th rib is shown. The aorta and esophagus are at hand medial to the end of the incision, and the main bronchus is readily accessible.

K. Entrance into the chest was through the periosteal bed of the 5th rib. Several sutures placed as shown to approximate the ribs and close the interspace are tied with the ribs held by the approximator. The continuous suture is then placed before the approximator is removed. The drawings of the section through the chest wall show the process and the end result—a strong closure without any risk of catching the intercostal nerve in the suture.

If the rib has been resected, we employ heavy pericostal sutures passed in from the interspace above, then "walked" under the rib below to pass out between the intercostal nerve and the rib, thus minimizing the risk of intercostal neuralgia (see pages 136–137, *Alternate Technique for Anterior Thoracotomy, B*).

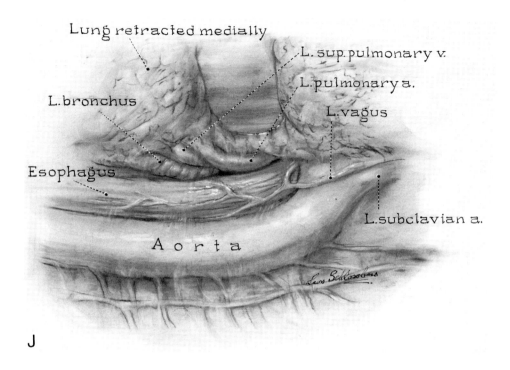

Lung retracted medially

L. sup. pulmonary v.

L. pulmonary a.

L. bronchus

L. vagus

Esophagus

L. subclavian a.

A o r t a

J

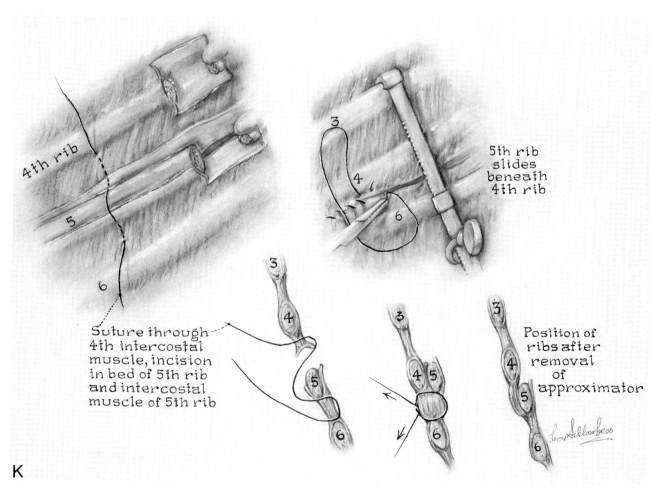

4th rib

5

6

5th rib
slides
beneath
4th rib

Suture through
4th intercostal
muscle, incision
in bed of 5th rib
and intercostal
muscle of 5th rib

Position of
ribs after
removal
of
approximator

K

L and M. Layer by layer closure of the muscles with interrupted nonabsorbable sutures is slightly more time-consuming than continuous absorbable suture closure, but more elegant and possibly more secure.

REFERENCE

1. Weinberg, J.A., and Kraus, A.R.: Intercostal incision in transpleural operations. J. Thorac. Surg. 19:769–778, 1950
   Advocacy of formal thoracotomy without rib resection.

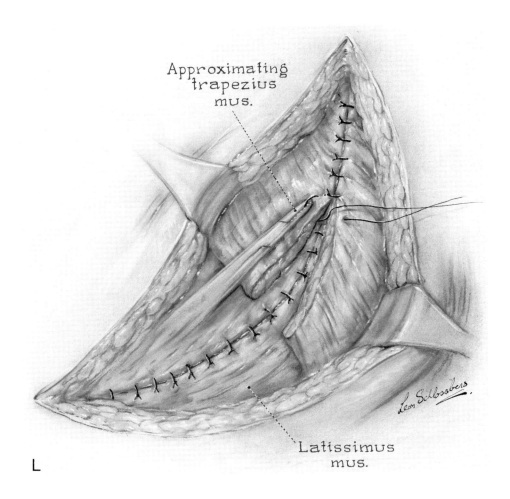

Approximating trapezius mus.

Latissimus mus.

L

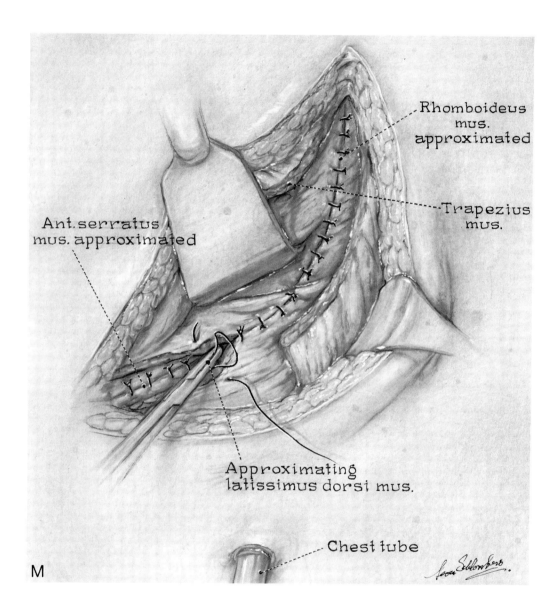

Rhomboideus
mus.
approximated

Trapezius
mus.

Ant. serratus
mus. approximated

Approximating
latissimus dorsi mus.

Chest tube

M

ANTERIOR (ANTEROLATERAL) THORACOTOMY

From the beginning of the early days of pneumonectomy, ligation and division of the patent ductus, and the Blalock operation for tetralogy of Fallot, a considerable group of surgeons preferred to do most of these intrathoracic procedures through an anterior thoracotomy. The anterior thoracotomy has the advantage that even fragile patients are not disturbed by the dorsal recumbent position, that a relatively small skin incision can provide wide access to the chest if the intercostal division is carried far posteriorly (making this essentially an anterolateral thoracotomy), and that the incision is quickly made and quickly closed. It has the disadvantage that exposure is not as ample as with posterolateral thoracotomy and that the tissues available for closure of the chest wall are relatively meager. It is particularly suited to resection of bullae and to upper lobectomy. As Alley pointed out, there was a "cult of wide exposure," in which the large posterolateral thoracotomy was used for virtually every intrapleural procedure. Since then, there has been a return to the anterior thoracotomy and, more recently, the wide employment of the axillary or lateral thoracotomy (see later), made possible by superior anesthesia and lighting and the realization of the specific requirements of exposure for safe performance in individual procedures, facilitated by the use of new technical aids such as staples and clips.

A. The fingers are slipped under the pectoralis major, which is divided with the fine needle–tipped electrocautery. Individual vessels may be clamped with the hemostat and coagulated.

B. The lower slips of the pectoralis minor are divided.

Alternatively, the attachments of the pectoralis to the ribs may be cut away and the muscle simply retracted.

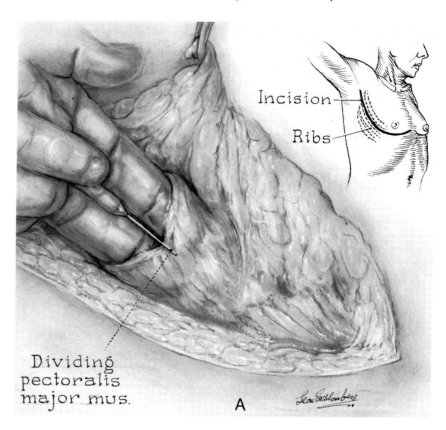

Incision

Ribs

Dividing
pectoralis
major mus.

A

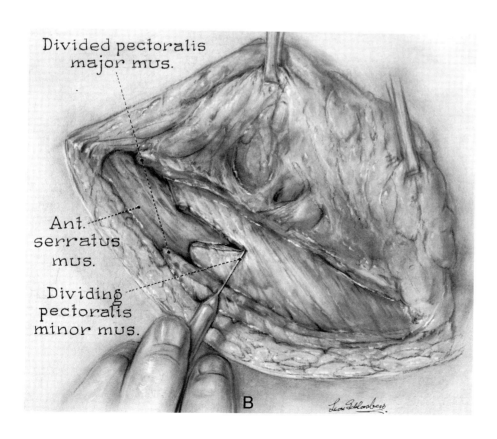

Divided pectoralis
major mus.

Ant.
serratus
mus.

Dividing
pectoralis
minor mus.

B

C. The incision is usually made in the 3rd interspace or through the bed of the 4th rib, as shown. The periosteum has been incised with the electrocautery and is shown being stripped away from the upper border of the rib.

D. Entrance into the pleural cavity is through the incised periosteal bed, exposed by wedging a Richardson retractor between the 3rd and 4th ribs. The precaution is taken of first inserting the finger and then spreading the interspace to make sure, if necessary by applying a moist stick sponge to the lung, that the lung is held safe from injury in making the longitudinal incision with scissor or cautery. The farther posterior the incision in the periosteal bed, the greater the exposure.

E. If it is found that more exposure is required, the internal mammary vessels are doubly ligated and divided and the 3rd, or 3rd and 4th, costal cartilages divided anteriorly, substantially increasing the exposure of the mediastinum and the anterior hilar structures. Cutting the cartilages with a modest obliquity facilitates their later resuturing.

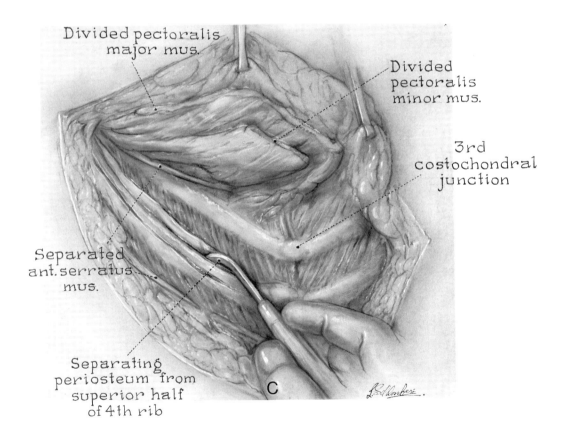

Divided pectoralis major mus.

Divided pectoralis minor mus.

3rd costochondral junction

Separated ant. serratus mus.

Separating periosteum from superior half of 4th rib

C

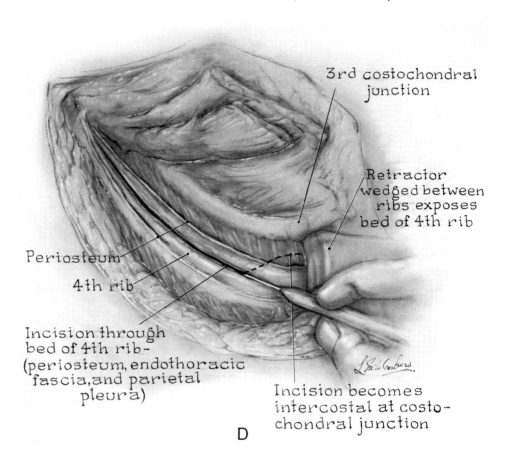

3rd costochondral junction

Retractor wedged between ribs exposes bed of 4th rib

Periosteum

4th rib

Incision through bed of 4th rib (periosteum, endothoracic fascia, and parietal pleura)

Incision becomes intercostal at costo-chondral junction

D

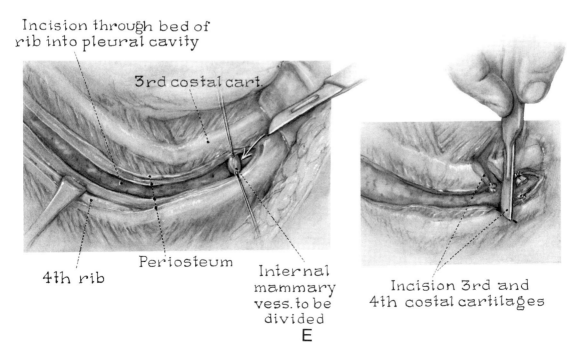

Incision through bed of rib into pleural cavity

3rd costal cart.

4th rib

Periosteum

Internal mammary vess. to be divided

Incision 3rd and 4th costal cartilages

E

ANTERIOR (ANTEROLATERAL) THORACOTOMY *(Continued)*

F. The exposure gained by an anterior thoracotomy is shown. Lung biopsy, blebectomy, upper lobectomy, and a variety of mediastinal dissections are easily performed through this incision. The hilar structures are satisfactorily accessible for other pulmonary resections including pneumonectomy, but the exposure, if the dissection is difficult or if trouble develops, is not always adequate.

G. Closure is achieved by placing the hooks of the Bailey rib approximators over the superior edge of the 2nd rib and the inferior edge of the 5th rib *(right)*; the 4th rib is placed beneath the 3rd rib and its intercostal muscle *(center and right)* as the approximator is tightened down. Simultaneously, the intercostal muscles of the 4th interspace bulge out, facilitating the placement of interrupted or continuous sutures from the 3rd intercostal muscle to the bulging, relaxed 4th intercostal muscles, over the 4th rib as shown at left and in the sagittal section. As the rib approximator is released, the 4th rib, as later seen on postoperative x-ray examination, assumes a near normal anatomical position. This type of closure provides a very safe first layer of closure in an area where tissues for closure are rather meager and avoids the need for the often painful pericostal sutures.

REFERENCE

1. Alley, R.D.: Thoracic surgical incisions and postoperative drainage. In: Cooper, P. (Ed.). *The Craft of Surgery.* New York, Little, Brown and Company, 1964, p. 196

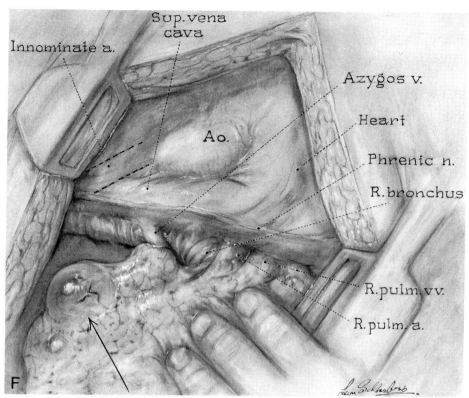

Innominate a.

Sup. vena cava

Azygos v.

Ao.

Heart

Phrenic n.

R. bronchus

R. pulm. vv.

R. pulm. a.

F

Bullous emphysema r. upper
lobe lung

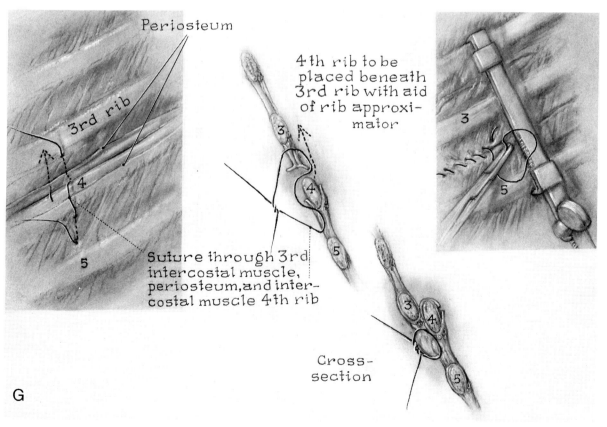

Periosteum

3rd rib

4

5

4th rib to be
placed beneath
3rd rib with aid
of rib approxi-
mator

3

4

5

3

5

Suture through 3rd
intercostal muscle,
periosteum, and inter-
costal muscle 4th rib

3

4

5

Cross-
section

G

ALTERNATE TECHNIQUE FOR ANTERIOR THORACOTOMY

A. An intercostal incision is made in the appropriate interspace, the ribs wedged apart with a retractor (not shown), and the interspace cut as far posteriorly as one can reach, with the scissors applied upon the upper border of the lower rib to avoid the intercostal vessels. The intercostal muscles and pleura may be further divided posteriorly by passing a blunt periosteal elevator, or the fingers, to the angle of the rib. It is this posterior extension of the anterior incision that provides maximal exposure. Medially, the incision is carried to the sternum, taking the internal mammary vessels as they are exposed—occasionally merely displacing them medially. As in the previous technique for anterior thoracotomy, increased exposure may be provided anteriorly by division of the 3rd, or 3rd and 4th, costal cartilages.

B. In the closure, transected costal cartilages are reapproximated with heavy through-and-through sutures of nonabsorbable material. Heavy pericostal sutures are introduced so as to come between the intercostal structures and the lower border of the lower rib (seen in enlarged cross section) to avoid postoperative intercostal neuralgia. The 3rd and 4th cartilages are shown to have been divided and are being resutured with stout nonabsorbable sutures. The intercostal muscles are then sutured. We prefer interrupted sutures of nonabsorbable material.

REFERENCES

1. Rienhoff, W.F., Jr.: Pneumonectomy. A preliminary report of operative technique in two successful cases. Bull. Johns Hopk. Hosp. 53:390–393, 1933
2. Gross, R.E.: A surgical approach for ligation of a patent ductus arteriosus. N. Engl. J. Med. 220:510–514, 1939
3. Gross, R.E., and Hubbard, J.P.: Surgical ligation of a patent ductus arteriosus: Report of first successful case. JAMA 112:729–731, 1939
4. Blalock, A., and Taussig, H.B.: The surgical treatment of malformations of the heart in which there is pulmonary stenosis or pulmonary atresia. JAMA 128:189–202, 1945
5. Blalock, A.: The technique of creation of an artificial ductus arteriosus in the treatment of pulmonic stenosis. J. Thorac. Surg. 16:244–255, 1947
6. Rienhoff, W.F., Jr., King, J.D.B., and Dana, G.W., Jr.: Surgical treatment of carcinoma of the lung. Evaluation of six hundred and ninety-nine cases from 1933 through 1956. JAMA 166:228–232, 1958

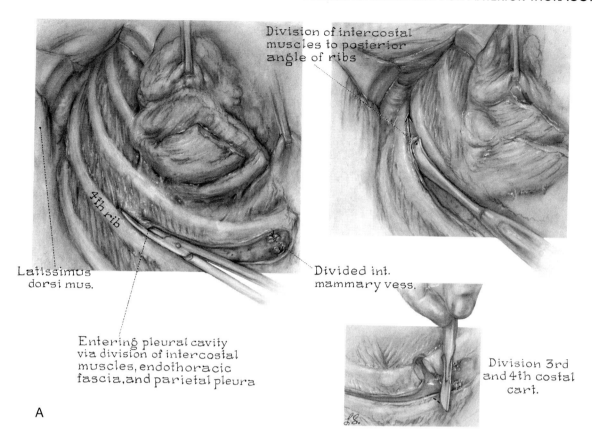

Division of intercostal
muscles to posterior
angle of ribs

4th rib

Latissimus
dorsi mus.

Divided int.
mammary vess.

Entering pleural cavity
via division of intercostal
muscles, endothoracic
fascia, and parietal pleura

Division 3rd
and 4th costal
cart.

A

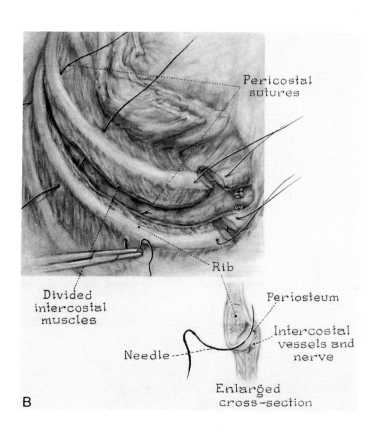

Pericostal
sutures

Rib

Divided
intercostal
muscles

Periosteum

Intercostal
vessels and
nerve

Needle

Enlarged
cross-section

B

LATERAL THORACOTOMY WITHOUT DIVISION OF MUSCLE (AXILLARY THORACOTOMY)*

A. With the patient properly braced in the lateral position and the arm supported at right angle (but no more, to avoid overstretching of the brachial plexus), a lateral, transverse incision is made, extending anteriorly below the breast. The chest wall incision thereafter, through the bed of the rib directly below the skin incision, is carried posteriorly and anteriorly by dividing the intercostal muscles, posteriorly along the superior border of the rib under the elevated latissimus dorsi and anteriorly under the pectoralis major.

For a pneumonectomy, the 4th or 5th rib bed is preferred; for excision of apical blebs, pleurectomy, upper lobectomy, and upper lobe biopsy, the 3rd rib bed; for dorsal sympathectomy, the 2nd rib bed.

The extension of the skin incision beyond the muscle borders of the latissimus dorsi and pectoralis major is essential to allow maximal spreading of the wound (center). The latissimus laterally and the pectoralis medially are elevated with retractors as the incision into the pleural cavity is extended. Occasionally (lower drawing), a short incision across the edge of the muscle will be necessary to allow the wound to be opened widely.

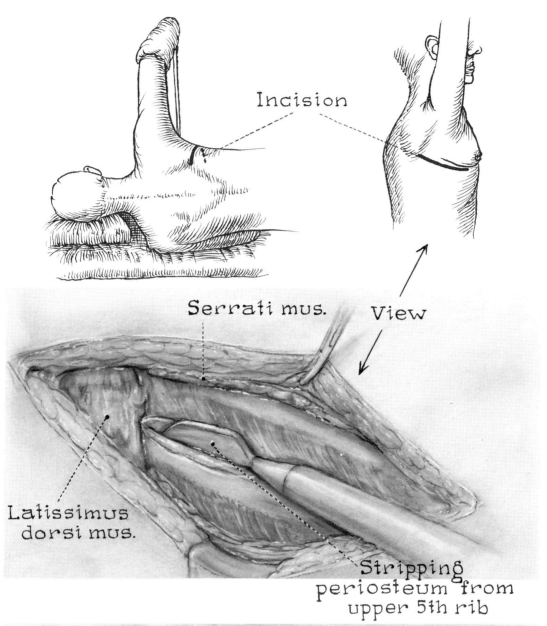

Incision

View

Serrati mus.

Latissimus
dorsi mus.

Stripping
periosteum from
upper 5th rib

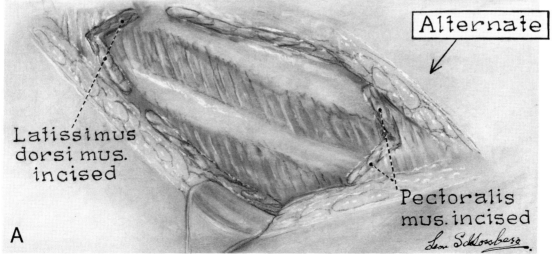

Alternate

Latissimus
dorsi mus.
incised

Pectoralis
mus. incised

A

Leon Schlossberg

LATERAL THORACOTOMY WITHOUT DIVISION OF MUSCLE
(Continued)

B. Shown is an incision through the periosteal bed of the 5th rib. The periosteum is incised with the electrocautery at the upper border of the rib and stripped away sufficiently to permit an incision through it, for most purposes for a much longer distance than shown.

C. A Richardson retractor, slid through the incision into the pleural cavity and then turned at right angles, wedges the ribs apart and simplifies extension of the incision in both directions. The intrathoracic exposure is determined by the length of this incision. For pneumonectomy the incision should be carried out posteriorly to the angle of the ribs and medially to the sternum. Posteriorly, the serratus and latissimus, and anteriorly the pectoralis, are elevated and preserved as the incision of the interspace progresses.

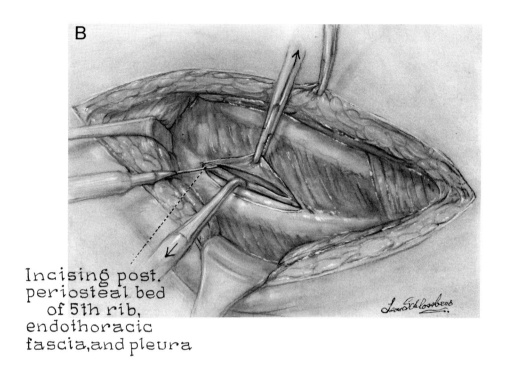

B

Incising post.
periosteal bed
of 5th rib,
endothoracic
fascia, and pleura

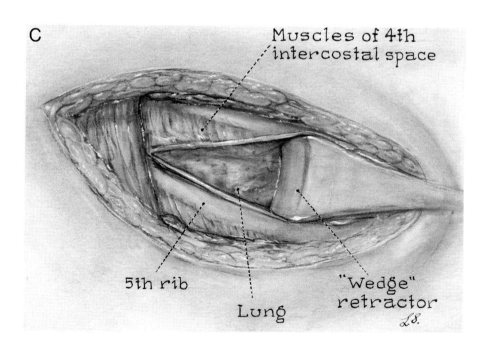

C

Muscles of 4th
intercostal space

5th rib

Lung

"Wedge"
retractor

D. The technique is shown of holding the lung away while the incision of pleura and intercostal muscles *(dotted lines)* is continued anteriorly and posteriorly behind the retracted pectoralis and latissimus. The cautery, scissors, or scalpel is used along the upper border of the rib, from within the chest cavity, to continue the initial periosteal bed incision as shown in *B*.

E. The exposure provides good access to the pulmonary hilum. The large, flat muscles anteriorly and posteriorly are readily stretched and retracted. If the intercostal incision is made the length of the interspace, the limiting factor may be the skin incision, which may need to be extended.

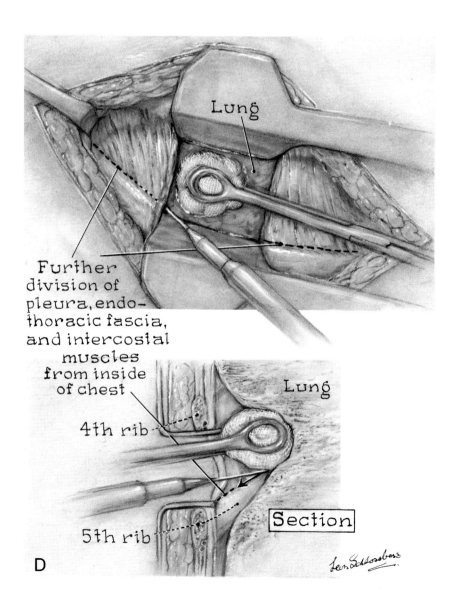

Lung

Further division of pleura, endothoracic fascia, and intercostal muscles from inside of chest

Lung

4th rib

5th rib

Section

D

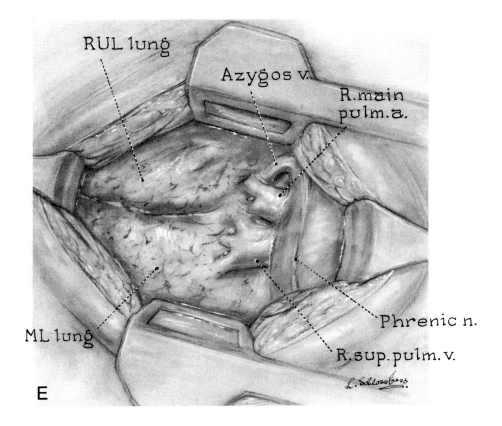

LATERAL THORACOTOMY WITHOUT DIVISION OF MUSCLE
(Continued)

F. The closure is achieved by overlapping the 4th rib and intercostal muscle over the 5th rib as the prongs of the Bailey rib approximator pull on the 3rd and 6th ribs. Sutures are placed as on pages 126–127, *Posterolateral Thoracotomy, K.*

G. The closure by overlapping the ribs is completed with a continuous suture from pleura and intercostal muscle of the 4th space to the buckled-up 5th intercostal muscle and periosteum. As the rib approximator is removed, the ribs return to a normal position.

Note: As for many operative approaches, this one has been discovered and rediscovered by surgeons in various places and at various times.

REFERENCES

1. Atkins, H.J.B.: Sympathectomy by the axillary approach. Lancet 1:538–539, 1954
   In an earlier "letter to the editor," Lancet December 17, 1949, p. 1152, Atkins said, "When Prof. R.H. Goetz, of Cape Town, visited this country last summer he persuaded me to adopt the periaxillary approach to the stellate and upper thoracic sympathetic ganglia." In the 1954 article, Atkins says, "the procedure was devised by W.G. Schulze and Prof. R.H. Goetz, at the Groote Schuur Hospital, Cape Town." A letter from Professor R.P. Hewitson, of the Groote Schuur Hospital in Cape Town, December 20, 1984, says, "Professor Cole Rous, who succeeded Professor Saint when he retired at the end of 1946, was doing sympathectomies through an anterolateral second rib approach. Naturally, this leaves an ugly scar, particularly in females, and so Bill Schulze in 1947 made the approach through the second rib entirely in the axilla. He says that Professor Goetz had no part in this but the latter was, as is well known, very interested in the sympathetic nervous system and its outflow from the chest. Schulze approached Goetz to describe the sympathetic anatomy, with the idea that he [Schulze] would describe his axillary approach in the same article—but Goetz never responded and so Schulze did not get around to publishing. Schulze went over to London for a period (to get his FRCS amongst other things) and demonstrated this approach to Hedley Atkins amongst others. . . ."
2. Noirclerc, M., Dor, V., Chauvin, G., Kreitman, P., Masselot, R., Balenbois, D., Hoyer, J., and Broussard, M.: La thoracotomie laterale large sans section musculaire. Ann. Chir. Thorac. Cardio-vasc. 12:181–184, 1973
3. Becker, R.M., and Munro, D.D.: Transaxillary minithoracotomy: The optimal approach for certain pulmonary and mediastinal lesions. Ann. Thorac. Surg. 22:254–259, 1976
4. Little, J.M.: Transaxillary transpleural thoracic sympathectomy. Surgical Techniques Illustrated 2:15–27, 1977
5. Linder, F., Jenal, G., and Assmus, H.: Axillary transpleural sympathectomy: Indication, technique, and results. World J. Surg. 7:437–439, 1983

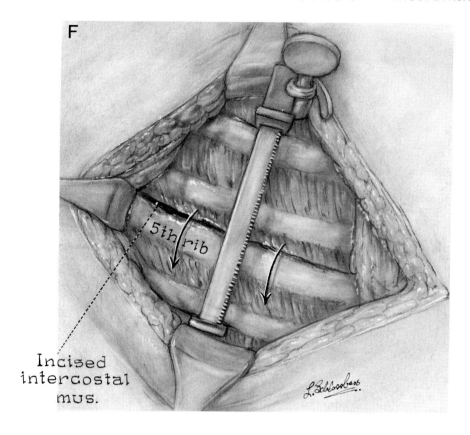

F

5th rib

Incised
intercostal
mus.

L. Schlossberg

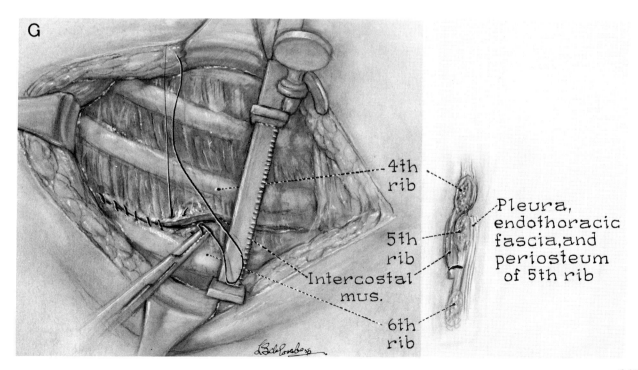

G

4th
rib

5th
rib

Intercostal
mus.

6th
rib

Pleura,
endothoracic
fascia,and
periosteum
of 5th rib

L. Schlossberg

145

TRAUMATIC INJURY OF SUBCLAVIAN VESSELS—
TECHNIQUES OF EXPOSURE

A. This diagram of the major blood vessels of the upper extremity shows that the right subclavian artery arises high in the thorax from the innominate artery, whereas the left subclavian artery takes origin directly from the aortic arch, thus at a lower and more posterior level. Both subclavian arteries course retropleurally from their origins in the mediastinum and rise slightly above the level of the clavicle in the base of the neck as they arch over the pleural apices. The lateral border of the 1st rib marks the transition of the subclavian artery into the axillary artery; similarly, the lateral border of the teres major muscle in the arm serves to mark the axillary-brachial transition. The three segments of the subclavian artery are defined by the anterior scalenus muscle; the artery lies deep to it. The first part of the subclavian artery, medial to the scalenus, gives rise to the thyrocervical trunk, internal mammary, and vertebral arteries. The three parts of the axillary artery are defined by relation to the pectoralis minor muscle, which crosses the vessel approximately at its midportion. The axillary artery gives origin to the thoracoacromial, lateral thoracic, humeral circumflex, and subscapular arteries.

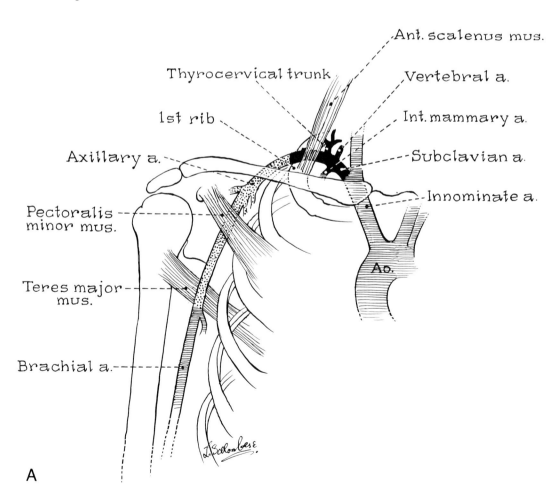

A

B. Exposure of the injured *right subclavian artery*, as obtained through a median sternotomy, gives an excellent view of the ascending aorta; proximal part of the aortic arch; innominate, right subclavian, and common carotid arteries; innominate veins; and superior vena cava. This incision allows control of the proximal part of the right subclavian artery. For wounds more distally situated in the subclavian artery, the incision may be extended further, into the right side of the neck, as indicated by the dotted line shown in the inset. The clavicle need not be divided. In the presence of massive, imminently fatal intrathoracic bleeding, a right anterolateral thoracotomy would have been made in the emergency department to provide initial control of hemorrhage (see *H*).

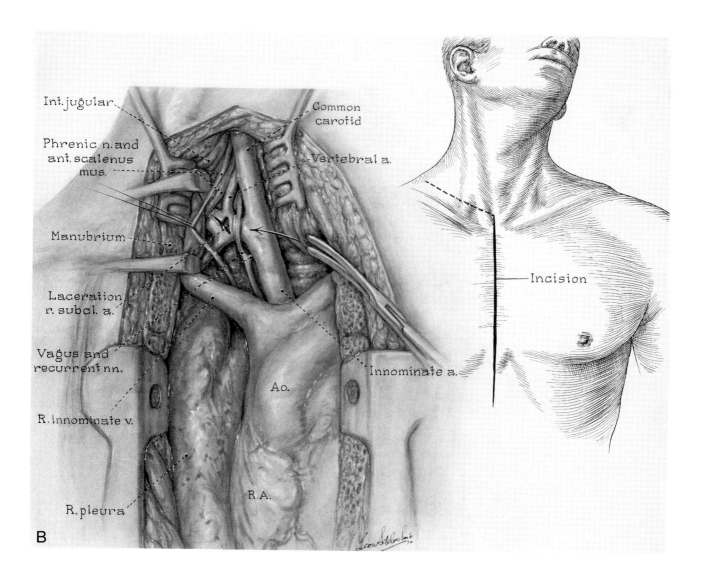

C. Exposure of a wound in the distal part of the right subclavian artery has been obtained through a median sternotomy with supraclavicular extension of the upper end of the incision into the soft tissues of the right side of the neck. The soft tissue incision has been extended far out above the right clavicle. The sternocleidomastoid, anterior scalenus, and strap muscles have been divided to expose the subclavian artery out to the point at which it passes over the 1st rib. The clavicle has not been divided or resected.

D. The *left subclavian artery* is not readily controlled through a median sternotomy. Exposure of the left subclavian artery is here shown through an anterolateral 3rd intercostal space incision. In the presence of massive intrathoracic bleeding, the incision is made in the emergency department for initial control of hemorrhage. Although this incision provides satisfactory exposure of wounds in the proximal part of the left subclavian artery, it is not adequate for repair of injuries in the distal portion of the left subclavian artery.

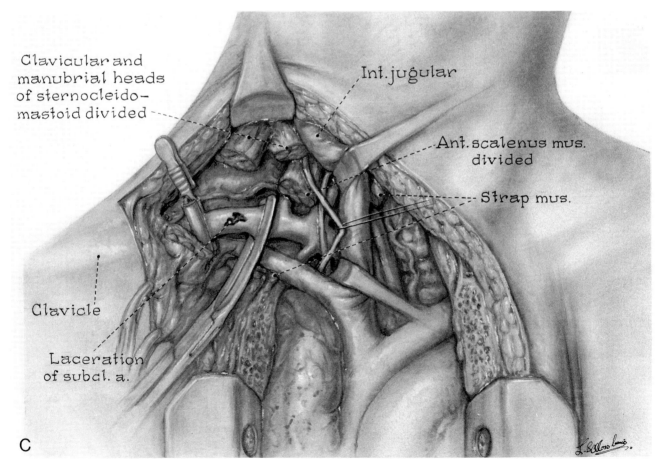

Clavicular and manubrial heads of sternocleidomastoid divided

Int. jugular

Ant. scalenus mus. divided

Strap mus.

Clavicle

Laceration of subcl. a.

C

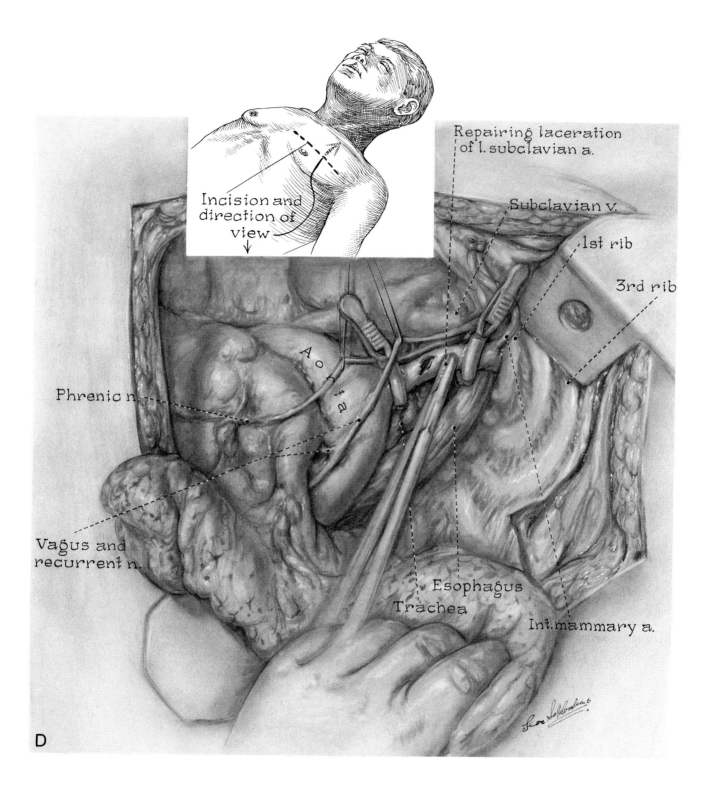

Incision and direction of view

Repairing laceration of l. subclavian a.

Subclavian v.

1st rib

3rd rib

Aorta

Phrenic n.

Vagus and recurrent n.

Esophagus

Trachea

Int. mammary a.

D

E. For exposure of the distal part of the left subclavian artery through a left supraclavicular incision, the sternocleidomastoid and anterior scalenus muscles have been
divided. Initial control of the proximal subclavian artery has been obtained through
the left anterolateral thoracotomy, and the intrathoracic portion of the artery has
been mobilized completely. For easy delivery into the supraclavicular incision, the
vertebral and internal mammary arteries are ligated and divided in the chest, at their
origin.

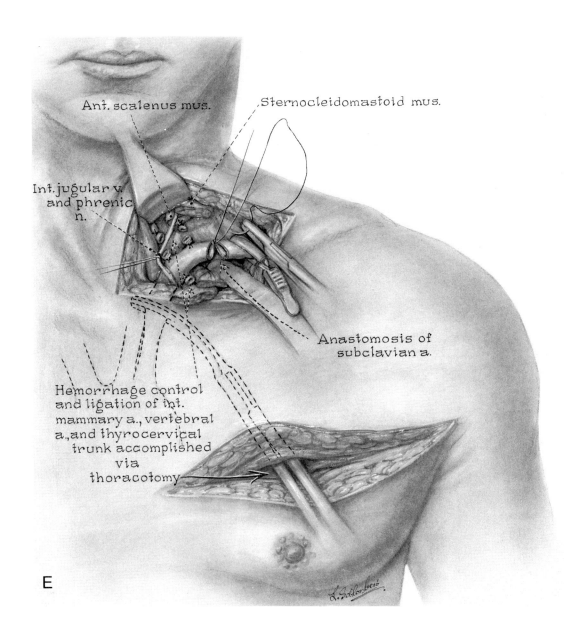

F. A posterolateral left thoracotomy for exposure of the aorta and intrathoracic left subclavian artery provides maximal exposure. The arm must be draped free so that if a supraclavicular incision is to be made, the patient can be rotated to a more nearly supine position and the arm brought down to the side.

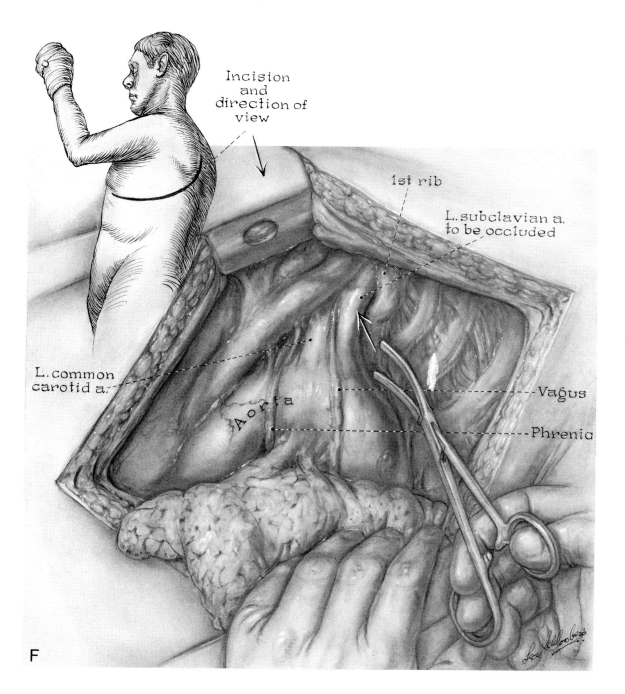

G. Once the subclavian artery is controlled through the posterolateral thoracotomy and mobilized, the patient is laid back and the arm brought down. A transverse supraclavicular incision, dividing the sternocleidomastoid and anterior scalenus muscles, provides access to the subclavian vessels.

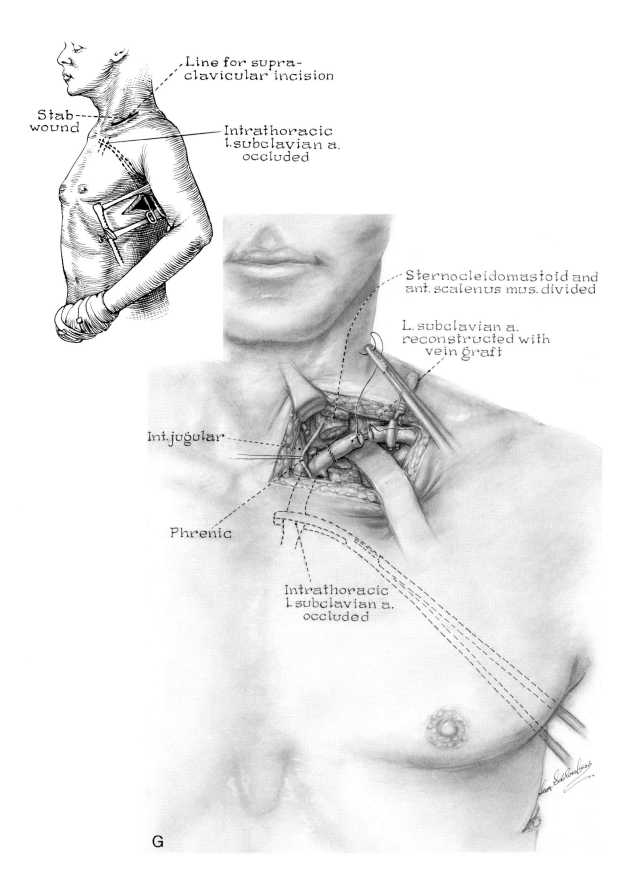

Line for supra-clavicular incision

Stab wound

Intrathoracic l. subclavian a. occluded

Sternocleidomastoid and ant. scalenus mus. divided

L. subclavian a. reconstructed with vein graft

Int. jugular

Phrenic

Intrathoracic l. subclavian a. occluded

G

H. Trapdoor incision for approach to subclavian vessels is shown in four views. (1) In this instance it is used for lifesaving control of hemorrhage from injury to the subclavian vessels by an in-driven fractured clavicle, since massive bleeding occurred each time the pack in the exploratory neck wound was removed. (2) A rapid 3rd interspace anterolateral thoracotomy allowed effective hemostatic compression by a pack placed against the cupola of the hemithorax. (3) The median sternotomy, connected to the 3rd interspace incision below and to the exploratory supraclavicular incision above, permitted wide retraction of the trapdoor flap. (4) The existing comminuted clavicular fracture made this approach appealing and provided magnificent exposure. Otherwise, a Gigli saw division of the clavicle would be required to permit this elevation of the trapdoor. This is a larger procedure than that shown in C, but the exposure is unequalled.

Figures *A* through *E* from Brawley, R.K., Murray, G.F., Crisler, C., and Cameron, J.L.: Management of wounds of the innominate, subclavian and axillary vessels. Surg. Gynecol. Obstet. 131:1130–1140, 1970, by permission of Surgery, Gynecology & Obstetrics.

Figures *F* and *G* from Schaff, H.V., and Brawley, R.K.: Operative management of penetrating vascular injuries of the thoracic outlet. Surgery 82:182–191, 1977, with permission.

Figure *H* adapted from Steenburg, R.W., and Ravitch, M.M.: Cervico-thoracic approach for subclavian vessel injury from compound fracture of the clavicle: Considerations of subclavian-axillary exposures. Ann. Surg. 157:839–846, 1963.

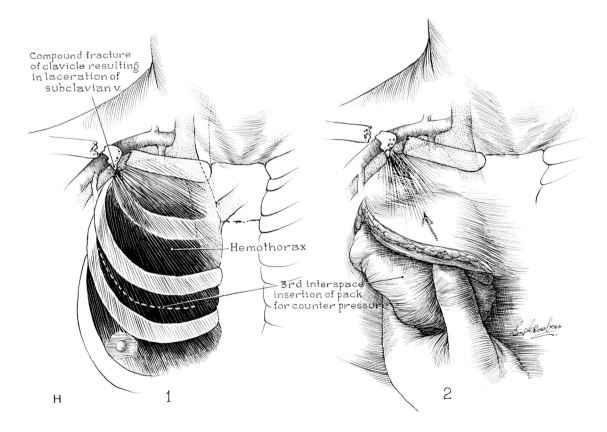

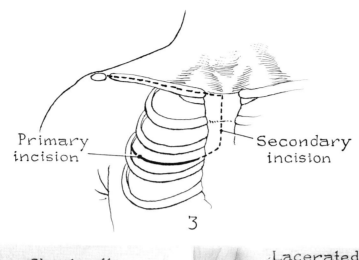

Primary incision

Secondary incision

3

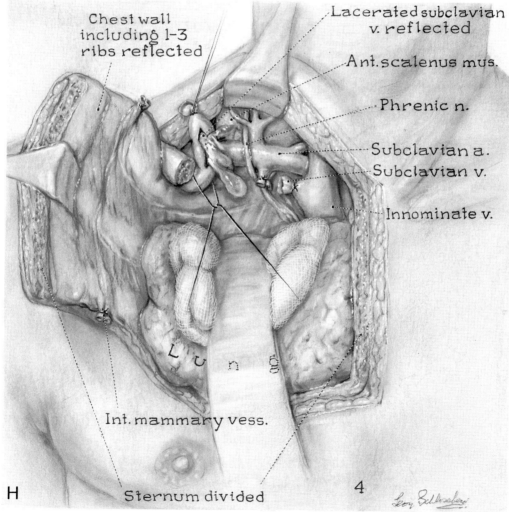

Chest wall including 1-3 ribs reflected

Lacerated subclavian v. reflected

Ant. scalenus mus.

Phrenic n.

Subclavian a.

Subclavian v.

Innominate v.

Int. mammary vess.

Sternum divided

H

4

155

The
Thoracic
Skeleton

The Thoracic Skeleton

The relationship of clavicle, scapula, and diaphragm to the rib cage, as well as the fusion of costal cartilages VIII through X, their attachment to the 7th cartilage, and its insertion onto the lower sternum, close to or fused with the 6th cartilage, is shown. The diaphragm (*dotted line*) rises to the 4th interspace on the right and the 5th on the left. Shown are the pleural fissures and the outline of the pericardium.

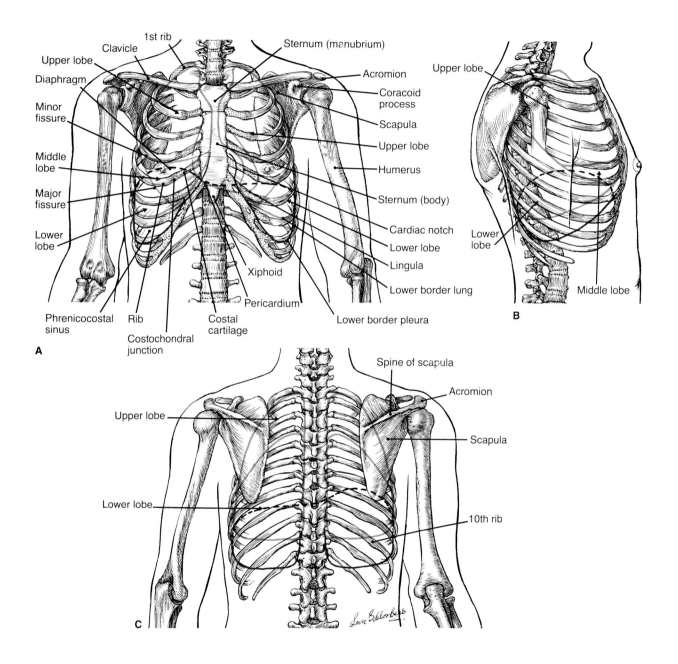

A

1st rib
Clavicle
Upper lobe
Diaphragm
Minor fissure
Middle lobe
Major fissure
Lower lobe
Phrenicocostal sinus
Rib
Costochondral junction
Costal cartilage
Xiphoid
Pericardium
Sternum (manubrium)
Acromion
Coracoid process
Scapula
Upper lobe
Humerus
Sternum (body)
Cardiac notch
Lower lobe
Lingula
Lower border lung
Lower border pleura

B

Upper lobe
Lower lobe
Middle lobe

C

Upper lobe
Lower lobe
Spine of scapula
Acromion
Scapula
10th rib

Diagnostic and Therapeutic Procedures

THORACENTESIS

A. The site for thoracentesis is the intersection of the suitable intercostal space with the longitudinal line running through the center of the pleural collection.

B. Anesthesia of skin and soft tissue is obtained with lidocaine (Xylocaine), 0.5 to 1.0%, by raising a skin wheal and progressively injecting the anesthetic as the needle is advanced until it is felt that the pleura has been infiltrated. Often the pleural fluid appears in the anesthesia syringe. The larger needle for fluid evacuation is placed by "shaving" the upper edge of the rib to gauge the distance into the pleural cavity, and it is maintained in position by the spring currently provided in commercially available thoracentesis sets. A clamp, grasping the needle at skin level, can fulfill the same purpose. The needle is connected to a syringe via a three-way stopcock that allows for aspiration and evacuation into a collecting flask or bag.

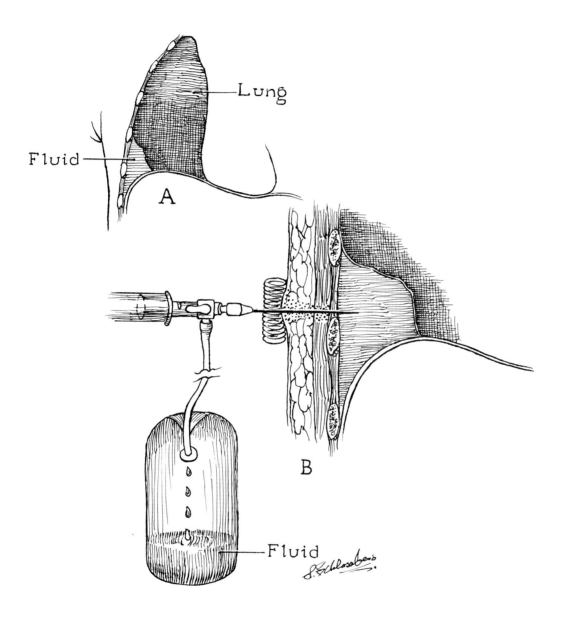

TUBE THORACOSTOMY

Basic Rules for Chest Tube Placement

1. For the comfort of the recumbent patient, chest tubes should not emerge from the skin between the posterior axillary line and the spine.
2. For drainage of air, the tube is most usefully inserted at the level of the anterior axillary line—2nd intercostal space. Nevertheless, fluid and air often coexist, and an anteriorly placed tube cannot be expected to drain fluid.
3. For drainage of fluid, the tube should be placed through the intercostal space that is at the level of the bottom of the collection, from midaxillary line to midclavicular line. In general, the lower and more posterior, the better.
4. Ideally, the tube tract should avoid the course of a possible thoracotomy incision.

Trocar and Cannula Technique

A. A large area of skin, subcutaneous tissue, and intercostal muscle is anesthetized to permit the painless introduction of the tube. The needle and anesthesia syringe are used for thoracentesis to confirm the location of fluid or air.
B. The skin is incised transversely, only sufficiently to allow insertion of the tube without binding against the skin edges.
C. We prefer to create the tract for the tube by using curved scissors, in preference to the clamp technique often recommended.
D. By closing the scissors and cutting the intervening soft tissues and then opening and spreading them, progress is made in the most comfortable way for the patient.
E. The plastic cannula-catheter and trocar are then advanced over the scissors, the superior rim of the rib is felt, and the trocar and cannula are advanced minimally into the collection.
F. As the trocar tip transmits the "give" of the parietal pleura, its point is pulled back and the soft end of the chest tube is advanced so that all holes are within the pleural cavity. It is now anchored to the skin with sutures and tape and connected to underwater drainage.

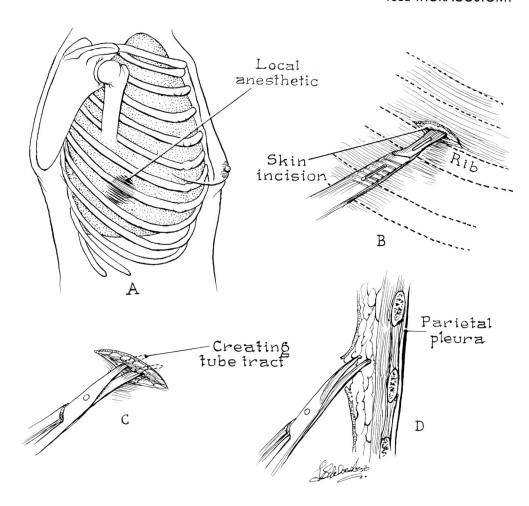

Local anesthetic

Skin incision

Rib

A

B

Creating tube tract

Parietal pleura

C

D

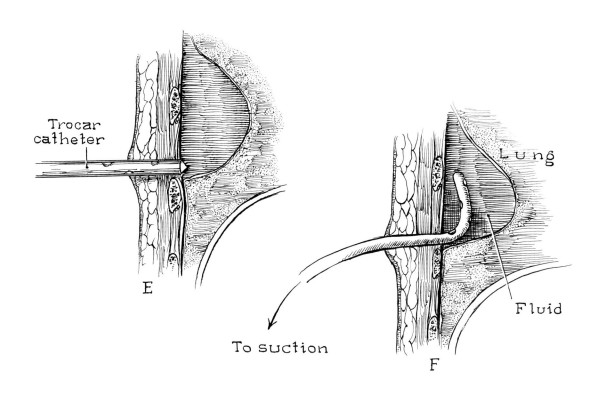

Trocar catheter

To suction

E

Lung

Fluid

F

TUBE THORACOSTOMY *(Continued)*

Clamp and Catheter Technique

This is in most cases the simplest method of introduction of a thoracostomy tube and utilizes materials available anywhere in the hospital.

A. Skin, fat, intercostal tissues, and pleura are infiltrated above the lowermost rib overlying the pleural collection.

B. Through a small incision a pointed clamp (Rankin) penetrates into the pleural collection.

C. The clamp may be inserted into a side hole of the catheter by stretching the catheter tautly to conform to the clamp, or

D. The drainage catheter may be held in the jaws of the clamp to conform as much as possible to the curve of the clamp.

E. The catheter head expands within the chest as the clamp is withdrawn and the catheter is fixed in place.

Clamp and catheter technique drawing from Rutherford, R.B., and Campbell, D.N.: Thoracic Injuries. In: *The Management of Trauma*, 1st Edition, W.F. Ballinger, R.B. Rutherford, and G.D. Zuidema (Eds.). Philadelphia, W.B. Saunders Company, 1968, with permission.

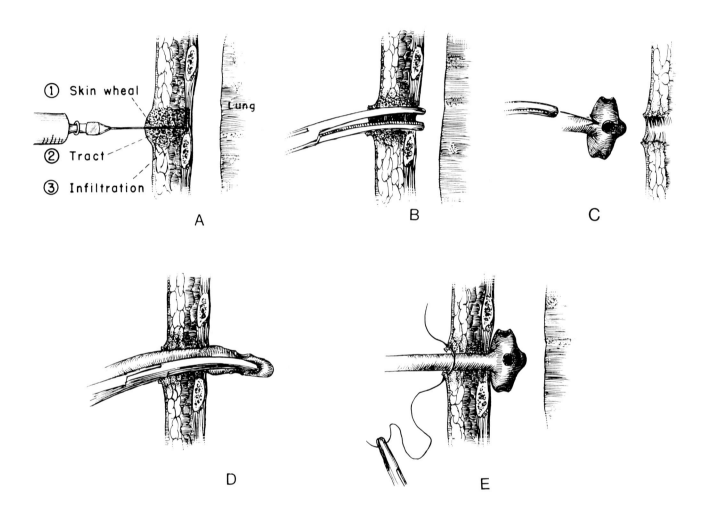

① Skin wheal

Lung

② Tract

③ Infiltration

A

B

C

D

E

INTERCOSTAL NERVE BLOCK

Intercostal nerve block is one of the basic and most effective measures in the alleviation of pain and respiratory distress from fractured ribs. The infiltration needle is walked down the dorsal surface of the rib, as far posteriorly as possible, until the needle passes over the lower border of the rib and is directed upward as close as possible to the nerve in its bed just above the lower border of the rib. The soft tissues are infiltrated with 0.5% Xylocaine and the nerves with 2% Xylocaine. The number of injection sites are borne in mind during determination whether to use 1 or 2 cc for each nerve.

From Rutherford, R.B., and Campbell, D.N.: Thoracic Injuries. In: *The Management of Trauma*, 1st Edition, W.F. Ballinger, R.B. Rutherford, and G.D. Zuidema (Eds.). Philadelphia, W.B. Saunders Company, 1968, with permission.

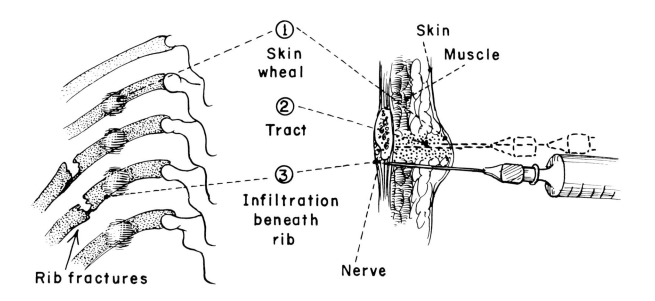

① Skin wheal

② Tract

③ Infiltration beneath rib

Rib fractures

Skin

Muscle

Nerve

NEEDLE ASPIRATION BIOPSY OF LUNG

The tumor is located by biplane chest x-ray or CT scan, and the procedure is performed under fluoroscopic or CT scan control.

Local anesthesia with 1% Xylocaine is established along the superior edge of the rib at the point on the chest wall closest to the lesion. A larger, sturdier (16 to 17 gauge) needle passed through the chest wall in the direction of the tumor is used as a cannula for the thinner biopsy needle.

The aspiration needle is advanced into the tumor under biplane fluoroscopy or CT scan. At each advance of the needle, the patient is asked to stop breathing. Material is aspirated at various depths in the tumor while the shielding, outside needle is kept in place with a clamp applied to it at skin level.

The material obtained is immediately processed for cytologic smear and for cell block if a large enough specimen has been harvested.

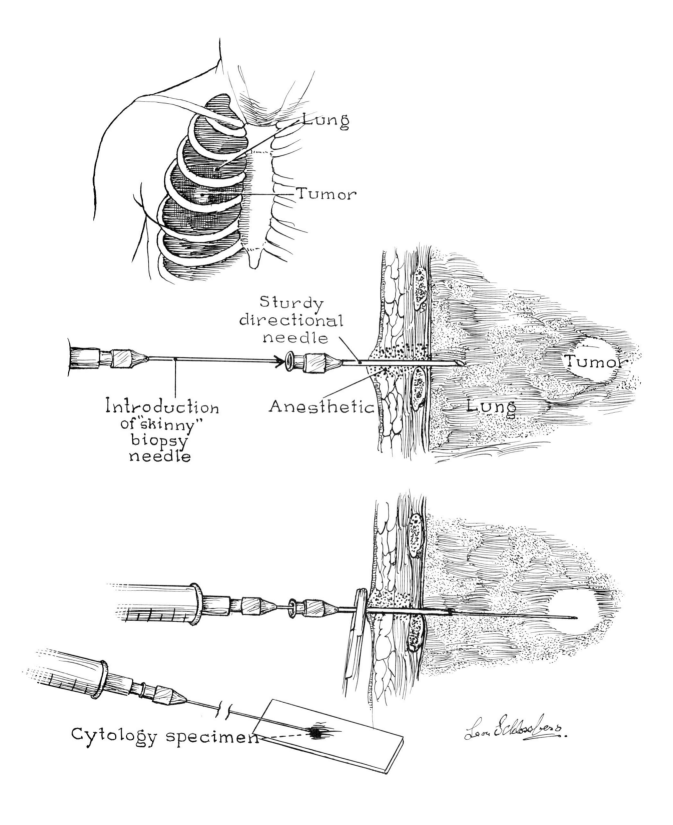

Lung

Tumor

Sturdy
directional
needle

Introduction
of "skinny"
biopsy
needle

Anesthetic

Tumor

Lung

Cytology specimen

PERICARDIOCENTESIS

Pericardiocentesis, whether for pericardial effusion or hemopericardium, is performed under local infiltration anesthesia. The approach through the left 4th interspace (a finger's breadth from the sternum to avoid the internal mammary artery) traverses a shorter course than the subxyphoid route, which may require a longer needle. On the other hand, the pericardium cannot be "missed" when the needle is inserted from below, and there is less likelihood of injuring a coronary vessel or entering the pleura.

For subxyphoid pericardiocentesis, the needle is directed upward in the midline or slightly to the right, inclined so as to pass a little posterior to the sternum. For the intercostal approach, the needle is directed medially, upward and posteriorly, as shown. For chronic pericardial effusion, a 16-gauge angiocath permits introduction of a plastic catheter into the pericardium, avoiding repeated aspirations, or providing continuous decompression until a fenestration of the pericardium is undertaken.

From Rutherford, R.B., and Campbell, D.N.: Thoracic Injuries. In: *The Management of Trauma*, 1st Edition, W.F. Ballinger, R.B. Rutherford, and G.D. Zuidema (Eds.). Philadelphia, W.B. Saunders Company, 1968, with permission.

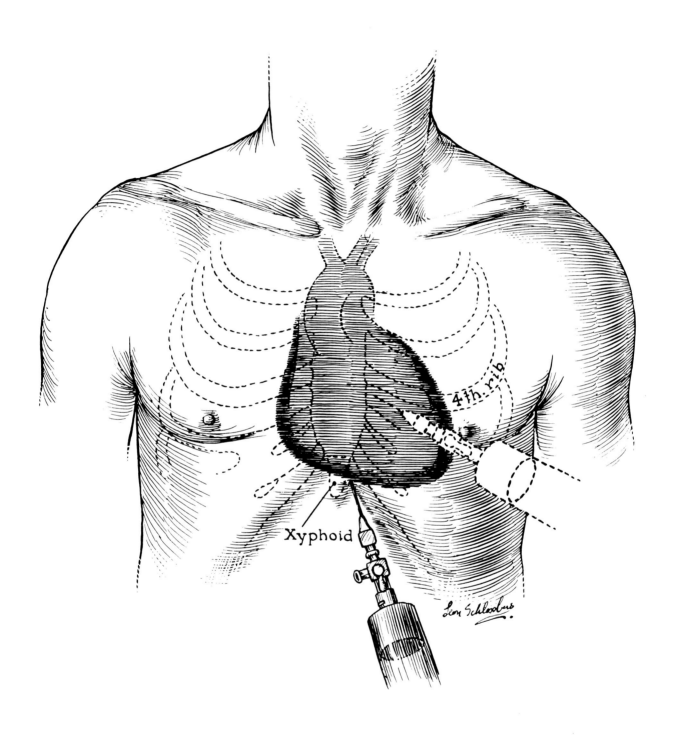

Xyphoid

4th rib

Leon Schlossberg.

PERICARDIAL WINDOW

A. The approach is through a vertical incision excising the xiphoid. The procedure can be performed under local anesthesia and sedation. If a nearly complete pericardiectomy for effusive disease is indicated, a thoracotomy is the procedure of choice.

B. The incision is carried down to the distal sternum and xiphoid. The upper third of the linea alba is incised. The peritoneum is not opened. The left costal arch is exposed. The xiphoid process and lower left costal arch are excised with a bone cutter or bites of a rongeur.

C. The diaphragm is incised in the midline down to the pericardial surface. Stay sutures are placed on either side of the projected pericardiotomy, and the pericardium is incised and drained. A specimen of pericardium is excised. If only a window· is indicated, a drainage catheter is sutured into place and brought out through a lateral stab wound. As the incision is closed, the pericardial edges are sutured to the extraperitoneal tissues to allow for continued drainage and absorption of fluid (not shown in these drawings). Alternatively, the pericardial window may be opened into the pleural cavity.

D. For a partial pericardiectomy, the resection of bone and cartilage is extended laterally and most of the anterior pericardium between both phrenic nerves is excised. A drain is sutured to the base of the excised pericardium at its diaphragmatic surface, and the edges of the pericardium are sutured to the subcutaneous tissue and the open upper linea alba.

The creation of a pericardial window to provide continuous internal drainage of chronic, usually malignant, pericardial effusion has found increasing use in recent years, as combined radio- and chemotherapy prolong the lives of affected patients.

The suggestion for a pericardial window was first made by Richérand in 1818.

REFERENCE

1. Richérand, Le Chevalier A.B.: Histoire d'une résection des côtes et de la plevre. Lue à l'Académie Royale des Sciences de l'Institut de France, le Lundi 27 Avril 1818, Paris. Paris: Caille et Ravier, 1818
   After performing a massive chest wall resection for tumor, Richérand, seeing the pericardium at the base of the granulating wound, suggested operative drainage of large accumulations of pericardial fluid, using the term "pericardial window."

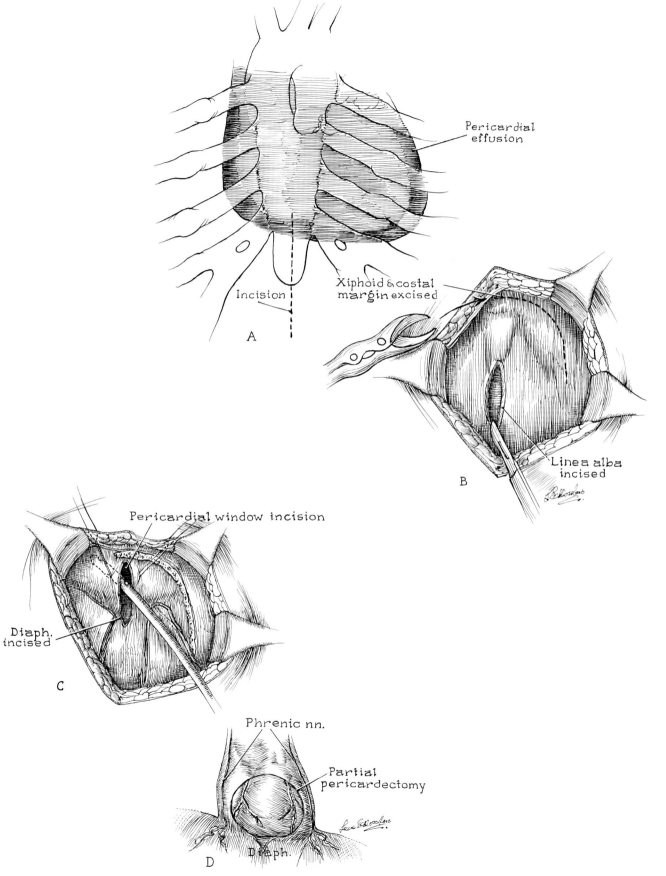

Pericardial
effusion

Incision

Xiphoid & costal
margin excised

A

Linea alba
incised

B

Pericardial window incision

Diaph.
incised

C

Phrenic nn.

Partial
pericardectomy

Diaph.

D

CARDIORRHAPHY FOR PENETRATING WOUNDS OF THE HEART

A. In the special circumstance of a lifeless or all but lifeless patient, a prepared surgeon, and an equipped emergency room, a swift anterolateral thoracotomy is made in the 4th left interspace. (In women the skin incision is in the inframammary crease.) If necessary, the sternum can be transected in continuity with the intercostal incision and the internal mammary vessels secured en route. In the usual circumstance of thoracotomy in a formal operating room, a median sternotomy is preferred.

B. The pericardium is opened widely, and clot and blood are evacuated. Bleeding will often have stopped, and it is as well to avoid dislodging clot from the myocardial wound until one is fully set for the repair.

C. While the finger occludes the cardiotomy, sutures on appropriately sized needles are passed behind the occluding finger, from one side of the wound to the other, and serially tied.

D. If the sutures in the myocardium tend to cut through or seem insecure, or if the ventricle is thin-walled, mattress sutures are placed through Teflon pledgets.

E. In the not rare circumstance in which the laceration is so close to a coronary vessel that there is no room for sutures between the vessel and the myocardial wound, mattress sutures (*dotted lines*) to the far side of the coronary vessels are passed under the vessels, coapting the wound edges without compromising the blood flow through the vessels.

F. For wounds of the atrium and great vessels, immediate tangential application of a vascular clamp controls the bleeding and permits safe suture. Attempts to sew a great vessel while using tamponade on the laceration with a finger invite tearing by the sutures of the wall of the distended vessel and enlargement of the wound. In gunshot wounds of the heart, as of the abdominal viscera, the "rule of twos" must be borne in mind, and for all but obviously guttered wounds, a wound of exit from the heart should be sought.

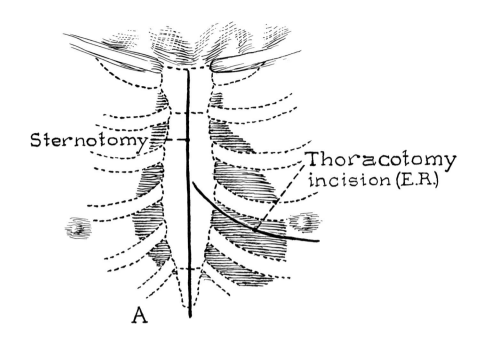

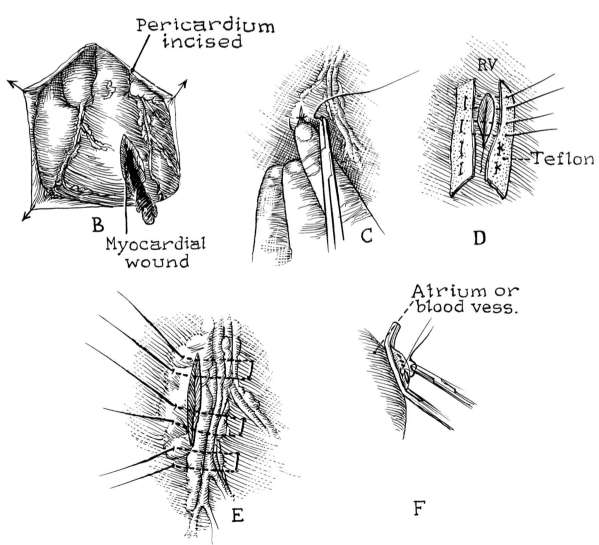

TEMPORARY SEAL OF OPEN TRAUMATIC OR INFECTED CHEST WOUND

A. A surgeon's glove is sterilely washed clear of all talcum powder. The wrist seam of the glove, the four fingers, and the tip of the thumb are cut off. The glove is incised along the ulnar, or 5th finger, edge.

B. A flat rubber sheet is thus obtained with a central tubular extension (the thumb), through which a chest tube of appropriate size is passed, glued in place, and held by circular ligatures reinforcing the seal.

C. The skin surrounding the chest wound or incision is cleaned with a fat- and mucus-dissolving agent and dried. Glue is applied to the patient's skin and the undersurface of the opened glove. The sheet of glove rubber is stretched and applied to the skin, the chest tube entering the pleural cavity.

The edges of the rubber sheet are secured to the skin with a quadrangular border of tape, and the chest tube is connected to a drainage collecting system. Suction is used as indicated.

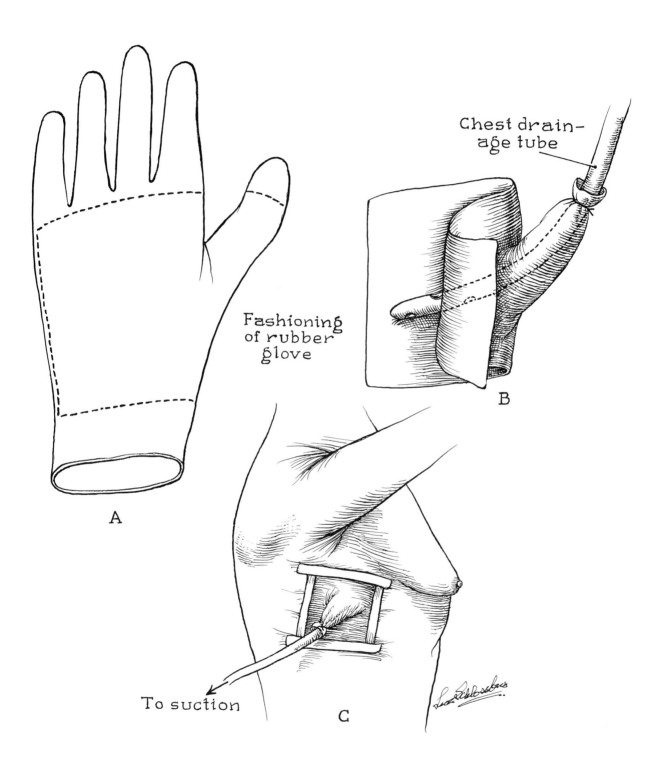

Chest drain-
age tube

Fashioning
of rubber
glove

A

B

To suction

C

MEDIASTINOSCOPY

General anesthesia is employed to eliminate coughing and the possibility of mediastinal air dissection through the bared trachea.

A. The path of the instrument is first cleared by blunt dissection with the finger, and the plane of dissection taken is directly on the trachea.

B. Although, with care, nodes to the right and left of the trachea and along the main bronchi may be seen and biopsied, deeper carinal nodes tend to be out of the field of view and beyond the reach of the instrument.

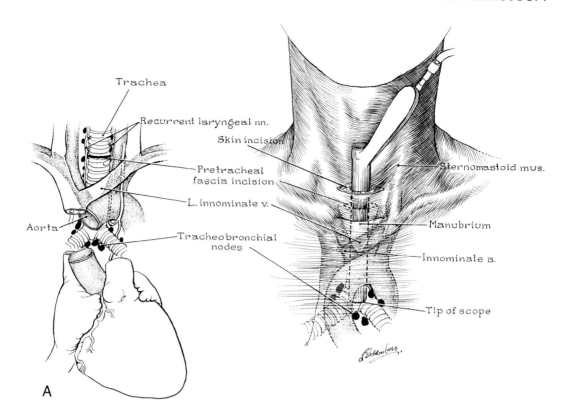

Trachea

Recurrent laryngeal nn.

Skin incision

Pretracheal fascia incision

L. innominate v.

Aorta

Tracheobronchial nodes

Sternomastoid mus.

Manubrium

Innominate a.

Tip of scope

A

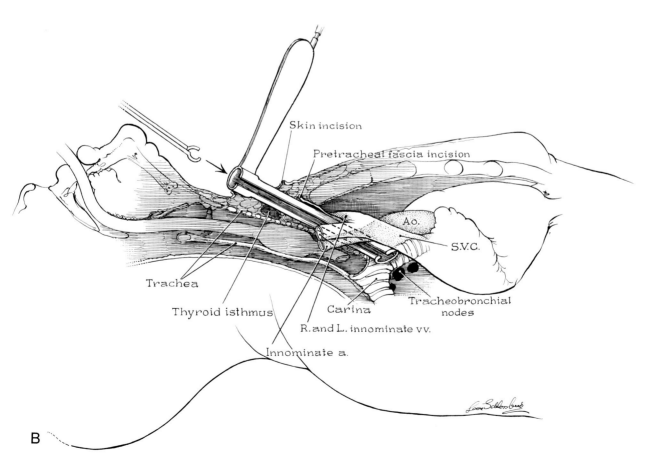

Skin incision

Pretracheal fascia incision

Ao.

S.V.C.

Trachea

Thyroid isthmus

Carina

Tracheobronchial nodes

R. and L. innominate vv.

Innominate a.

B

MEDIASTINOSCOPY *(Continued)*

C. The drawing shows dramatically the magistral structures that are sequentially brought in view at the end of the mediastinoscope. Instances of injury to each of these have been reported. As in any endoscopic procedure, gentle and deliberate passage of the instrument under clear vision and without use of force minimizes the risk of damage from the instrument itself. The greater hazard is of attempted biopsy of an incompletely identified "lymph node," which has turned out to be an innominate artery, pulmonary artery, or bronchus in instances known to us—and this obviously does not exhaust the possible list. The advantage of mediastinoscopy compared with that of mediastinotomy lies in its exposure of both sides of the trachea and main bronchi, of special importance in left lower lobe lesions that metastasize to both left and right tracheobronchial nodes. However, direct biopsies of pulmonary lesions and of node metastases in the aortic window below the arch of the aorta are not possible.

Figures *A* and *B* courtesy of Dr. R. Robinson Baker (unpublished drawings).

REFERENCES

1. Harken, D.E., Black, H., Clauss, R., and Farraud, R.E.: A simple cervicomediastinal exploration for tissue diagnosis of intrathoracic disease. N. Engl. J. Med. 251:1041–1044, 1954
2. Radner, S.: Suprasternal node biopsy in lymphspreading intrathoracic disease. Acta Med. Scand. 152:413–415, 1955
3. Carlens, E.: Mediastinoscopy: A method for inspection and tissue biopsy in the superior mediastinum. Dis. Chest 36:343–352, 1959
4. Steele, J.D., and Marable, S.A.: Cervical mediastinotomy for biopsy. J. Thorac. Surg. 37:621–624, 1959
5. Pearson, F.G.: Mediastinoscopy. A method of biopsy in the superior mediastinum. J. Thorac. Cardiovasc. Surg. 49:11–21, 1965
6. Trinkle, J.K., Bryant, L.R., Hiller, A.J., and Playforth, R.H.: Mediastinoscopy—experience with 300 consecutive cases. J. Thorac. Cardiovasc. Surg. 60:297–300, 1969

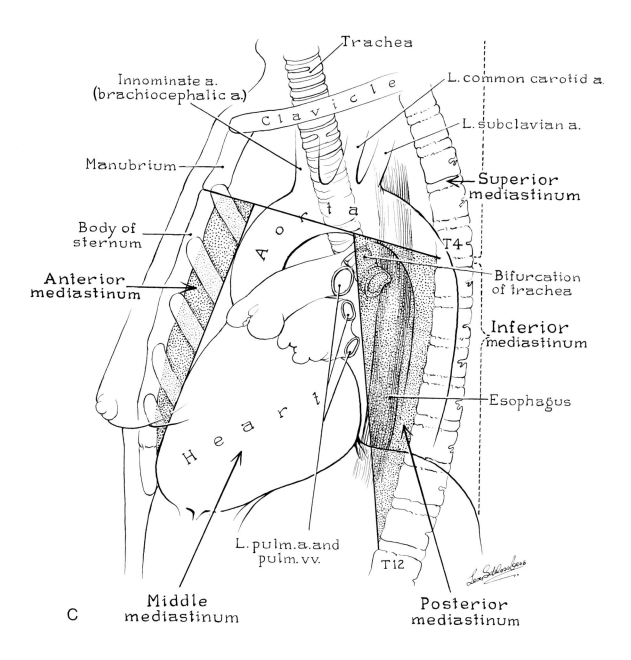

Trachea

Innominate a.
(brachiocephalic a.)

Clavicle

L. common carotid a.

L. subclavian a.

Manubrium

Superior
mediastinum

T4

Body of
sternum

Aorta

Bifurcation
of trachea

Anterior
mediastinum

Inferior
mediastinum

Heart

Esophagus

L. pulm. a. and
pulm. vv.

T12

C

Middle
mediastinum

Posterior
mediastinum

183

MEDIASTINOTOMY*

   The procedure is performed under general, endotracheal inhalation anesthesia, so that the lungs can be expanded if the pleura is entered.

A. In general, the approach is through the bed of the 2nd costal cartilage, but it may be through the bed of the 3rd cartilage if the lesion to be biopsied is seen in that location on x-rays or CT.

B. The perichondrium overlying the cartilage is incised and stripped; the costal cartilage is removed by transection at the costochondral and chondrosternal junctions.

C. After incision of the perichondrium posteriorly, the internal mammary vessels are dissected free and drawn laterally by traction loops. The anterior mediastinal reflection of the pleura is dissected from under the sternum, medial to the mammary vessels, and displaced laterally.

D. The anterior and posterior mediastinum are now entered by blunt dissection so that enlarged nodes or thymus can be liberated.

E. An enlarged individual node, or fat pad containing small nodes, is dissected, the stalk or vascular bundle clipped, and the lesion removed.

F. On the left side, mediastinotomy of the 2nd or 3rd cartilage allows for biopsies below the arch of the aorta, in the aortic window, and along the left main bronchus, an advantage over mediastinoscopy for lesions of this area.

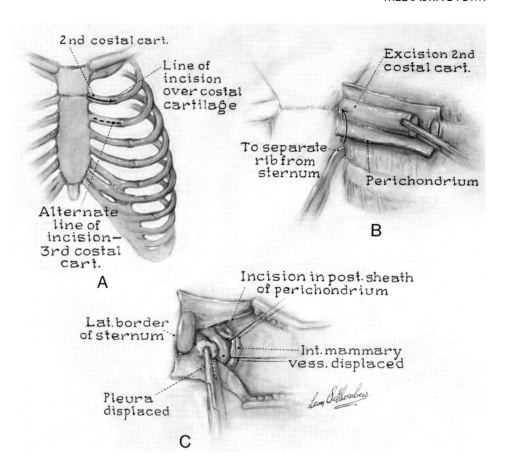

2nd costal cart.

Line of incision over costal cartilage

Alternate line of incision— 3rd costal cart.

A

Excision 2nd costal cart.

To separate rib from sternum

Perichondrium

B

Incision in post. sheath of perichondrium

Lat. border of sternum

Int. mammary vess. displaced

Pleura displaced

Leon Schlossberg

C

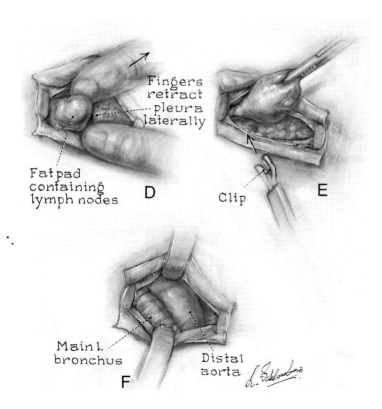

Fingers retract pleura laterally

Fat pad containing lymph nodes

D

Clip

E

Main l. bronchus

Distal aorta

L. Schlossberg

F

G. Another advantage is the possibility of extending the mediastinotomy by resecting the anterior portion of the 2nd or 3rd rib and performing a limited anterior thoracotomy for biopsy of superior and anterior lesions of the lung that have defied diagnosis by other means.

H. After excision of the anterior portion of the rib, the pleura is opened and biopsy of the anterior and apical segments of the upper lobe becomes possible. At this point, it may be decided to extend the incision into a formal thoracotomy for a definitive resection.

I. On the right side, the same approach is possible through the bed of the 2nd or 3rd costal cartilage. Internal mammary vessels and anterior pleural reflection are displaced laterally.

J. The anterior-superior mediastinum is entered between the pleura laterally and the ascending aorta and superior vena cava medially. Inferiorly, the cardiac pulsations are palpable through the pericardium, and deep to the vena cava the trachea and origin of the right main bronchus are palpated. Lymph nodes in this area are teased out by blunt instrument and finger dissection. The lung, seen through the thin pleura, can be biopsied as shown in *G* and *H*.

---

*Note: The various anatomical structures encountered in a left or right mediastinotomy are shown here through the eyes of an anatomist. In fact, the approach provides a very limited exposure from the standpoint of an explicit visual inspection and is performed by careful finger palpation as a confined "well" is created in depth, allowing for progressive widening and placement of deep, narrow retractors. Although light-carrying retractors and specula can be useful, the surgeon often "carries his eyes at his finger tips" and should be confident in his ability to differentiate, by palpation, organs, tissue textures, and resistances that allow for dissection in avascular planes. Mediastinotomy has advantages in the approach to the aortic arch on the left and the potential for direct lung biopsy, but it is limited by the fact that the carina and crossover metastases from the left lower lobe to the right mediastinum cannot be exposed, and mediastinoscopy is preferable in such instances. Mediastinotomy presents the advantage that in the event of injury to a major vascular structure, control can be readily achieved through extension of the original incision.

REFERENCES

1. Chamberlain, J.M.: In discussion of Pearson, F.G.: Mediastinoscopy: A method of biopsy in the superior mediastinum. J. Thorac. Cardiovasc. Surg. 49:11–21, 1965
2. McNeill, T.M., and Chamberlain, J.M.: Diagnostic anterior mediastinotomy. Ann. Thorac. Surg. 2:532–539, 1966

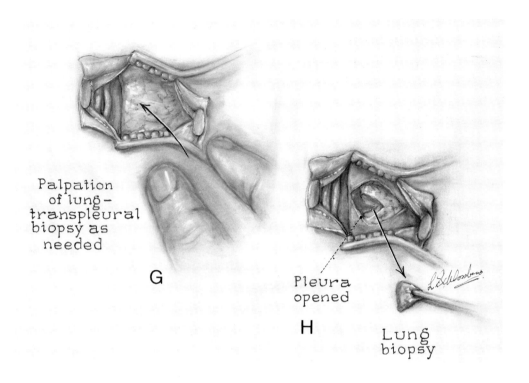

Palpation
of lung-
transpleural
biopsy as
needed

G

Pleura
opened

H

Lung
biopsy

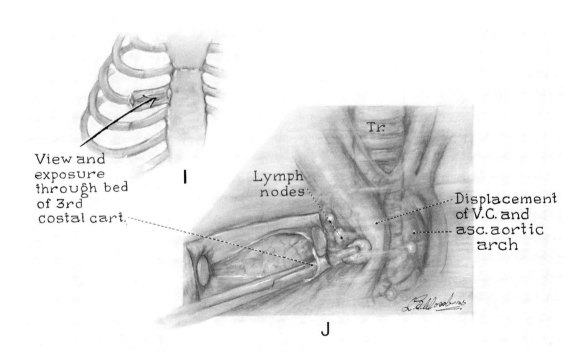

View and
exposure
through bed
of 3rd
costal cart.

I

Tr.

Lymph
nodes

Displacement
of V.C. and
asc. aortic
arch

J

Pulmonary Resections

Pulmonary Resections

SEGMENTAL ANATOMY OF THE LUNG

In the earlier days of frequent segmental resections of the lung for tuberculosis, lung abscess, and bronchiectasis, a detailed knowledge of the segmental anatomy of the lung was of importance to the surgeon in planning dissections. Today, with the widespread adoption of stapling techniques and the "conservative resection" (see *Segmental and Atypical Pulmonary Resections*), which spares pulmonary tissue by staying well within or cutting across anatomical segmental boundaries, the sublobar anatomy of the lung has, for the most part, lost its significance so far as the technique of operation is concerned, although it is still of interest in terms of the precise localization of lesions by routine chest radiographic examination, tomography, bronchography, and CT. In those areas of the world where bronchiectasis is still a common surgical problem, segmental anatomy retains some importance, although the old-time finger dissection resection along the intersegmental line is not likely to be performed. In the patient requiring multiple atypical resections, the definition and pattern of lung tissue removed by an intersegmental, transegmental, or mostly segmental approach is of importance.

From DeLand, F.H., and Wagner, H.N., Jr.: *Atlas of Nuclear Medicine.* Volume II. Philadelphia, W.B. Saunders Company, 1970, with permission.

REFERENCES

1. Brock, R.C.: *The Anatomy of the Bronchial Tree.* London, Oxford University Press, 1946
   The classic study of segmental anatomy
2. Chamberlain, J.M., Storey, C.F., Klopstock, R., and Daniels, C.F.: Segmental resection for pulmonary tuberculosis. J. Thorac. Surg. 26:471–485, 1953
3. Boyden, E.A.: *Segmental Anatomy of the Lungs.* New York, McGraw-Hill Book Company, 1955
4. Kimel, V.M.: Resectional therapy for pulmonary tuberculosis at Sunmount 1950–1957, 807 cases. III. An evaluation of the techniques of reconstruction of the lung in segmental resections. J. Thorac. Cardiovasc. Surg. 39:405–408, 1960
5. Amosov, N.M., and Berezovsky, K.K.: Pulmonary resection with mechanical suture. J. Thorac. Cardiovasc. Surg. 41:325–335, 1961
   Discussion of "economical (non-anatomic) resection"
6. Young, W.G., Jr., and Moor, G.F.: The surgical treatment of pulmonary tuberculosis. In: *Gibbon's Surgery of the Chest,* 4th Edition, D.C. Sabiston, Jr., and F.C. Spencer (Eds.). Philadelphia, W.B. Saunders Company, 1983
   Page 622—lovely drawings of the old, classical finger dissection technique of segmental dissection
7. Steichen, F.M., and Ravitch, M.M.: *Stapling in Surgery.* Chicago, Year Book Medical Publishers, Inc., 1984

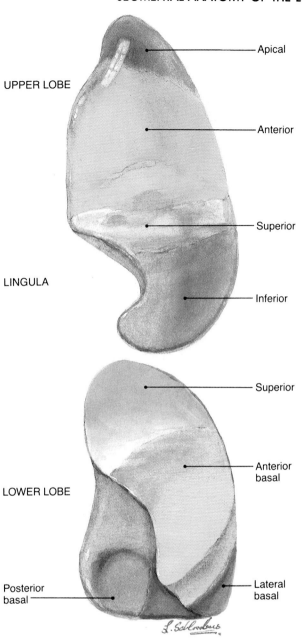

UPPER LOBE

Apical

Anterior

Superior

LINGULA

Inferior

Superior

Anterior
basal

LOWER LOBE

Posterior
basal

Lateral
basal

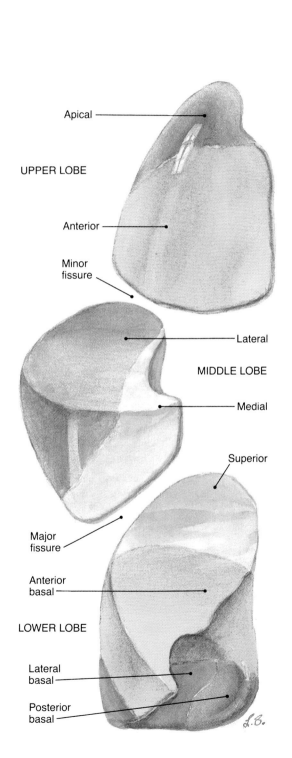

Apical

UPPER LOBE

Anterior

Minor
fissure

Lateral

MIDDLE LOBE

Medial

Superior

Major
fissure

Anterior
basal

LOWER LOBE

Lateral
basal

Posterior
basal

SEGMENTAL ANATOMY OF THE LUNG *(Continued)*

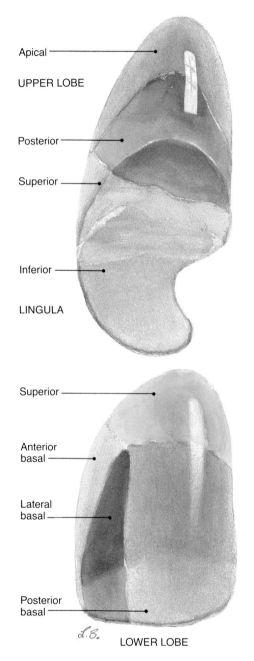

Apical

UPPER LOBE

Posterior

Superior

Inferior

LINGULA

Superior

Anterior basal

Lateral basal

Posterior basal

L.B.

LOWER LOBE

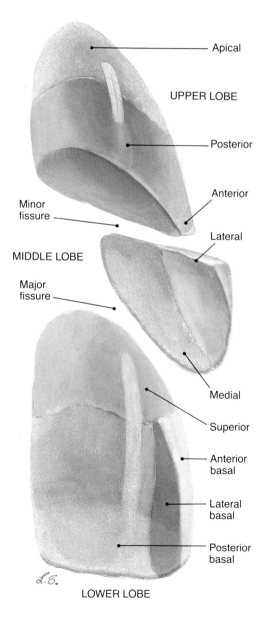

Apical

UPPER LOBE

Posterior

Anterior

Minor fissure

Lateral

MIDDLE LOBE

Major fissure

Medial

Superior

Anterior basal

Lateral basal

Posterior basal

L.B.

LOWER LOBE

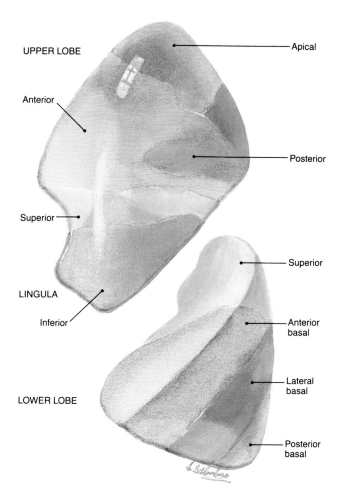

UPPER LOBE

Apical

Anterior

Posterior

Superior

LINGULA

Inferior

Superior

Anterior
basal

Lateral
basal

LOWER LOBE

Posterior
basal

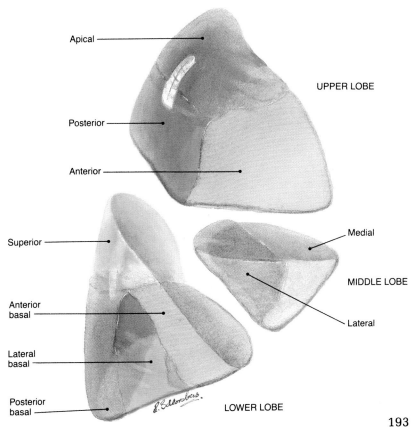

Apical

Posterior

Anterior

UPPER LOBE

Superior

Medial

MIDDLE LOBE

Anterior
basal

Lateral

Lateral
basal

Posterior
basal

LOWER LOBE

193

LUNG BIOPSY

Amputation of the Apex

The TA 55 or TA 90 stapler, depending upon the size required, is slid across the apex behind the lesion, the staples are driven home, and the specimen is cut away on the edge of the stapler, with the result shown. Stapling of parenchyma is more secure than suturing with respect to both bleeding and air leak, and it almost never produces a local hematoma. The same technique is applicable to the tip of the lingula and appropriately shaped portions of lobar edges. No sutures are needed.

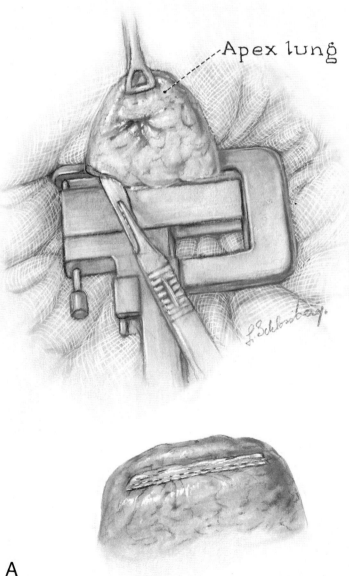

A

Tangential Excision of a Metastatic Nodule

The jaws of the TA instrument are placed behind the nodule-containing portion of the lung, the tissue is stapled, and the specimen is cut away on the edge of the stapler. The inset shows the curved pattern assumed by the straight staple line as the lung expands. This technique has enormously simplified the aggressive pursuit of multiple pulmonary metastases and minimizes both the amount of lung parenchyma sacrificed and the complications of multiple biopsies. No sutures are needed.

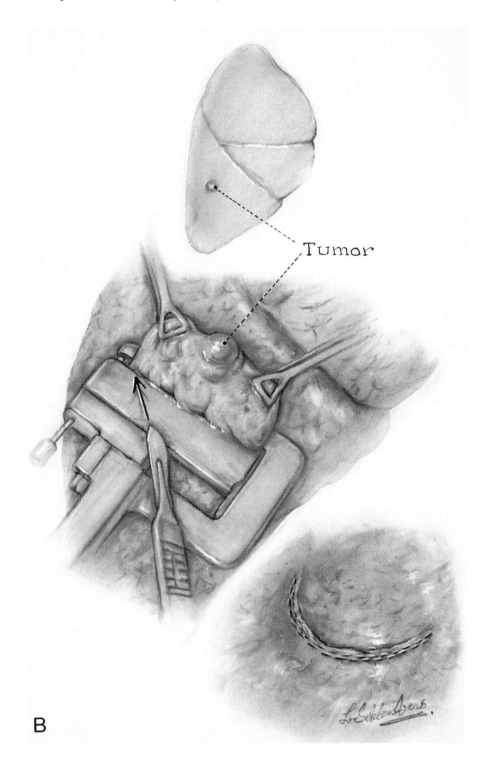

Tumor

B

Wedge Excision with the GIA Stapler

A nodule, which is near a convenient edge of lung, can be excised by two applications of the GIA. The overlapping staple line has proved to be quite secure. This technique is useful for open lung biopsy of any area but is not needed for the apex of a lobe or the tip of the lingula, which can be amputated by a single application of the TA stapler as shown previously. No sutures are required.

REFERENCES

1. Steichen, F.M., and Ravitch, M.M.: *Stapling in Surgery.* Chicago, Year Book Medical Publishers, 1984
2. Ravitch, M.M.: Intersecting staple lines in intestinal anastomoses. Surgery 97:8–14, 1985

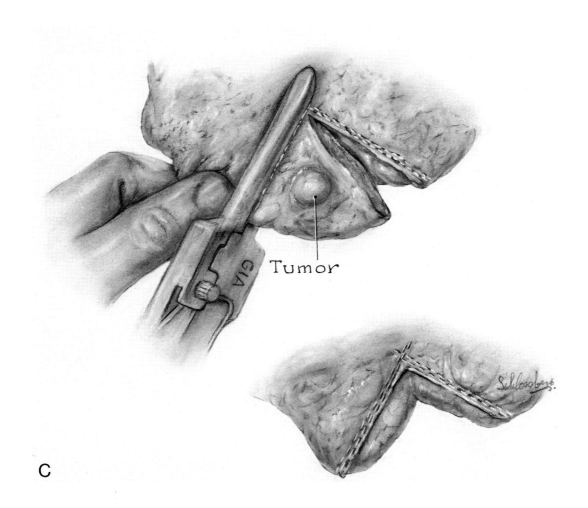

Tumor

C

RESECTION OF GIANT BULLA

The TA 90 instrument is simply placed across the lung just below the base of the large bulla. After placement of the staple line, the bulla is amputated. A hemostatic and airtight closure of the remaining lung tissue results. In the amputation of the apex (shown previously) or stapled transections of greater thicknesses of lung, the virtual elimination of bleeding and air leaks is offset, to a small degree, by some compression of pulmonary parenchyma in suturing together opposite surfaces of the lung—a more than acceptable trade-off. Bullae, however, expand out of the lung, and coaptation of the pulmonary tissue at the base of the bulla actually restores the normal situation. No sutures are required.

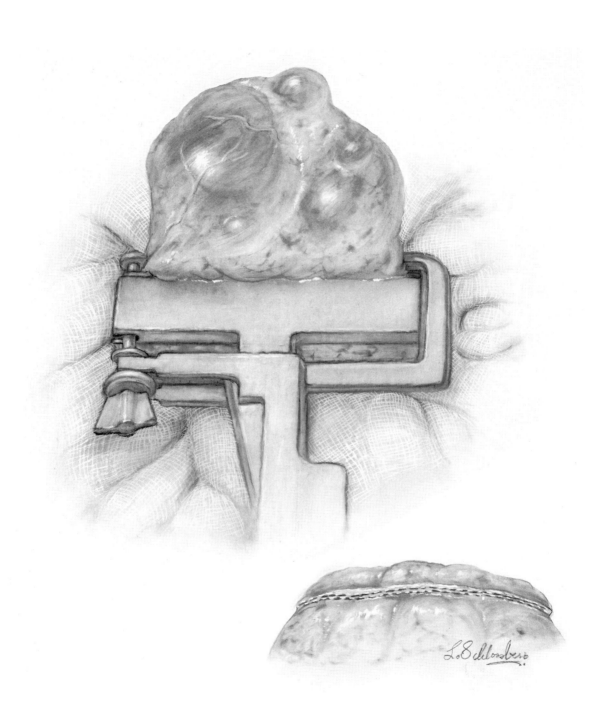

SEGMENTAL AND ATYPICAL PULMONARY RESECTIONS

With the advent of mechanical sutures, the classical anatomical segmental resection has become a technique of the past, although some of its features, such as preliminary ligation of the segmental artery, the bronchus, and, rarely if ever, the vein, may still be useful. The former technique of blunt dissection along intersegmental planes resulted in oozing of blood, sometimes in significant amounts, and occasional prolonged leakage of air. With stapling techniques, besides removing the equivalent of a segment, it is now possible to perform a resection of less than the segmental unit or more—intra- and intersegmental resections.

Apical-Posterior Segmentectomy, Left Upper Lobe

The mediastinal pleura overlying the convexity of the left main pulmonary artery has been opened, and the apical-posterior artery, the 1st branch, has been divided between ligatures.

The TA 90 stapler (1) is now applied across the base of the apical-posterior segment, and the pulmonary tissue is divided (2) along the edge of the stapler.

For increased security, the bronchial and venous stumps may at times be suture-ligated in the staple line.

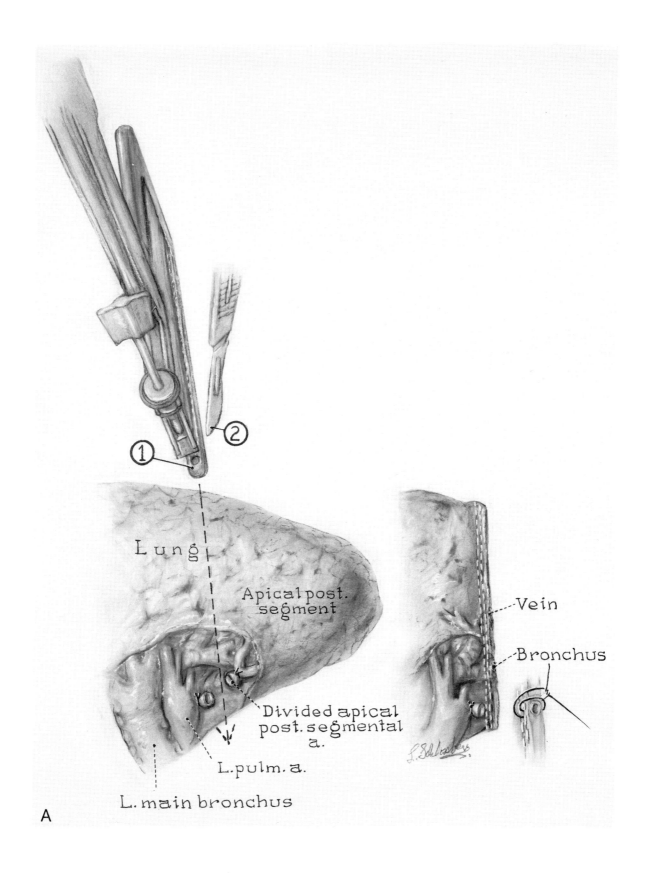

① ②

Lung

Apical post.
segment

Divided apical
post. segmental
a.

L. pulm. a.

L. main bronchus

Vein

Bronchus

A

Superior Segmentectomy, Right Lower Lobe*

The superior segmental artery, immediately opposite the origin of the middle lobe artery (see pages 230–233, *Right Middle Lobectomy, A*), is exposed through the posterior aspect of the oblique fissure and transected between ligatures. The corresponding bronchus, running parallel and posterior to the arterial branch, is transected and closed at its takeoff from the intermediate bronchus.

The TA 90 stapler (1) is applied across the base of the superior segment, at the margin of the aerated lung, and the specimen is amputated (2) peripheral to the stapler, with the result shown at the right.

Venous branches in the staple line may be suture-ligated, although this is usually not necessary.

---

*The detail shows only the lower lobe.

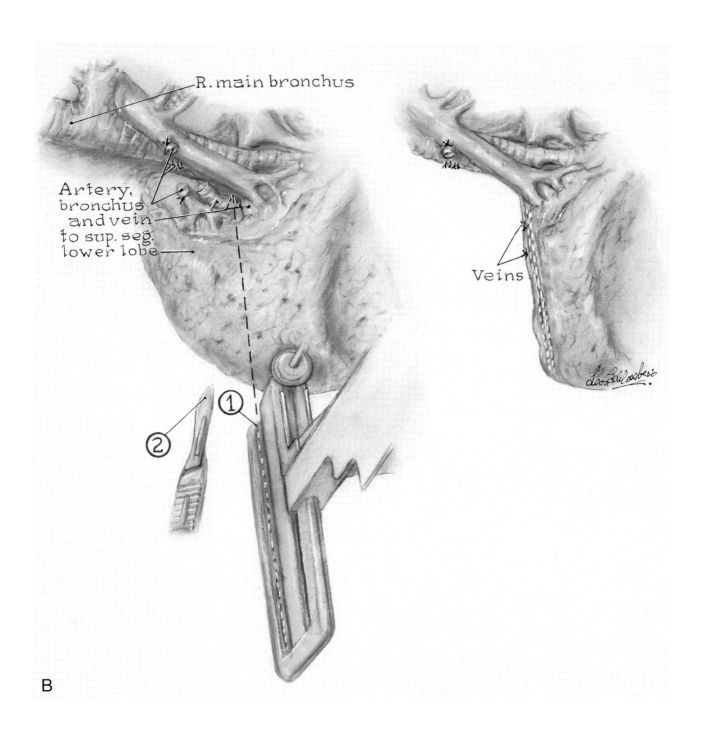

R. main bronchus

Artery,
bronchus
and vein
to sup. seg.
lower lobe

① ②

Veins

B

PULMONARY RESECTION—TREATMENT OF THE ARTERY

A. The artery in every case is best exposed by dissection directly upon its adventitia. Once the plane is opened up by the scissors, as shown, dissection is pursued, either entirely with the scissors, or

B. By a twisting, rotating motion of the gauze dissector at the end of a long clamp, which traps the fine areolar fibers and pushes them *toward* the mediastinum. In general, sharp dissection is safest, particularly when inflammation has scarred and toughened the perivascular tissues.

C and D. Treatment of the pulmonary arteries in a right upper lobectomy is shown. Ligature of the main stem of the superior division of the pulmonary artery and separate ligature of its branches provide secure proximal control. Failing this, a transfixion suture of the upper lobe artery is preferred. It is always worth the time to ligate the vessels on the parenchymal side, as shown. The artery is divided between the proximal and distal ligatures.

E. For the main pulmonary artery, stapling is by all odds the safest and simplest technique; the artery is tied on the lung side.

F. The artery was transected on the edge of the stapler *before* the instrument was released.

G. Equally safe but somewhat more time-consuming is over-and-over suture, distal to a vascular clamp.

    The technique of dissecting, securing, and dividing the veins is essentially the same.

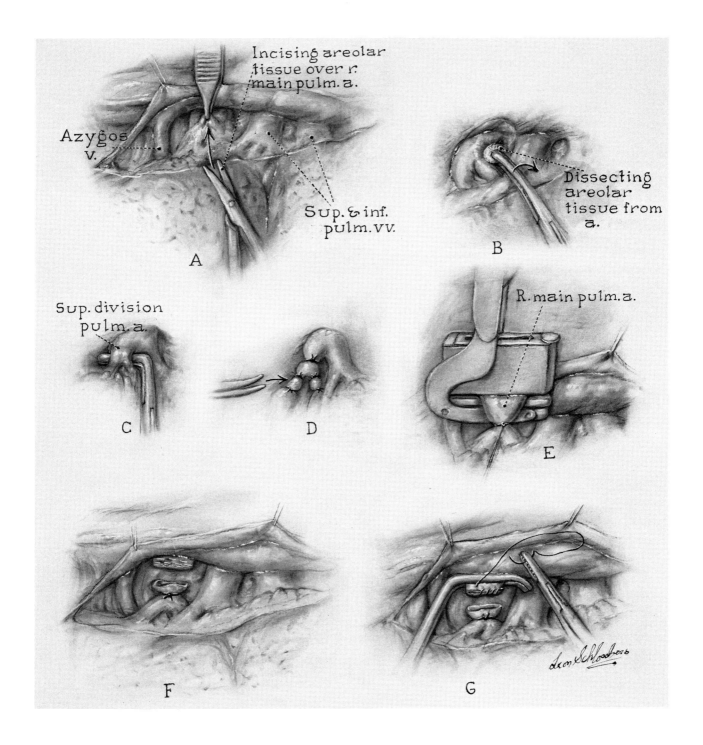

Incising areolar tissue over r. main pulm. a.

Azygos v.

Sup. & inf. pulm. vv.

A

Dissecting areolar tissue from a.

B

Sup. division pulm. a.

C

D

R. main pulm. a.

E

F

G

PULMONARY RESECTION—TREATMENT OF THE BRONCHUS

The ideal treatment of the bronchus is a no-stump closure. The healing of bronchus, whether stapled or sutured, depends on its own circulation, not the circulation of the mediastinal tissues. For this reason, and because any length of bronchial stump acts as a sump, inviting infection and breakdown, a no-stump closure is sought in every instance. With the stapler, as shown in C, this is quite easily accomplished by placing it parallel to and against the parent bronchus or the trachea. If one clamps the bronchus and applies sutures as shown in D, a minimal stump cul de sac is unavoidable. Whether the bronchus sutures are placed over the end as shown or as mattress sutures either in the axis of the bronchus or transverse to that is a matter of individual preference.

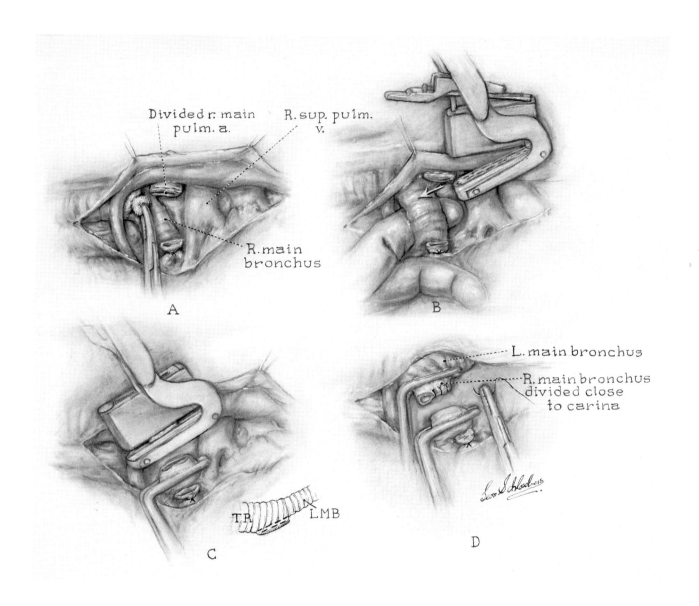

Divided r. main pulm. a.

R. sup. pulm. v.

R. main bronchus

A

B

C

TR   LMB

L. main bronchus

R. main bronchus divided close to carina

D

THE THORACIC VISCERA SEEN IN TRANSPARENCY THROUGH THE CHEST WALL

A. Anteroposterior.

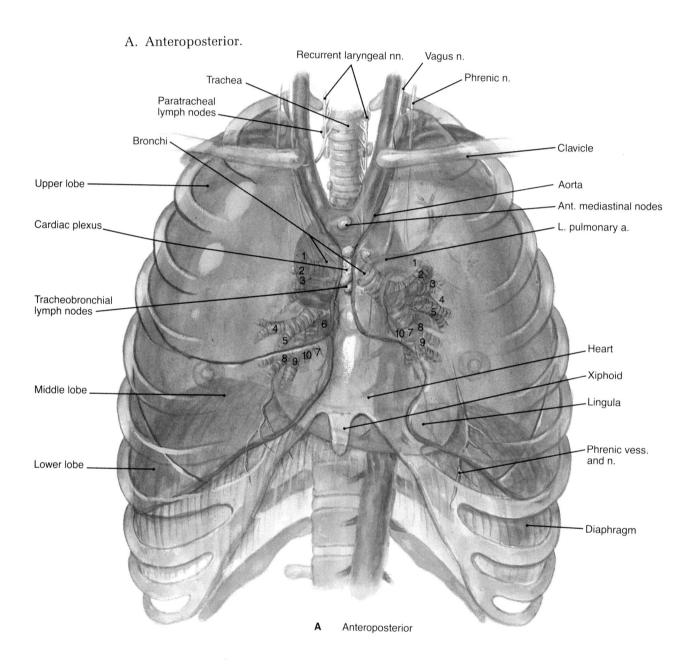

A   Anteroposterior

LEFT ANTERIOR VIEW

Upper lobe
1. Apical
2. Anterior
3. Posterior
4. Superior Lingular
5. Inferior Lingular

Lower lobe
6. Superior
7. Medial Basal
8. Anterior Basal
9. Lateral Basal
10. Posterior Basal

B. Left lateral.

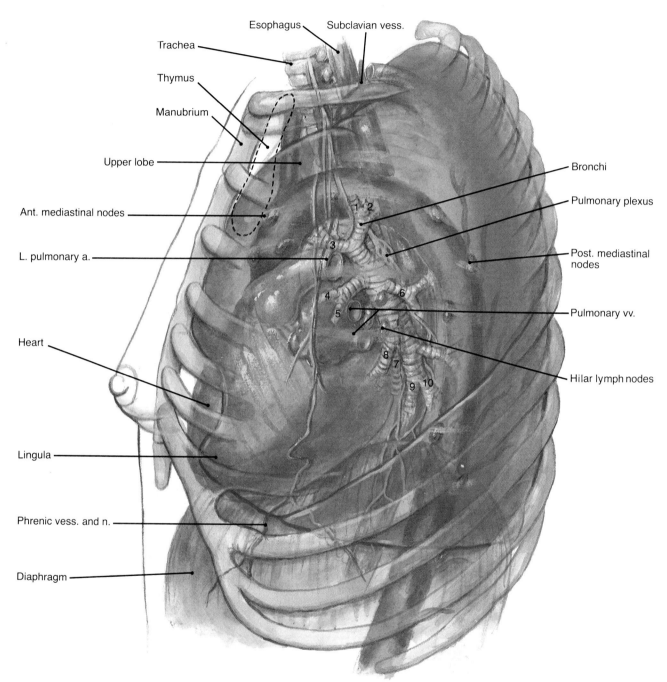

Esophagus

Subclavian vess.

Trachea

Thymus

Manubrium

Upper lobe

Ant. mediastinal nodes

L. pulmonary a.

Heart

Lingula

Phrenic vess. and n.

Diaphragm

Bronchi

Pulmonary plexus

Post. mediastinal nodes

Pulmonary vv.

Hilar lymph nodes

B   Left lateral

LEFT LATERAL VIEW
Upper lobe
1. Apical
2. Anterior
3. Posterior
4. Superior Lingular
5. Inferior Lingular

Lower lobe
6. Superior
7. Medial Basal
8. Anterior Basal
9. Lateral Basal
10. Posterior Basal

C. Right lateral.

The artist's technique permits one to see the relationships of the fissures to the chest wall and of the great vessels, the bronchi, the pulmonary veins, the recurrent laryngeal nerves, the phrenic nerves, the lymphatics, the intercostal nerves, and the sympathetic trunk.

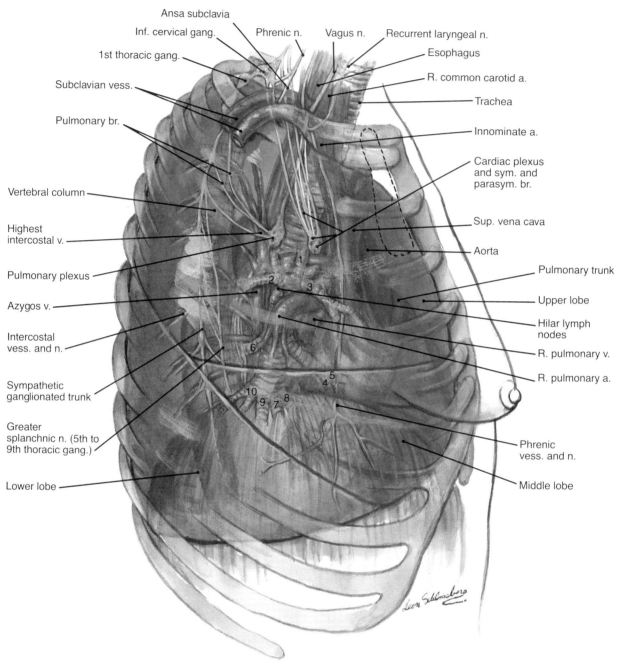

C Right lateral

RIGHT LATERAL VIEW

Upper lobe
1. Apical
2. Posterior
3. Anterior

Middle lobe
4. Lateral
5. Middle

Lower lobe
6. Superior
7. Medial Basal
8. Anterior Basal
9. Lateral Basal
10. Posterior Basal

Pneumonectomy and Lobectomy

The color renditions of the pulmonary and lobar anatomy demonstrate the topographic relationships of the bronchi, arteries, and veins. The views shown are for the most part those seen by the surgeon on dissection. For the sake of anatomical clarity, dissection is shown carried out from the hilum well beyond the dissection needed by the surgeon. The nerve plexuses, lymph nodes, lymphatic vessels, and areolar tissue have been deleted to permit sharper definition of the bronchovascular structures. The area included in the white ovals is all that the surgeon sees, dissecting only enough to be certain of the identification of the structures to be divided and of handling them safely. In the course of operation the surgeon may, in pneumonectomy, work alternately from in front and behind. This is true of some lobectomies, in which some of the dissection may also be made in the interlobar fissure. Without an elaborate sequence of illustrations, it would not be feasible to show all of these possibilities.

There are almost innumerable variations of the distribution of the lobar and, particularly, the segmental arteries and veins. We have shown what we believe to be the commonest patterns, and others are mentioned in the text.

The nomenclature of the bronchi, vessels, and segments is that of Jackson and Huber.

REFERENCE

1. Jackson, C.L., and Huber, J.F.: Correlated applied anatomy of the bronchial tree and lungs with a system of nomenclature. Dis. Chest 9:319–326, 1943

HILUM OF THE RIGHT LUNG

Anterior Aspect

On the right, the main bronchus and the pulmonary vascular trunks are seen to emerge from the mediastinum from behind the superior vena cava and the right atrium. The right pulmonary artery originates from the main pulmonary artery to the left of the midline and is therefore relatively long. The azygos vein lies above the upper edge of the lung root, and as it passes into the superior vena cava, it arches above the right main bronchus. The phrenic nerve, seen on the anterior surface of the superior vena cava, descends on the lateral surface of the pericardium. The main bronchus, the most superior hilar structure, is followed in order by the pulmonary artery and the pulmonary veins. The bronchus is most posterior; the artery is anterior and inferior to it. The superior pulmonary vein lies inferior to the pulmonary artery and still more anteriorly. The inferior pulmonary vein, the lowest major hilar structure, lies on a plane somewhat posterior to that of the superior vein. The pulmonary ligament as it reaches the hilum encompasses the inferior pulmonary vein. As the bronchus and the vessels divide into lobar and segmental branches, they spread out tridimensionally, entwining like vines on a trellis. For the right upper lobe and its segments, the bronchial and arterial branches maintain the same relationships as in the pulmonary hilum. The veins are not strictly segmental in distribution. The venous trunk from the upper lobe is made up of apical-anterior, inferior, and posterior tributaries. It will be seen that one or more middle lobe veins drain into the upper lobe vein.

The right upper lobe bronchus arises from the right main bronchus 1.5 cm or so beyond the tracheal bifurcation and divides into three segmental branches—apical, anterior, and posterior. The right pulmonary artery divides into superior and inferior trunks. The superior, the first branch of the right pulmonary artery, divides into the apical and anterior segmental arteries of the upper lobe. The artery to the posterior segment of the right upper lobe, arising from the inferior trunk, curves around the anterior surface of the intermediate bronchus to run along the lateral border of this bronchus deep in the interlobar fissure, lateral to the bronchus of the middle lobe.

The bronchial and arterial structures to the middle and lower lobes are in planes posterior and lateral to that of the superior pulmonary vein and are most readily approached posterolaterally through the interlobar fissures. The superior pulmonary vein lying in front of and inferior to the inferior pulmonary artery trunk is usually formed by three tributaries from the right upper lobe—apical-anterior, inferior, and posterior—and two from the right middle lobe; these last tributaries often form a single trunk before joining the superior pulmonary vein.

Although the inferior pulmonary vein can be exposed from in front, a procedure facilitated by dividing the inferior pulmonary ligament, the vein lies more posteriorly than the superior vein and is hidden by the overhanging lower lobe. The inferior vein is formed by a collecting trunk of veins from the superior segment of the lower lobe, emerging from behind the basal bronchus, and by three or four basal veins, often joining into one or two short common segments before entering the main inferior vein.

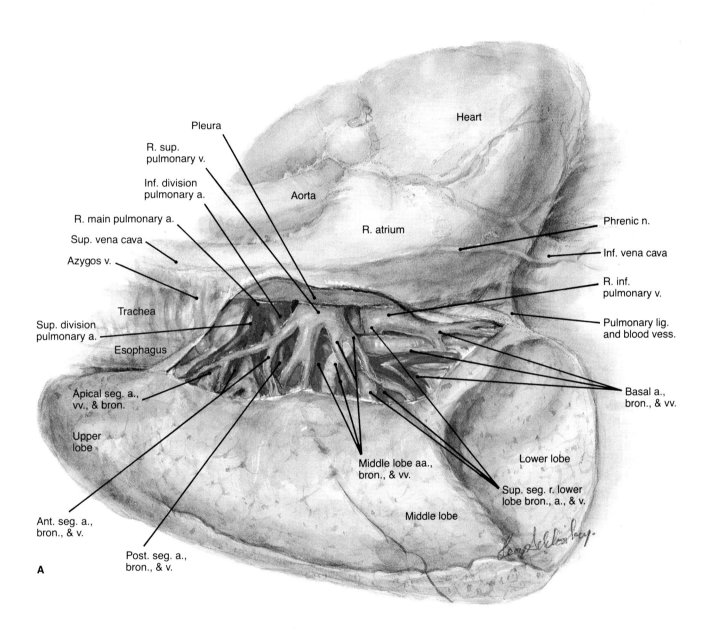

Pleura

R. sup.
pulmonary v.

Inf. division
pulmonary a.

R. main pulmonary a.

Sup. vena cava

Azygos v.

Trachea

Sup. division
pulmonary a.

Esophagus

Apical seg. a.,
vv., & bron.

Upper
lobe

Ant. seg. a.,
bron., & v.

Post. seg. a.,
bron., & v.

Heart

Aorta

R. atrium

Phrenic n.

Inf. vena cava

R. inf.
pulmonary v.

Pulmonary lig.
and blood vess.

Basal a.,
bron., & vv.

Middle lobe aa.,
bron., & vv.

Lower lobe

Sup. seg. r. lower
lobe bron., a., & v.

Middle lobe

A

HILUM OF THE RIGHT LUNG *(Continued)*

Posterior Aspect

The azygos vein is shown above the upper border of the hilum. The right upper lobe bronchus originates from the lateral aspect of the right main bronchus and in this view hides the superior trunk of the right pulmonary artery and the entire superior pulmonary vein.

The inferior trunk of the right pulmonary artery, not readily seen from in front, passes around the lower edge of the right upper lobe bronchus, giving off a branch to the posterior segment of the right upper lobe. During operation this branch can be reached from the anterior approach after the superior vein has been divided, or it can be approached laterally through the minor fissure. The inferior arterial trunk then passes on anterior to the intermediate bronchus—the common bronchial trunk of the middle and lower lobes—and lateral to the right middle lobe bronchus.

The bronchial arteries and veins are closely applied to the walls of the lobar bronchi. The dorsal branches are seen clearly in this view.

In its interlobar course, the inferior trunk of the pulmonary artery supplies the middle lobe by branches to the lateral and medial segments, originating and running lateral and slightly superior to the corresponding middle lobe bronchi. Posterolaterally and directly opposite the origin of the middle lobe arteries is the origin of the artery to the superior segment of the lower lobe. The arterial supply to the basal segments of the lower lobe is composed of a tuft of four terminal arteries. All the arterial branches originate superiorly and run anterolaterally along the corresponding lower lobe segmental bronchi.

The lobar and segmental arterial and bronchial relationships are best exposed by opening the posterior aspects of the interlobar fissures.

The inferior pulmonary vein, best exposed from a posteroinferior approach after dividing the pulmonary ligament, is formed by tributaries from the superior segment and all the basal segments of the right lower lobe. The tributaries from the superior segment join the inferior vein as a single trunk after crossing the basal bronchus posteriorly. The basal veins emerge from the lobe between the corresponding segmental bronchi and join the inferior vein either separately or in two trunks.

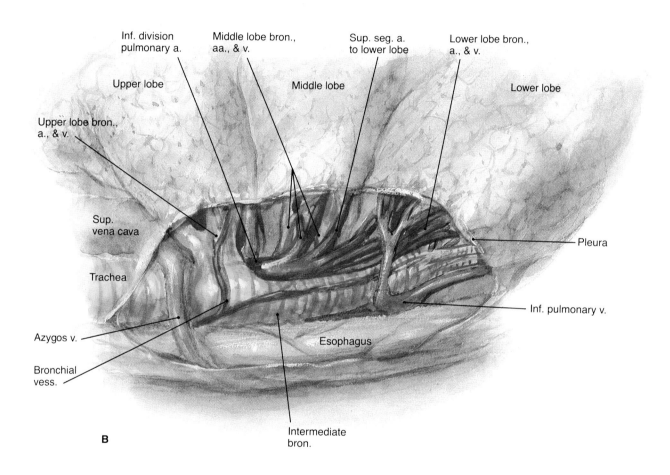

Inf. division
pulmonary a.

Middle lobe bron.,
aa., & v.

Sup. seg. a.
to lower lobe

Lower lobe bron.,
a., & v.

Upper lobe

Middle lobe

Lower lobe

Upper lobe bron.,
a., & v.

Sup.
vena cava

Pleura

Trachea

Inf. pulmonary v.

Azygos v.

Esophagus

Bronchial
vess.

Intermediate
bron.

B

Anatomical Variations in Vascular, Bronchial, and Parenchymal Architecture of the Right Lung

The lobar and segmental bronchi correspond to the classical description by Jackson and Huber in practically all patients, with the minor, clinically unimportant exception that there may be a second independent bronchus to the superior segment of the lower lobe interposed between the superior and basal segments and best recognized at bronchoscopy. Very rarely an accessory right upper lobe bronchus may be found originating from the trachea. In addition to the three segmental arteries to the upper lobe—the ascending posterior branch subject to great variation in size—there may be a recurrent artery originating from the apical-anterior stem or from the apical branch above the right upper lobe bronchus, supplying a portion of the posterior segment. Similarly, the anterior segment may receive an anterior ascending artery from the interlobar portion of the inferior pulmonary artery trunk. Very rarely, the posterior segment may receive recurrent branches from the anterior segmental artery, or the middle lobe arteries, or even from the superior segmental artery of the right lower lobe.

If the middle lobe arteries originate from a common trunk, there often is then a small accessory artery to the medial segment. Very exceptionally, small branches from the middle lobe or its medial segmental artery may ascend into the anterior interlobar surface of the right upper lobe.

Uncommonly, two separate superior segmental arteries of the right lower lobe may be found. The veins from the various bronchopulmonary segments show the greatest variation in pattern from the anatomy of the arteries and bronchi, which are closely related, and venous anomalies are much more frequent than arterial anomalies. Veins run peripherally below the visceral pleura and in intersegmental planes, in contrast to bronchi and arteries, which are centrally located. Communicating veins cross incomplete or fused fissures.

REFERENCES

1. le Roux, B.T.: Anatomical abnormalities of the right upper bronchus. J. Thorac. Cardiovasc. Surg. 44:225–227, 1962
2. Milloy, F.J., Wragg, L.E., and Anson, B.J.: The pulmonary arterial supply to the right upper lobe of the lung based upon a study of 300 laboratory and surgical specimens. Surg. Gynecol. Obstet. 116:34–41, 1963
3. Wragg, L.E., Milloy, F.J., and Anson, B.J.: Surgical aspects of the pulmonary arterial supply to the middle and lower lobes of the lungs. Surg. Gynecol. Obstet. 127:531–537, 1968

RIGHT PNEUMONECTOMY

A. The right chest has been opened through a posterolateral incision. Depressing the lung posteriorly exposes, from in front, the major structures of the right hemithorax. The pulmonary ligament is divided to gain additional mobility, and a vessel in it generally merits ligation or coagulation.

B. *Top*: The mediastinal pleura is incised and the fatty and areolar tissue overlying the right main pulmonary artery is cleared, exposing the arterial wall. The safest plane for dissection is immediately upon the arterial adventitia, best done with the scissors, freeing the artery circumferentially. *Bottom*: A peanut dissector is shown holding back the superior vena cava to expose the anterior surface of the right pulmonary artery. Alternatively, the azygos vein may be divided and ligated and the central end drawn medially by a clamp to achieve the same exposure. Right-angle clamps to pass the ligature are used only once the vessel has been cleared circumferentially. In general, scissors are safer than blunt dissectors unless the adherence of periarterial tissues is quite loose.

C. The main pulmonary artery has been tied on the specimen side and occluded proximally with a double row of fine vascular staples placed with one application of the stapling instrument. The artery is then divided with the scalpel on the edge of the stapler.

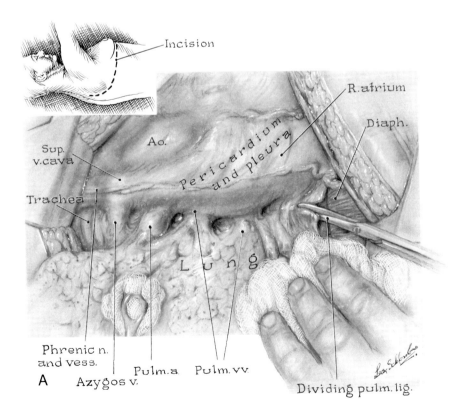

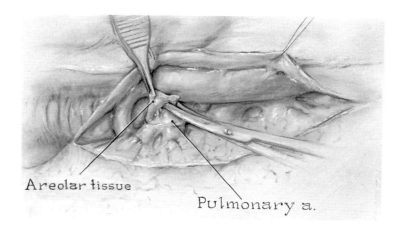

Areolar tissue

Pulmonary a.

Mediastinal pleura incised

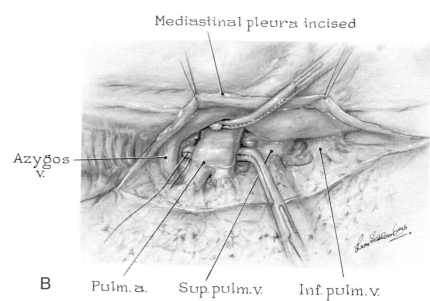

Azygos v.

B

Pulm. a.   Sup. pulm. v.   Inf. pulm. v.

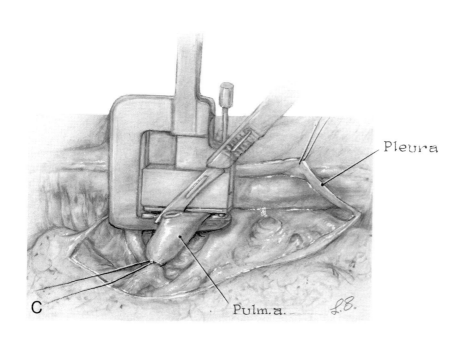

Pleura

C

Pulm. a.

RIGHT PNEUMONECTOMY *(Continued)*

D. The superior pulmonary vein has been similarly liberated by scissors and peanut dissection and will be transected between the peripheral ligature shown and the double row of centrally placed vascular staples, with the stapler introduced as shown by the arrow.

E. In pneumonectomy, the inferior pulmonary vein can be easily reached from the anterior aspect. It is shown having just been closed with staples and divided. The right main bronchus is now dissected up to the carina and occluded distally with a bronchial clamp. The stapling instrument is placed flush with the origin of the right main bronchus from the trachea, without encroaching on the tracheal lumen and without leaving any bronchial stump.

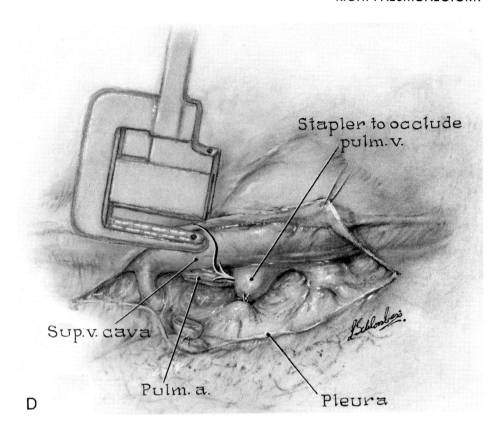

Stapler to occlude
pulm. v.

Sup. v. cava

Pulm. a.

Pleura

D

E

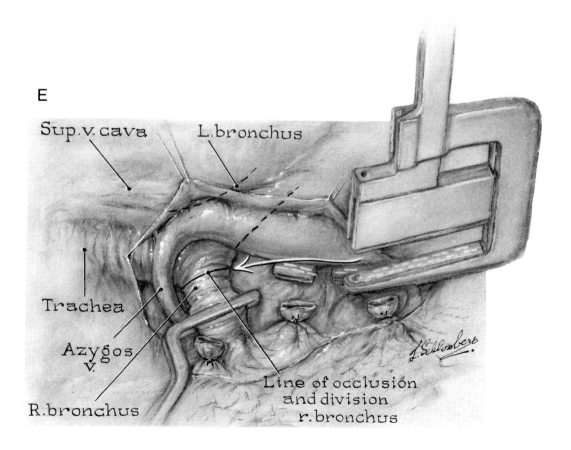

Sup. v. cava   L. bronchus

Trachea

Azygos
v.

R. bronchus

Line of occlusion
and division
r. bronchus

F. Following the stapling, the right main bronchus is transected, again using the stapler as a guide for the scalpel, and the specimen is removed.

G. In pneumonectomy, as opposed to lobectomy, the bronchus is usually closed over with pleura. The lowermost portion of the sutured mediastinal pleura is left open for drainage.

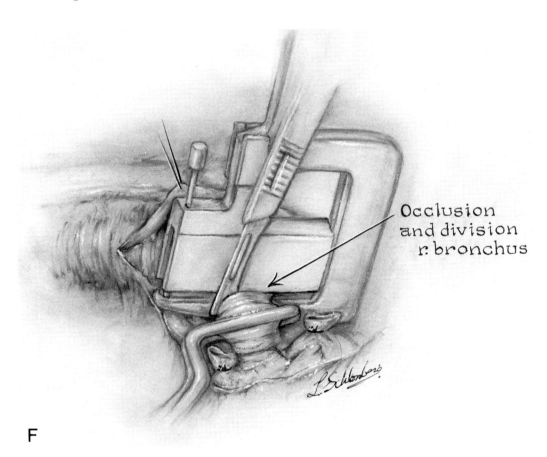

Occlusion and division r. bronchus

F

G

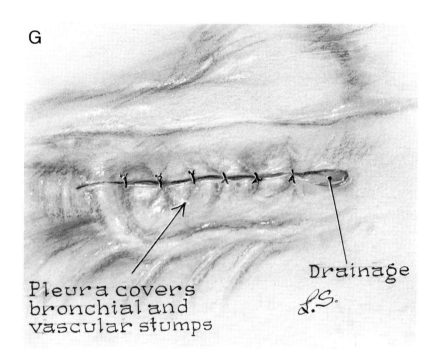

Pleura covers
bronchial and
vascular stumps

Drainage

L.S.

RIGHT UPPER LOBECTOMY

The anatomical structures entering the hilum of the lobe and requiring to be secured and transected are (1) the superior arterial trunk with its apical and anterior segmental branches; (2) the posterior segmental artery, originating from the inferior pulmonary trunk; (3) the tributaries to the superior pulmonary vein, from the apical-anterior, inferior, and posterior branches, sparing the veins from the middle lobe; and (4) the right upper lobe bronchus.

In addition, interlobar adhesions or incomplete fissures must be divided.

The mediastinum has been opened anteriorly, and the upper lobe and remaining lung have been retracted down and back. The azygos vein is seen at the upper limit of the dissection. The main pulmonary artery is identified behind the vena cava, and dissection is carried peripherally to expose the superior and inferior pulmonary arterial trunks. The superior pulmonary arterial trunk, with its branches to the anterior and apical segments, is exposed and severed between transfixion ligatures. The transection may be, as shown, between two ligatures placed on the long common stem or, if the common stem is short, between a proximal ligature on the stem and individual distal ligatures on the two branches. The superior lobe vein has been identified medially and cleared laterally, exposing its three tributaries. Care must be taken of the posterior branch lying deep to the apical-posterior and inferior veins. The middle lobe veins entering the superior pulmonary vein must be identified and spared. The vein may be secured as shown with a double application of the stapler or, commonly, between the stapler centrally and a suture ligature peripherally. At times it is simpler to ligate separately each of the tributaries peripherally. The artery to the posterior segment, arising from the inferior arterial trunk, is now readily exposed and is shown transected between two transfixion ligatures. The incomplete fissure may be completed at this point or after the division of the bronchus. To complete the fissure now (A), an opening is created through the hilum, front to back, in the angle formed between the upper and intermediate bronchi. The appropriate size TA stapler can be positioned as shown, with the retaining pin passing through this opening, or the instrument can be applied in the opposite direction, with the lower jaw passed down through the opening from the medial aspect to the posterior surface of the hilum. The upper lobe is cut away on the upper border of the stapler and the stapler removed. The GIA stapler may be used for the same purpose.

At times it is anatomically and technically difficult from the anterior approach to expose the artery to the posterior segment. It is then best to enter the oblique fissure between the upper and lower lobes posteriorly, identify the artery from this approach, and transect it between ligatures. Dissection of the posterior segmental artery is often the most difficult step in an upper lobectomy. The tunnel for placing the TA 90 stapler should not be developed until the artery has been secured.

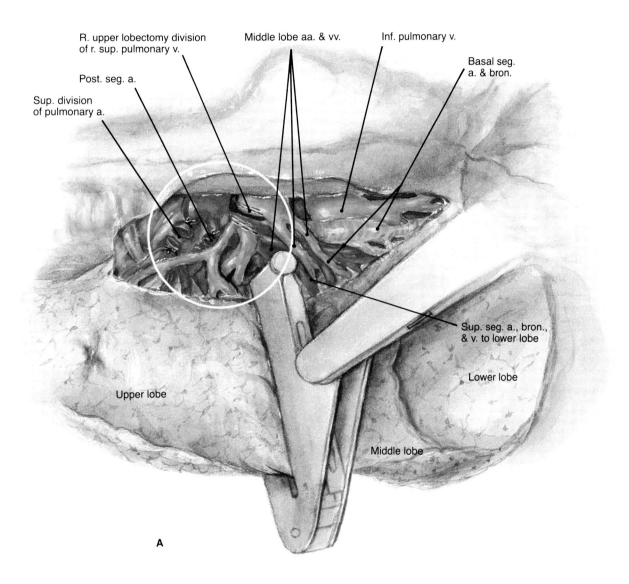

R. upper lobectomy division
of r. sup. pulmonary v.

Middle lobe aa. & vv.

Inf. pulmonary v.

Basal seg.
a. & bron.

Post. seg. a.

Sup. division
of pulmonary a.

Sup. seg. a., bron.,
& v. to lower lobe

Lower lobe

Upper lobe

Middle lobe

A

RIGHT UPPER LOBECTOMY *(Continued)*

At this point (*B*), with the lung lobe lifted forward and exposed from the posterior aspect, it is seen that the bronchus is all that remains to be divided. The bronchial artery may be ligated separately or the bronchus may be stapled and divided first to see whether or not the staples in the bronchus have secured the bronchial artery. The stapler is applied flush with the main bronchus so there will be no bronchial stump. The division of the incomplete fissure may be delayed until this point, when the specimen is essentially simply held up and the stapler applied along the line between air-containing and collapsed lung.

Occasionally, the approach to the posterior segmental artery from behind and above is made difficult by scar or obliterated interlobar fissures. In such cases, the artery to the posterior segment is not secured until after the bronchus has been transected. The interlobar portion of the inferior trunk of the pulmonary artery lies anterior and inferior to the bronchial stump deep in the fissure, covered by visceral pleura. Any branch passing from this artery into the upper lobe must be the posterior segmental artery. On rare occasions, an additional upper and smaller anterior branch can also be discovered. The incomplete fissure can now be safely stapled, applying the TA 90 or the GIA stapler at the line of demarcation between collapsed and inflated lung.

REFERENCE

1. Milloy, F.J., Wragg, L.E., and Anson, B.J.: The pulmonary arterial supply to the right upper lobe of the lung based upon a study of 300 laboratory and surgical specimens. Surg. Gynecol. Obstet. 116:34–41, 1963

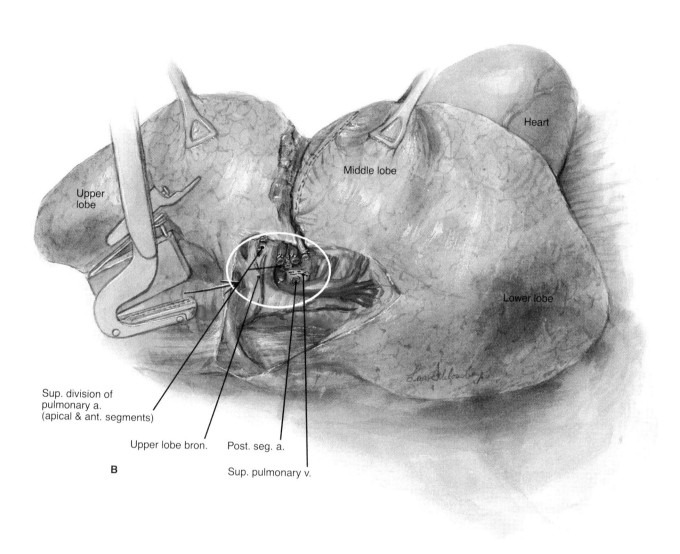

Upper
lobe

Middle lobe

Heart

Lower lobe

Sup. division of
pulmonary a.
(apical & ant. segments)

Upper lobe bron.

Post. seg. a.

Sup. pulmonary v.

B

RIGHT LOWER LOBECTOMY

The anatomical structures involved in the dissection for a right lower lobectomy are (1) the arterial branches of the superior and basal segments of the right lower lobe, all originating from the inferior pulmonary trunk; (2) the inferior pulmonary vein and its tributaries; (3) the superior and basal segmental bronchi; (4) the inferior pulmonary ligament; and (5) a possible incomplete oblique fissure.

The pulmonary artery and its branches to the right lower lobe are accessible deep in the posterior aspect of the oblique fissure and are exposed by incising the visceral pleura in the floor of the fissure. This approach is simplified by opening the triangular extension of the fissure floor into the horizontal fissure. The oblique fissure is incised anteriorly, and the entire artery, its branches, and the bronchus to the right lower lobe are identified and dissected out. The superior segmental artery, above and anterior to its bronchus, can be found arising from the posterolateral aspect of the inferior pulmonary arterial trunk opposite the middle lobe arterial trunk or the lowermost middle lobe artery. Both arteries should be clearly identified and dissected out to avoid injury to the middle lobe artery. Very rarely, the posterior ascending segmental artery to the upper lobe may originate from the superior artery of the lower lobe, in which case, ligation of the superior artery must be appropriately distal. Dissection of the peripheral course of the superior segmental artery into the right lower lobe will uncover the short common trunk of the remaining inferior pulmonary arterial trunk giving off a tuft of basal segmental arteries. It is often possible by an oblique application of the vascular stapler, preserving the middle lobe artery anteriorly, to close off the arterial trunk leading to both the superior and basal segmental arteries. At other times, the anatomical arrangement requires separate treatment of the superior segmental artery.

The bronchial anatomy of the right lower lobe corresponds to the arterial distribution. Most often it is safer to transect and suture separately the takeoff of the bronchus to the superior segment, as pictured.

The illustration indicates a stapled closure of the artery below the origin of the middle lobe arteries. The posterior segmental artery to the upper lobe is hidden in this view and is somewhat proximal to the right middle lobe artery. The peripheral ends of the superior segmental artery and the common trunk to the basal segments have been separately ligated. The bronchus to the superior segment of the lower lobe has been separately divided and sutured at its origin from the intermediate bronchus, opposite the origin of the middle lobe bronchus, and the distal end has been ligated. The stapler is shown being applied to the bronchial stem leading to the basal segments, without infringing on the takeoff of the middle lobe bronchus anteriorly. At other times, the distal intermediate bronchus is of sufficient length to permit an oblique application of the stapler, so as to include the superior and basal segmental bronchi in this staple closure, while sparing the orifice of the middle lobe bronchus. At this point, the vein is equally accessible from in front or behind and requires only to be stapled and divided.

If the lower lobe vein is treated first, the lobe is retracted anteriorly and superiorly and the inferior pulmonary ligament divided. The artery contained in it must be separately ligated or coagulated. The inferior pulmonary vein is then exposed from below and behind and can be closed (inset) with vascular staples and transected after ligation of the peripheral tributaries. In such an approach, the bronchus is treated last, in the same fashion as described previously.

If the oblique fissure is incomplete anteriorly, separation from the middle lobe is readily achieved by the application of a row of staples, placed either before or after the inferior pulmonary vein has been secured.

REFERENCE

1. Wragg, L.E., Milloy, F.J., and Anson, B.J.: Surgical aspects of the pulmonary arterial supply to the middle and lower lobes of the lungs. Surg. Gynecol. Obstet. 127:531–537, 1968

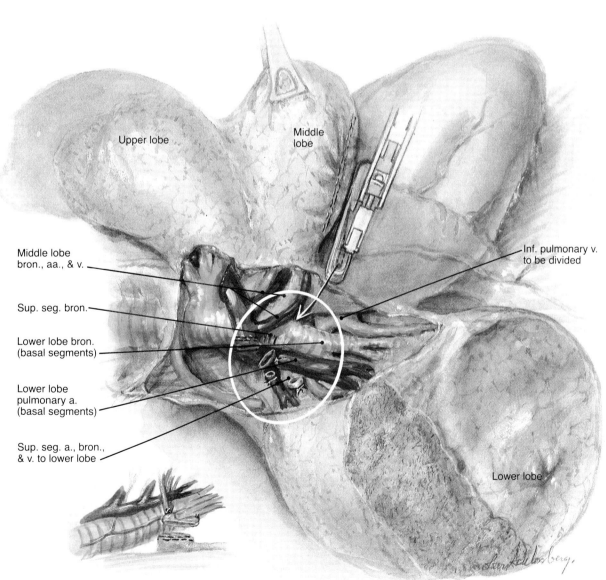

Upper lobe

Middle lobe

Middle lobe bron., aa., & v.

Sup. seg. bron.

Lower lobe bron. (basal segments)

Lower lobe pulmonary a. (basal segments)

Sup. seg. a., bron., & v. to lower lobe

Inf. pulmonary v. to be divided

Lower lobe

RIGHT MIDDLE LOBECTOMY

The anatomical components involved in right middle lobectomy are (1) a common arterial stem, or more often two arteries, arising from the inferior pulmonary trunk in its interlobar course; (2) the lobar bronchus, represented by a short common trunk and segmental divisions to the medial and lateral segments; and (3) the middle lobe vein, formed by corresponding segmental branches, joining the vein of the upper lobe to form the superior pulmonary vein.

The horizontal and oblique fissures vary in degrees of incompleteness.

Resection of the right middle lobe requires careful dissection of the inferior pulmonary trunk in its interlobar passage. Edward Churchill, in the early days of individual ligation and dissection lobectomies, once said that this dissection was so difficult that an isolated lobectomy of the middle lobe probably should not be attempted. The potential for injury to the ascending posterior segmental artery of the upper lobe, as well as to the artery of the superior segment of the lower lobe, make this operation somewhat more demanding than upper and lower lobectomies. The operation is best performed through a posterolateral thoracotomy to provide access to both the anterior and posterior aspects of the root of the lung. Dissection is begun in the oblique fissure between the middle and lower lobes by retracting the middle and upper lobe upward and the lower lobe downward. The interlobar portion of the pulmonary artery is identified in the depths of the oblique fissure. The arterial supply to the middle lobe is single, or, more commonly, two separate arteries are found originating from the anterior surface of the inferior arterial trunk, in a crowded little area directly opposite the artery to the superior segment of the lower lobe, which takes origin at the same level from the posterior surface and no more than a centimeter distal to the somewhat more lateral origin of the ascending posterior segmental artery of the upper lobe. The middle lobe artery or arteries are divided between ligatures or transfixion sutures.

The bronchus, best exposed from behind by drawing the lobe forward, is stapled and amputated as flush with the intermediate bronchus as possible.

The oblique fissure, between the middle and lower lobes, is usually well developed, whereas the horizontal fissure, between the upper and middle lobes, is often totally obliterated by adhesions or parenchymal tissue bridges between the two lobes.

A. The lobar arterial branches and bronchus have been divided. The middle lobe vein is carefully identified anteriorly, and a finger is put through the hilum so as to permit stapled completion of the fissure. This has already been done for the oblique fissure and is shown being performed for the horizontal fissure, with the retaining pin passing through the tunnel created by blunt dissection. The TA 55 stapler can as well be applied in the opposite direction, with its heel to the intermediate bronchus and the open end of the jaws at the free edge of the lung. By the same token, the anastomosing stapler, the GIA instrument, can be used to place two rows of staples on both sides of the division created by operation of its knife.

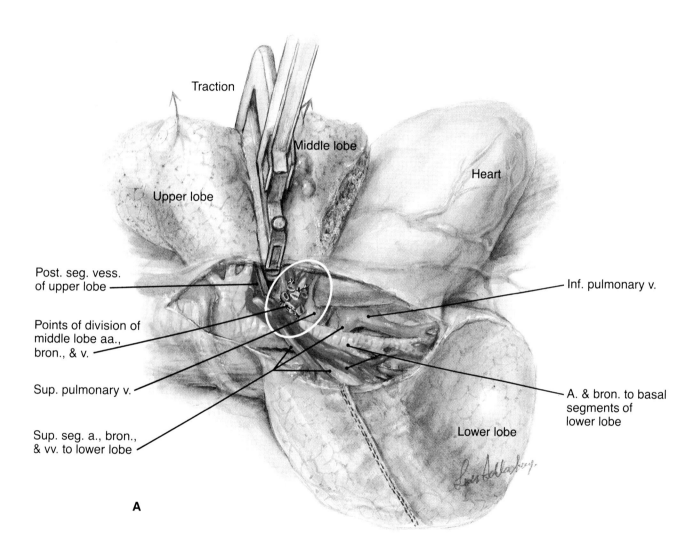

Traction

Middle lobe

Upper lobe

Heart

Post. seg. vess.
of upper lobe

Inf. pulmonary v.

Points of division of
middle lobe aa.,
bron., & v.

Sup. pulmonary v.

A. & bron. to basal
segments of
lower lobe

Lower lobe

Sup. seg. a., bron.,
& vv. to lower lobe

A

RIGHT MIDDLE LOBECTOMY *(Continued)*

B. The middle lobe vein has been stapled and divided, and only the division of a few tags of parenchymal tissue and parietal pleura around the hilum remain to be performed.

REFERENCES

1. Churchill, E.D., and Belsey, R.: Segmental pneumonectomy in bronchiectasis. The lingula segment of the left upper lobe. Ann. Surg. 109:481–499, 1939
2. Wragg, L.E., Milloy, F.J., and Anson, B.J.: Surgical aspects of the pulmonary arterial supply to the middle and lower lobes of the lungs. Surg. Gynecol. Obstet. 127:531–537, 1968

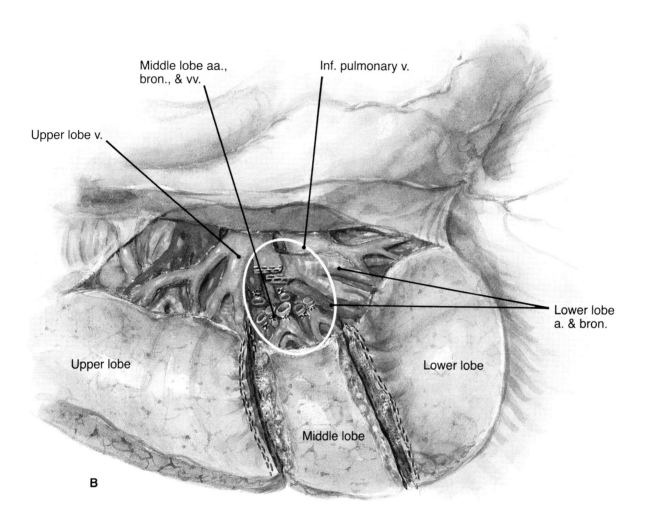

Upper lobe v.

Middle lobe aa.,
bron., & vv.

Inf. pulmonary v.

Lower lobe
a. & bron.

Upper lobe

Lower lobe

Middle lobe

B

233

HILUM OF THE LEFT LUNG

Anterior Aspect

There is a certain similarity between the anatomy of both lung roots, inasmuch as the left main bronchus is again the most posterior structure, entirely hidden by the more anterior and minimally superior left main pulmonary artery. The superior and inferior pulmonary veins are the most anterior structures and enter the left atrium caudad to the course of the left main artery. The root of the left lung emerging from under the arch of the aorta lies in front of the descending aorta. As on the right side, from the anterior aspect, the artery winds around the upper lobe bronchus into an anterior and lateral position. But in contrast to the right side, this change in course occurs superior to the left upper lobe bronchus and not inferior to it. The arterial supply to the left upper lobe is comparable to that on the right side, if one takes the left upper lobe and lingula to be the equivalents of the right upper and middle lobes. However, the arteries to the left upper lobe proper vary more in their origins, number, and relationships than do those of the right upper lobe.

The left pulmonary artery crosses over the superior aspect of the left upper lobe bronchus so that the arterial branches to the upper lobe are best exposed from above and laterally, and the arteries to the lingula and the lower lobe are best exposed from below. As shown, the veins are the first major vascular structures to be encountered in dissecting from the front.

The veins from the left upper lobe are superficial, spread out on one plane, and have no deep posterior tributary at the hilum, in contrast to the situation on the right side. Usually three or four trunks form the superior pulmonary vein: one clearly originates inferiorly from the confluence of two lingular veins and the most superior one is formed by the veins from the apical-posterior segment. The anterior segment is drained by two veins that join the apical-posterior vein. All these veins collect blood from the anterior and mediastinal surfaces of their segments (again in contrast to the right side, where there is a separate posterior deep collecting vein). The central and posterior portions of the segments are drained by veins running in intersegmental planes to the anterior trunks.

The left inferior pulmonary vein is almost in the same plane as the superior vein. It is formed by the tributaries from the superior segment (emerging from behind the lower lobe bronchus) and the basal segments. A small inferior lingular vein may occasionally empty into the inferior pulmonary vein.

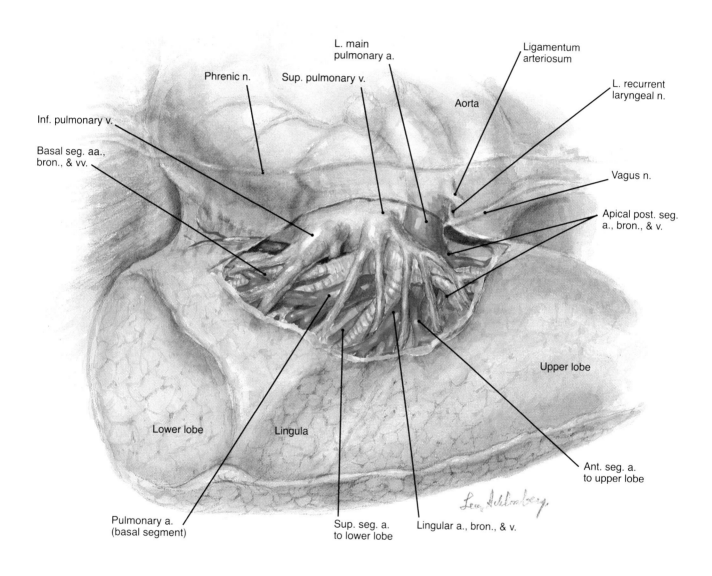

L. main
pulmonary a.

Ligamentum
arteriosum

Phrenic n.

Sup. pulmonary v.

Aorta

L. recurrent
laryngeal n.

Inf. pulmonary v.

Basal seg. aa.,
bron., & vv.

Vagus n.

Apical post. seg.
a., bron., & v.

Upper lobe

Ant. seg. a.
to upper lobe

Lower lobe

Lingula

Pulmonary a.
(basal segment)

Sup. seg. a.
to lower lobe

Lingular a., bron., & v.

HILUM OF THE LEFT LUNG *(Continued)*

Posterior Aspect

The most lateral structure is the convexity of the pulmonary artery as it winds around the upper lobe bronchus and courses downward into the interlobar fissure. The bronchial structures, the most posterior in the mediastinum (as on the right), are sandwiched between veins and the arterial branches. The four to seven arterial branches to the upper lobe may originate individually or have common trunks. Most constant is the apical-posterior trunk, with two branches arising from the anterior surface of the artery. The rendition here shows two separate arteries. This very short apical posterior trunk hides the anterior segmental artery that originates inferiorly to it from the anterior surface of the pulmonary artery, either before or at the level of the crossing of the left upper lobe bronchus by the pulmonary artery. For the surgeon, this is an inconvenient and potentially dangerous anatomical relationship. Usually there is a smaller, individual artery to the posterior subsegment that originates from the lateral aspect of the downward-coursing artery. The two lingular arteries to the superior and inferior segments may be individual, may come from a common lingular arterial trunk, or at times may join with the anterior segmental artery into an anterolingular trunk that arises from the interlobar portion of the pulmonary artery. The lingular arteries or their common trunk (without the anterior artery when it has a separate origin) arise after the pulmonary artery has passed into the posterior interlobar fissure, slightly below and posterior to the lingular bronchus. The arterial branches to the left lower lobe arise from the interlobar portion of the pulmonary artery. The highest branch, to the superior segment of the lower lobe, arises opposite the common lingular trunk or lowest lingular artery, from the posterolateral aspect of the interlobar artery. The pulmonary artery then branches into a tuft of four basal arteries that lie anterolateral to the corresponding segmental bronchi.

As on the right side, the inferior pulmonary vein is best exposed from below and laterally, after division of the inferior pulmonary ligament. Most of the tributaries contributing to the vein emerge from the lobe posterior to their respective segmental bronchi, except in the case of the anteromedial segment. Again, the venous patterns are less constant than the bronchial and arterial segmental relationships. Usually the inferior vein is formed from three trunks: one from the superior segment and two from the basal segments.

Anatomical Variations in Vascular, Bronchial, and Parenchymal Architecture of the Left Lung

On rare occasions, the segmental bronchi of left upper and lower lobes take origin from the left main bronchus like spokes from the hub of a wheel.

The frequent variation in origin, arrangement, and number of the left upper lobe arteries has been described. As can be the case on the right side, the superior segment of the left lower lobe may be supplied by two individual arteries.

The most frequently encountered arrangement for the superior vein has been described. Occasionally, the inferior lingular vein drains into the inferior pulmonary vein.

REFERENCES

1. Milloy, F.J., Wragg, L.E., and Anson B.J.: The pulmonary arterial supply to the upper lobe of the left lung. Surg. Gynecol. Obstet. 126:811–824, 1968
2. Wragg, L.E., Milloy, F.J., and Anson, B.J.: Surgical aspects of the pulmonary arterial supply to the middle and lower lobes of the lungs. Surg. Gynecol. Obstet. 127:531–537, 1968

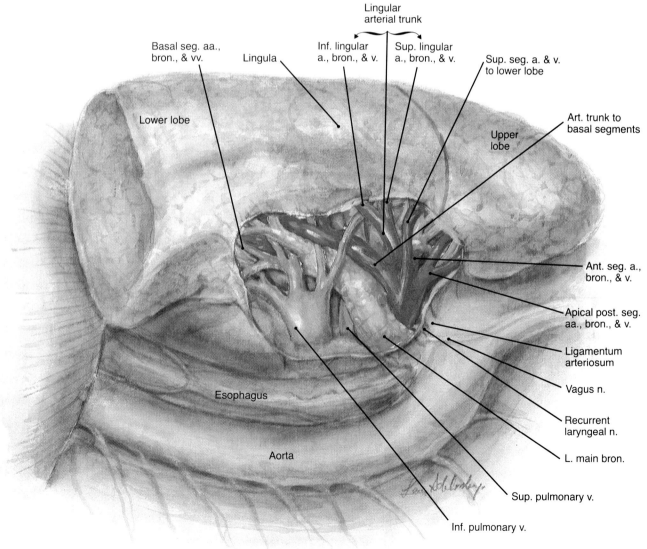

LEFT PNEUMONECTOMY

A. The left hemithorax has been entered through a posterolateral incision. Depressing the lung posteriorly exposes the hilum anteriorly. The pulmonary ligament is divided, and any vessels in it are secured.

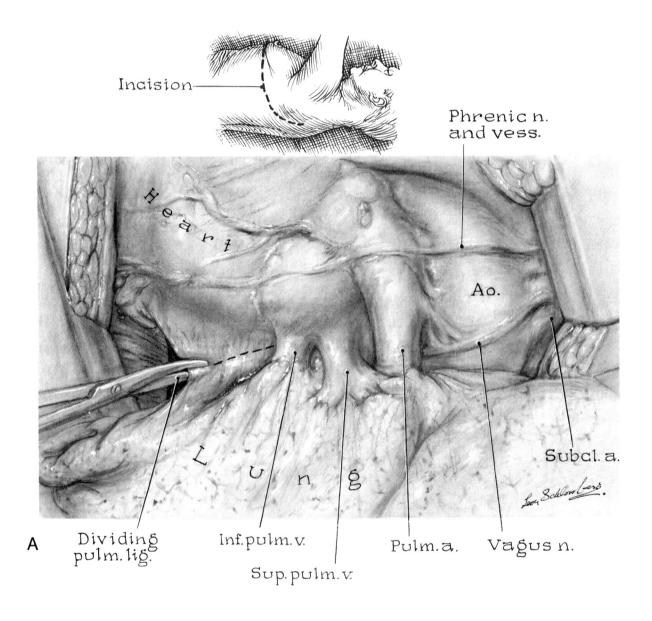

Incision

Phrenic n. and vess.

Heart

Ao.

Subcl. a.

L u n g

A Dividing pulm. lig.

Inf. pulm. v.

Sup. pulm. v.

Pulm. a.

Vagus n.

B. *Top*: The mediastinal pleura has been incised and the left main pulmonary artery cleared, respecting the left vagus and recurrent laryngeal nerves. The index finger, passed behind the artery, is used to guide the stapler into place. *Bottom*: The pulmonary artery has been divided between the double row of fine vascular staples and a peripheral ligature. The end result of the stapling procedure is shown here. Structures are always divided *with the instrument in place,* using it as a guide for scalpel or scissors, so as not to encroach accidentally on the staple closure. The fibrous ligamentum arteriosum is left intact proximal to the closure of the pulmonary artery.

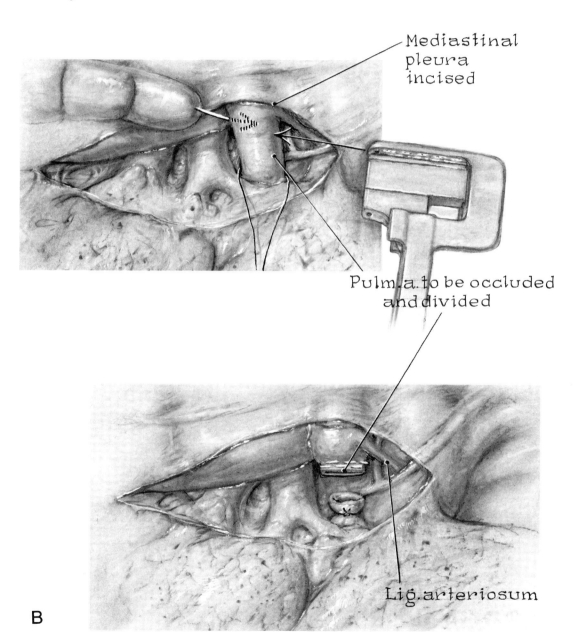

Mediastinal pleura incised

Pulm. a. to be occluded and divided

Lig. arteriosum

B

C. *Top:* With the superior and inferior pulmonary veins similarly dissected and divided between a central staple closure and a peripheral ligature, the left main bronchus is now dissected. *Bottom:* The left index finger pressing against the right side of the trachea displaces the lower trachea and carina to the left, to facilitate displacement of the left main bronchus from under the arch of the aorta and permit the exact placement of the stapler on the origin of the bronchus, flush with the trachea. The temptation to pull on the lung and bronchus to place the stapler must be resisted. The instrument is brought to the tissues and not vice versa, since structures stapled when on the stretch may leak. The stapling and transection of the bronchus are performed as illustrated for right pneumonectomy.

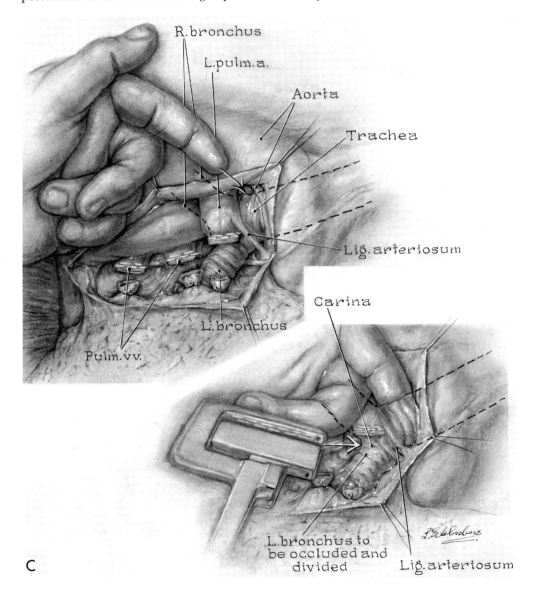

C

D. *Top:* The stapled closures are shown. The staple line occluding the left main bronchus has now retracted into the mediastinum, behind the pulmonary artery stump. Trachea and right main bronchus are outlined in the mediastinum. *Bottom:* In a pneumonectomy, the bronchial stump and, as much as possible, the vascular stumps are covered with a flap of pleura.

For suppurative disease, the bronchus is frequently attacked first, working from behind, with the lung lifted forward. The great advantage of the staplers is that, in pneumonectomy for inflammatory disease and a "frozen hilum," if a tunnel can be created under any hilar structure, it can be stapled, clamped, and divided much more safely and with less of the dangerous dissection than in the clamp and suture technique. Each subsequent structure is even more easily dealt with.

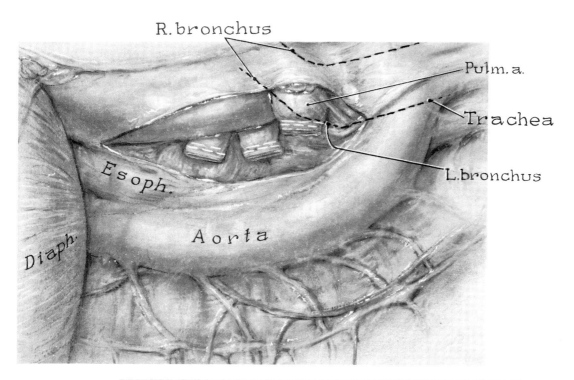

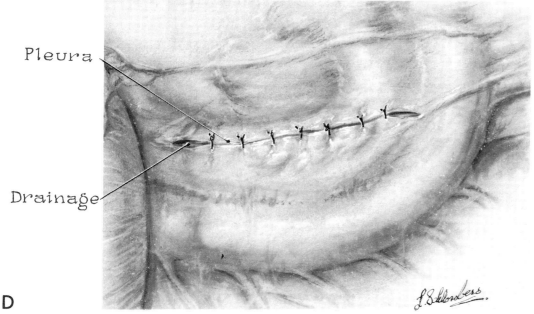

D

LEFT INTRAPERICARDIAL PNEUMONECTOMY

In the presence of hilar carcinoma of the lung precluding extrapericardial division of the pulmonary veins, pneumonectomy can often be safely accomplished as shown.

A. The left pulmonary artery has been stapled and divided and the pericardium opened.
B. A finger is slipped behind the atrium, and the tip of the lower jaw of the stapler (TA 55) is pressed against the finger tip and advanced as the finger is withdrawn.
C. The veins have been occluded within the pericardium, and the stapler is closed and activated on the atrium itself. The atrium is divided on the edge of the stapler, leaving a disc of atrium attached to the veins. The posterior pericardium is now incised (not shown) to complete the liberation of the veins, and there remains only the division and stapling of the bronchus—which may, alternatively, be done from behind before the vessels are divided—and such mediastinal node dissection as is elected.

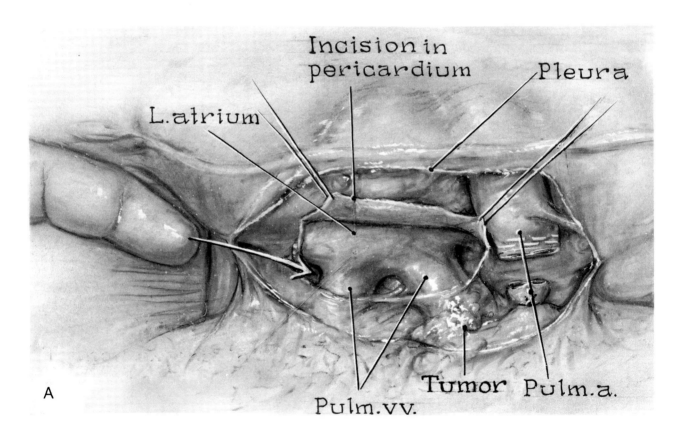

A

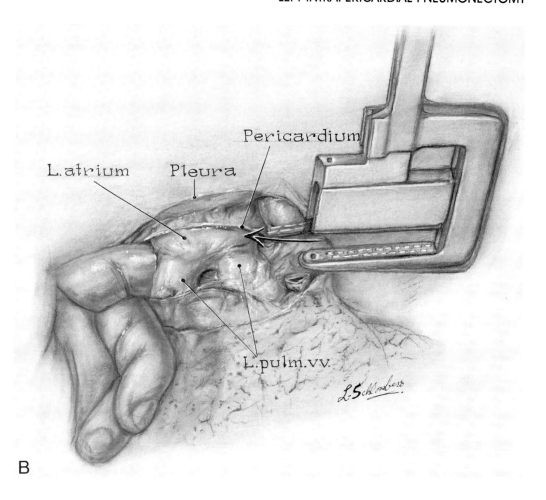

B

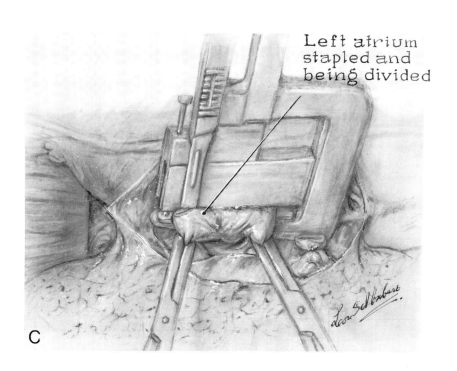

C

243

LEFT UPPER LOBECTOMY

The anatomical structures involved in resection of the left upper lobe are (1) the upper lobe arterial branches, which may be four to seven in number; (2) the superior pulmonary vein and its tributaries; (3) the upper (apical-posterior and anterior) and the lower (lingular) bronchial divisions; and (4) a possible incomplete fissure.

The upper lobe is retracted anteriorly and downward and the mediastinal pleura is incised to uncover the convexity of the left pulmonary artery in its course around the left main bronchus. The apical-posterior arteries, the uppermost branches of the left pulmonary artery, may arise from a common stem (*principal drawings*), which is usually very short, or they may originate separately, as shown in the inset at B. They take their origin from the convex anterosuperior surface of the main pulmonary artery. If there is a common apical-posterior stem, great care must be exercised in the dissection, since the artery to the anterior segment of the left upper lobe is often placed on the anterior surface of the concavity of the main artery, only a few millimeters distal and inferior to the apical-posterior trunk or to a single independent apical segmental branch. An attempt at tying or stapling the short common trunk of the apical-posterior arteries too close to its origin from the main artery may result in its avulsion, with the predictable consequences. As with the dissection of the right middle lobe arterial supply, this is an area requiring technical precision.

After securing the arteries to the apical-posterior and anterior segments, the interlobar space is entered posteriorly by retracting the upper lobe anteriorly. The artery is further liberated as it circles around the upper lobe bronchus posterolaterally and then takes a course anterolateral to the lower lobe bronchus. The remaining segmental branches to the upper lobe are encountered serially as they originate from the lateral and anterior surface of the main artery. Very often there is a second small independent artery to the posterior subsegment, followed by two arteries to the lingula. The lowest of these takes an anterior course arising opposite the posterolateral origin of the artery to the superior segment of the lower lobe. At times the superior lingular branch, or a common lingular arterial trunk, and the anterior segmental artery may have a short common stem and share the same origin. The lower artery to the lingula, as shown in the inset in B, arises from the pulmonary artery (anteriorly) distal to the origin (posteriorly) of the artery to the superior segment of the lower lobe. Each of these arterial branches is best secured with a manual ligature followed by transection, although we have at times been able to apply the vascular stapler to a large common apical-posterior stem and closely adjoining anterior segmental artery. If this is done, great care should be taken to avoid any levering by the stapler, to protect the convexity of the main pulmonary artery from injury.

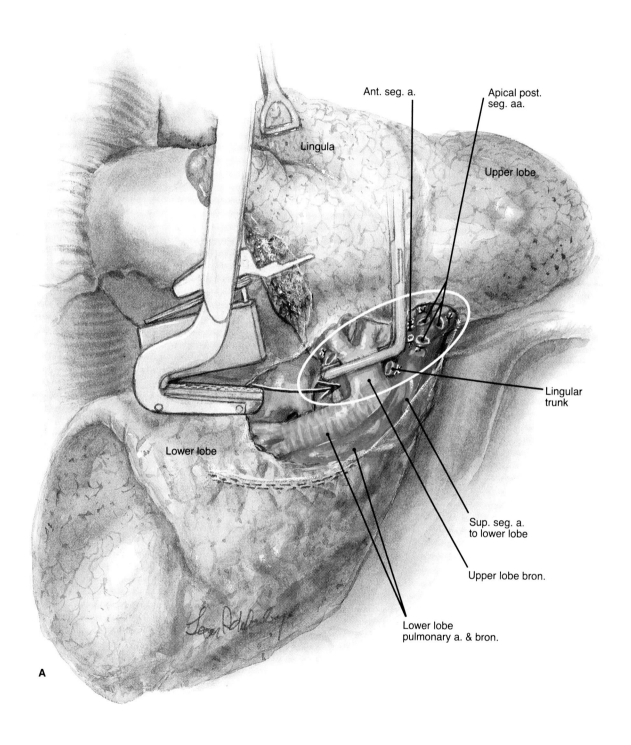

Lingula

Ant. seg. a.

Apical post. seg. aa.

Upper lobe

Lingular trunk

Lower lobe

Sup. seg. a. to lower lobe

Upper lobe bron.

Lower lobe pulmonary a. & bron.

A

LEFT UPPER LOBECTOMY *(Continued)*

After all arterial branches to the left upper lobe have been secured (A) the procedure is continued by dissecting and closing the bronchus next and securing the superior vein last, or by dissecting and securing the vein followed by the bronchus as the last structure to be treated. If the bronchus is dissected first, care should be taken to protect the vein anterior to it. After the bronchus has been freed, it can be closed either by a line of staples or by interrupted manual sutures. Both techniques are illustrated. In either case, the closure should be flush with the parent bronchus.

In order to expose the vein and its tributaries, the upper lobe is displaced posteriorly and the mediastinal pleura is incised over the vein. If the bronchus has been treated first, this maneuver is relatively easy. If the bronchus is still attached and the vein is to be secured after the arteries have been disposed of, the dissection of the vein from the bronchus requires some care. The superior vein is best secured with a vascular staple line (B). If the fissure is incomplete anteriorly, it can be transected superior to a staple line applied at the demarcation between upper and lower lobes, either at the end of the procedure or in mid course after all of the arterial branches have been secured.

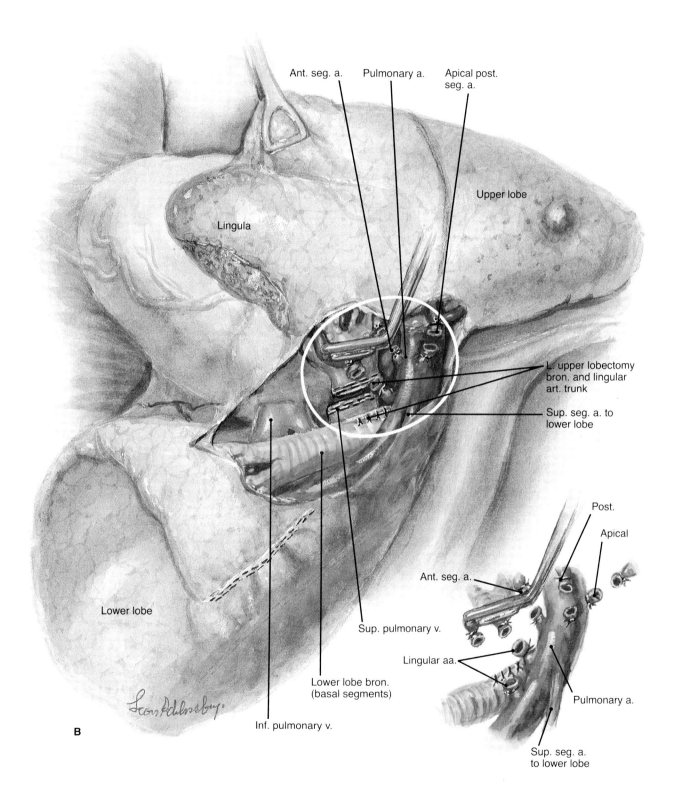

Ant. seg. a.

Pulmonary a.

Apical post.
seg. a.

Upper lobe

Lingula

L. upper lobectomy
bron. and lingular
art. trunk

Sup. seg. a. to
lower lobe

Sup. pulmonary v.

Lower lobe bron.
(basal segments)

Lower lobe

Inf. pulmonary v.

Post.

Apical

Ant. seg. a.

Lingular aa.

Pulmonary a.

Sup. seg. a.
to lower lobe

B

LEFT LOWER LOBECTOMY

The anatomical structures involved in left lower lobectomy are (1) the superior and basal segmental arteries—terminal branches of the main pulmonary artery; (2) the inferior pulmonary vein and its tributaries; (3) the superior and basal segmental bronchi; and (4) the pulmonary ligament.

The arterial branches to the lower lobe arise from the distal pulmonary artery deep in the fissure, so that the mid and posterior portions of the fissure must be opened to expose the arteries to the lower lobe. As shown in this illustration and in the illustration of left upper lobectomy (previous plate), the superior segmental artery to the lower lobe generally arises from the posterior surface of the pulmonary artery, somewhat proximal to the origin, from the anterior surface, of the artery to the lingula. It is usually necessary, therefore, to secure the superior segmental artery separately and then to approach the common trunk of the arteries to the basal segments. The origin of the artery to the superior segment is shown ligated and that of the basal arterial trunk, stapled. The vascular stapler is shown being brought to the already clamped pulmonary vein.

As on the right side, the basal segmental bronchial branches correspond to their arterial counterparts. In order to close the bronchial stem of the lower lobe as closely as possible to the lower border of the left upper lobe bronchus without interfering with its lumen, it is important to retract superiorly the left main arterial stump and the lowermost lingular artery. The bronchial stapler can then be applied obliquely, usually taking with it the origin of the bronchus to the superior segment. At times the bronchus to the superior segment has to be closed separately, and only the common stem to the basal segments can be closed with staples.

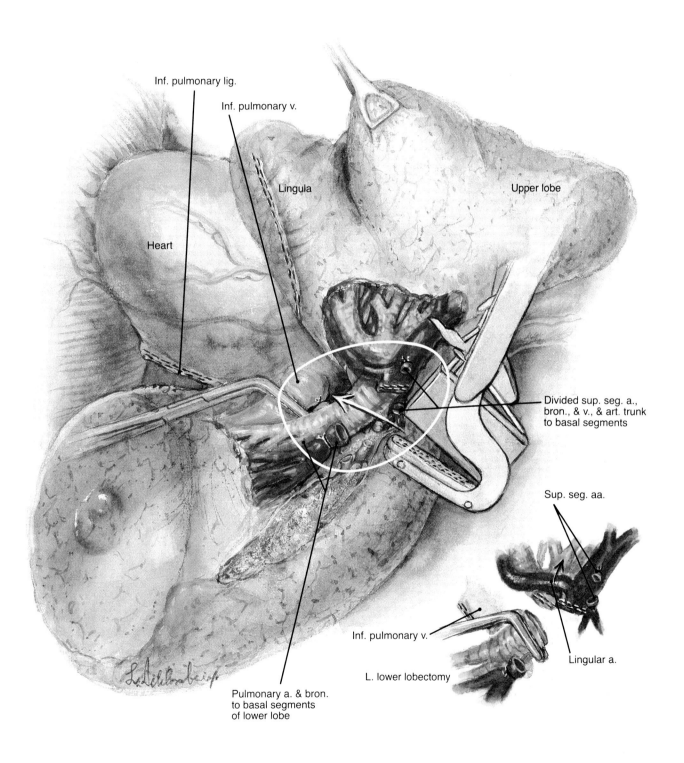

Inf. pulmonary lig.

Inf. pulmonary v.

Lingula

Upper lobe

Heart

Divided sup. seg. a.,
bron., & v., & art. trunk
to basal segments

Sup. seg. aa.

Inf. pulmonary v.

Lingular a.

L. lower lobectomy

Pulmonary a. & bron.
to basal segments
of lower lobe

Miscellaneous Pulmonary Resections

TRANSPERICARDIAL APPROACH TO THE RIGHT MAIN BRONCHUS

In cases of empyema and bronchial fistula after right pneumonectomy, the problem of operating through contaminated tissue via right thoracotomy can be solved by a transpericardial approach through virgin tissues.

A. This exposure is gained by median sternotomy and wide open pericardiotomy. The vena cava and aorta are separated by sharp dissection.

B. Incision of the posterior pericardium now exposes the retropericardial portion of the right pulmonary artery. The carina and right and left main bronchi are visible. Although at times it may be possible to depress the pulmonary artery and gain access to the right main bronchus above it, it has usually been found more effective to divide the pulmonary artery. The artery is elevated by blunt dissection behind it.

C. Stapling and division of the artery has been accomplished, in this case by two applications of the TA 30 stapling instrument with fine vascular staples. The stump of the right main bronchus is exposed, together with the origin of the fibrous fistulous tract.

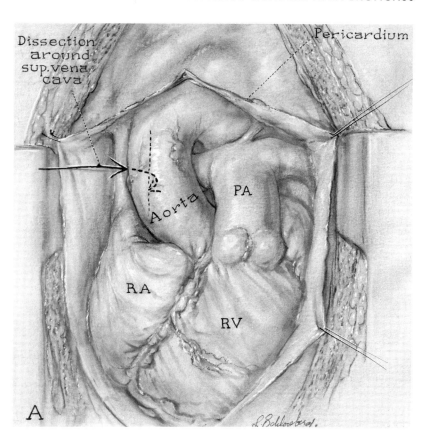

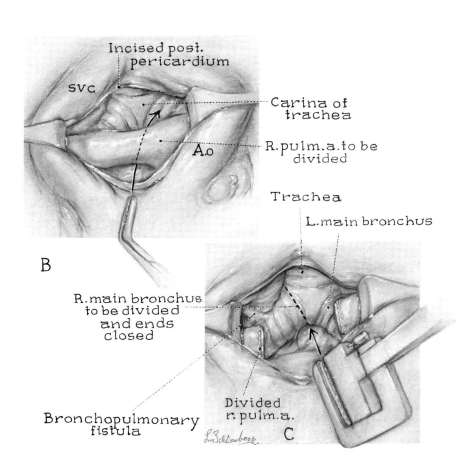

D. Blunt dissection, tunnelling under the bronchus, provides a channel for application of the TA 30 or TA 55 instrument, depending upon the circumstances, to staple the bronchus flush with the trachea. In the example shown, the distal end of the bronchus has been stapled as well and is being covered over with a flap of posterior pericardium. The preferred approach, if the bronchial stump is long, is to staple both ends; if short, to staple the tracheal end and suture the distal end. Some surgeons have chosen to suture the tracheal end and staple the distal end, and others have chosen the reverse approach. In any case, properly undertaken, the entire operation is performed through clean and uncontaminated tissues. For extra assurance, the sternohyoid muscle may be brought down and sutured over the proximal bronchial stump.

Although it is possible to treat a bronchial fistula after left pneumonectomy by a similar technique, access to the left main bronchus is not quite as readily gained as this illustration would suggest. Transpericardial amputation of the left main bronchus has been successfully performed, but there is increasing preference for right thoracotomy and approach to the left main bronchus in the mediastinum, from behind.

REFERENCES

1. Abruzzini, P.: Trattamento chirurgico delle fistole del bronco principale consecutive a pneumonectomia per tubercolosi. La Chir. Torac. 3:165–171, 1961
2. Petrovsky, B., Perelman, M., and Kuzmichev, A.: *Resection and Plastic Surgery of Bronchi.* Translated from the Russian by L. Aksenova, M.D. Moscow, Mir Publishers, 1968, pp. 202–221
3. Bogusch, L.K., Travin, A.A., and Semenenkow, J.L.: *Transperikardiale Operationen an den Hauptbronchien und Lungengefässen.* Translated from the Russian. Stuttgart, Hippokrates Verlag, 1971
   Magnificent illustrations and detailed instructions for transpericardial division of right and left bronchi. All from Moscow.
4. Virkkula, L., and Eerola, S.: Use of omental pedicle for treatment of bronchial fistula after lower lobectomy. Scand. J. Thor. Cardiovasc. Surg. 9:287–290, 1975
5. Baldwin, J.C., and Mark, J.B.D.: Treatment of bronchopleural fistula after pneumonectomy. J. Thorac. Cardiovasc. Surg. 90:813–817, 1985

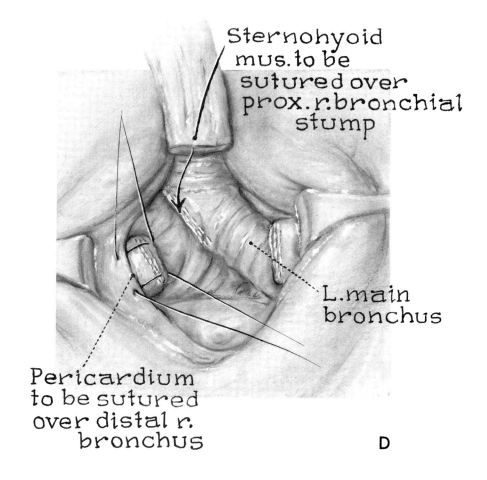

Sternohyoid
mus. to be
sutured over
prox. r. bronchial
stump

L. main
bronchus

Pericardium
to be sutured
over distal r.
bronchus

D

EN BLOC RIGHT UPPER LOBECTOMY AND CHEST WALL RESECTION—LOBECTOMY SECOND—PLEURAL TENT

A. The approach is through a right posterolateral incision and the periosteal bed of the unresected 5th rib. The tumor is shown located in the apex of the right upper lobe posteriorly, and it invades a posterior segment of the 3rd rib as well as the 2nd and 3rd intercostal spaces. Sliding the hand under the scapula before the chest has been opened permits assessment of possible extension of tumor beyond the immediate rib cage. Within the pleural cavity, the limits of the invasion of the chest wall and the state of hilar and mediastinal nodes are explored to determine operability and to define the required limits of resection. In this case, the hilar dissection of the right upper lobe will be easier once greater mobility has been provided by isolating and freeing the attached segment of chest wall.

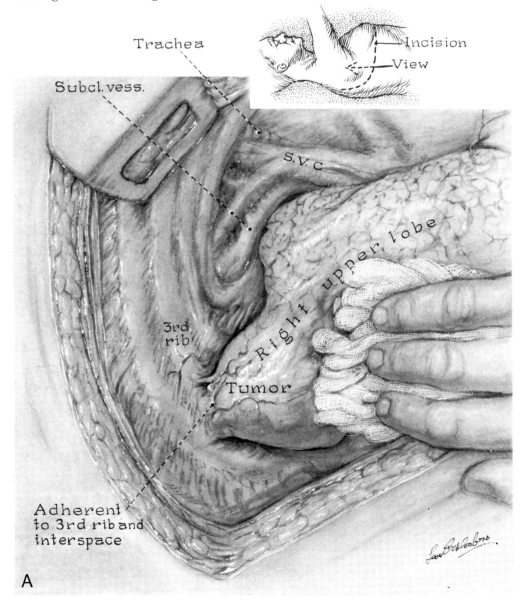

B. The margins of resection should include an uninvolved rib and interspace above and below. On either side of the tumor, there should be a safe 8- to 10-cm margin. Posteriorly, therefore, the transection of ribs must at times be flush with the vertebral bodies, through the costotransverse joints or by taking the transverse processes as well. At the selected sites of rib transection, the periosteum is incised and elevated from the ribs circumferentially. The transections start with the lowest, each preceded by ligation and transection of the intercostal vessels.

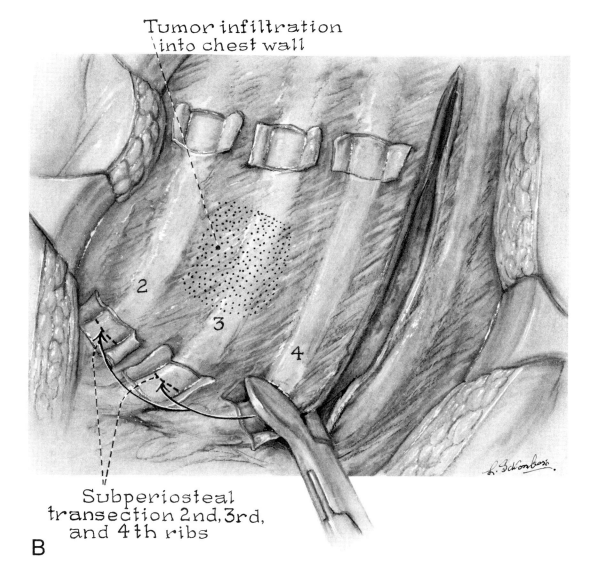

Tumor infiltration into chest wall

Subperiosteal transection 2nd, 3rd, and 4th ribs

B

C. The 2nd, 3rd, and 4th ribs, as well as the corresponding intercostal structures, have been divided. The periosteum of the 1st rib is incised, as well as the insertion of the posterior scalenus muscle on the 2nd rib. The periosteum of the 1st rib is depressed to allow incision through the rib bed. The 1st intercostal muscles are thereby taken with the specimen.

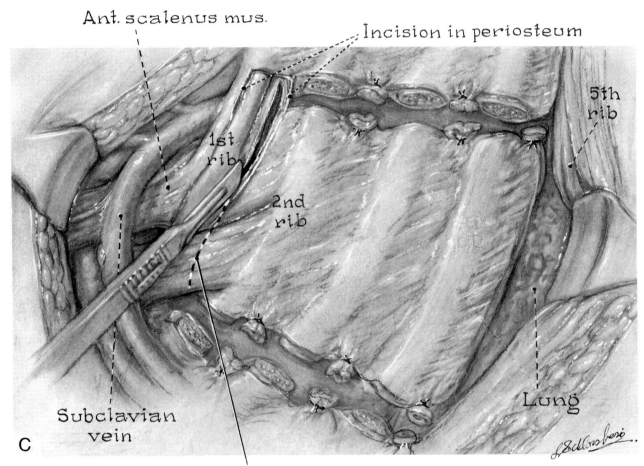

Ant. scalenus mus.

Incision in periosteum

5th rib

1st rib

2nd rib

Subclavian vein

C

Division of post. scalenus mus.

Lung

D. Dissection of the hilum anteriorly and superiorly identifies the vascular structures of the right upper lobe. The superior vena cava is displaced medially. The azygos vein is cephalad to the dissection. In this case, a large common trunk for the anterior and apical segmental arteries of the right upper lobe is divided between a staple line centrally and a manual ligature or transfixion suture peripherally. When the segmental arteries have separate origins, they are ligated or transfixed manually. If the middle lobe vein has not been identified earlier, it is exposed now to be sure of preserving its drainage, which in the usual case is into the central section of the upper lobe vein.

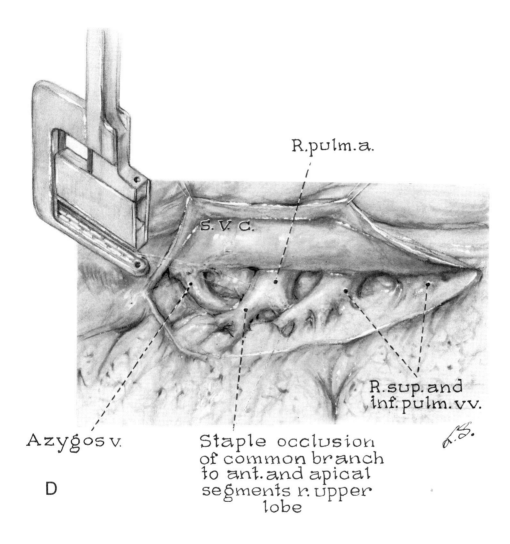

R.pulm.a.

S.V.C.

R.sup. and
inf. pulm. vv.

Azygos v.

Staple occlusion
of common branch
to ant. and apical
segments r. upper
lobe

D

E. *Top:* The vein from the right upper lobe is divided between a staple line centrally and a manual ligature on the pulmonary side, leaving intact the vein from the right middle lobe.

Not shown in these drawings is the ligature and division of the artery to the posterior segment of the right upper lobe. This artery is approached through the lesser fissure, at the level of the posterior tip of the middle lobe.

Bottom: The bronchus is approached anteriorly, or posteriorly by shifting forward the lobe and attached chest wall. It is closed with a double, staggered staple line and transected along the edge of the stapler, with the pulmonary end of the bronchus secured with a clamp.

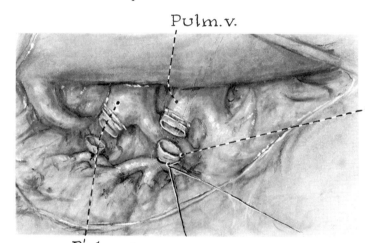

Pulm.v.

Ligation and division veins to the upper lobe

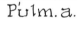

Pulm. a.

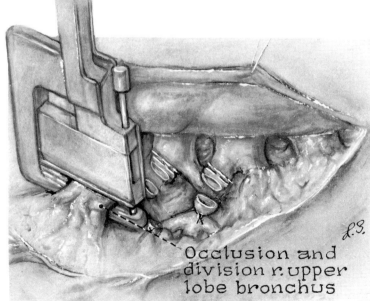

Occlusion and division r. upper lobe bronchus

E

F. A bridge of lung tissue, making for an incomplete lesser fissure, is about to be stapled on the middle lobe side and transected along the upper lobe side, using the upper edge of the stapler as a guide. Brief hyperinflation will bring the junction of uninflated and distended lung into sharp relief. The stapler is applied along the line so demonstrated.

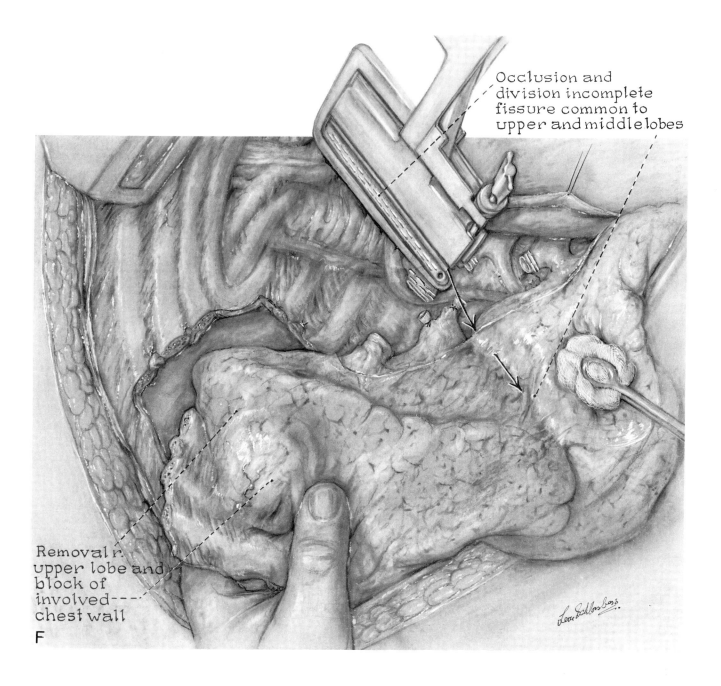

Occlusion and division incomplete fissure common to upper and middle lobes

Removal r upper lobe and block of involved chest wall

F

G. Reconstruction is then begun with development of a pleural tent, to keep the middle and lower lobes from overexpanding and herniating into the chest wall defect and to prevent an intrapleural space problem if they do not. Two flaps are raised, one from the superior mediastinum and one from the lateral-superior aspect of the chest.

H. The pleural flaps are rotated to cover middle and lower lobes and are sutured together and to the edge of the hilar-mediastinal pleura as well to the edge of the pleura remaining along the course of the 5th rib.

Not shown are the usual "piecrusting" of the pleural tent and the placement of two chest tubes, one below and one above the tent. The scapula will cover the modest posterior and superior chest wall defect (see later, *En Bloc Left Upper Lobectomy and Chest Wall Resection—Lobectomy First*), and prosthetic or other reconstruction is not required unless the resection has extended beyond the borders of the scapula. The muscles and fascia on the deep surface of the scapula are anchored with carefully and strategically placed sutures to the soft tissues beyond the edges of the chest defect. The incision is then closed as usual.

REFERENCES

1. Bell, J.W.: Management of the postresection space in tuberculosis. III. Role of pre- and postresection thoracoplasty. J. Thorac. Surg. 31:580–592, 1956
   Pleural tent
2. Miscall, L., Duffy, R.W., Nolan, R.B., and Klopstock, R.: The pleural tent as a simultaneous tailoring procedure in combination with pulmonary resection. Am. Rev. Tuberculosis and Pulmonary Diseases 73:831–852, 1956

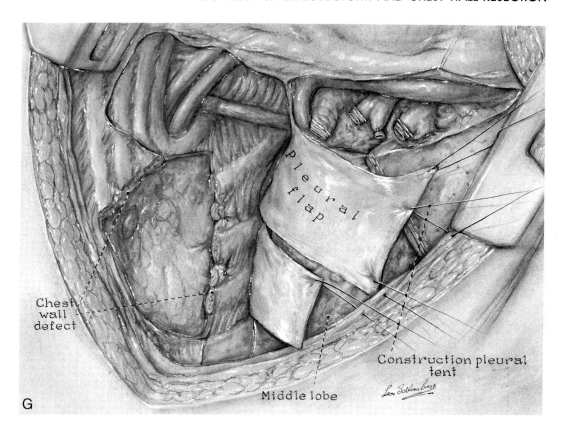

Chest wall defect

pleural flap

Construction pleural tent

Middle lobe

G

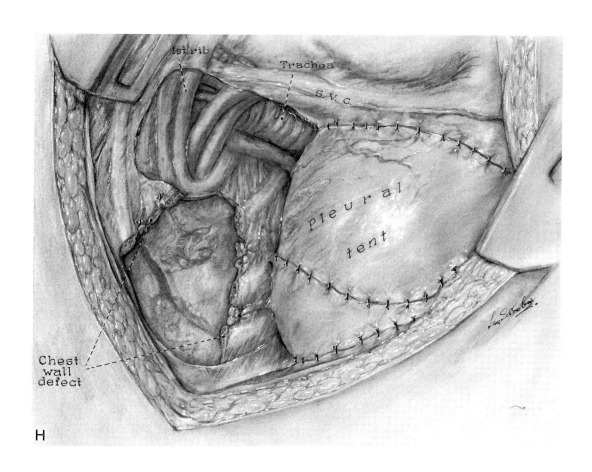

1st rib

Trachea

s.v.c.

pleural tent

Chest wall defect

H

EN BLOC LEFT UPPER LOBECTOMY AND CHEST WALL RESECTION—
LOBECTOMY FIRST

A. The chest is best entered through the standard posterolateral incision, but through the rib bed beyond the first normal rib below the lowest rib involved by tumor. Through the thoracotomy, the situation is assessed for extent and operability. The hilar structures are dissected, divided, and secured, in this case for left upper lobectomy (see pages 244–247, *Left Upper Lobectomy*), and any incomplete fissure is stapled and divided so that the lobe remains attached only to the chest wall.

The indicated ribs, here the 3rd, 4th, and 5th, are divided posteriorly with the bone cutters after subperiosteal exposure and suture ligature of the intercostals (not shown). A Gigli saw is shown passed into the chest anteriorly through the thoracotomy opening and out the interspace above the highest rib to be removed. The chest wall can be divided with great swiftness in this way, and with the intercostal arteries already secured posteriorly, the bleeding from the anterior ends in the moment before they are controlled is not major. Alternatively, the intercostal vessels are serially ligated and divided and the ribs sectioned successively. With the electrocautery, the incision is continued in the interspace above the highest rib being resected and is carried posteriorly to the line of transection of the ribs and down through the soft tissues at the posterior rib divisions, completing the liberation of the specimen.

B. *Left*: The treatment of the resultant defect varies with the section of chest wall removed. Anteriorly, with serratus and pectoralis directly attached to the chest wall and necessarily resected, some type of prosthetic reconstruction is required. The intact latissimus dorsi can cover a modest sized posterolateral defect without other measures and, as shown in this instance, the scapula will cover the defect for resections down to and including the 6th rib. If the 7th rib is removed, there is a risk that the scapula may be caught beneath it, and one may choose to amputate the tip of the scapula to prevent this.

Right: The scapula with its underlying and overlying muscles has been replaced, completely covering the defect, and the rhomboids have been reapproximated. Sutures are shown being placed in the divided ends of the trapezius, after which the closure of the latissimus completes the repair of the chest wall.

After Paone, J.F., Spees, E.K., Newton, C.G., Lillemoe, K.D., Kieffer, R.F., and Gadacz, T.R.: An appraisal of en bloc resection of peripheral bronchogenic carcinoma involving the thoracic wall. Chest 81:203–207, 1982.

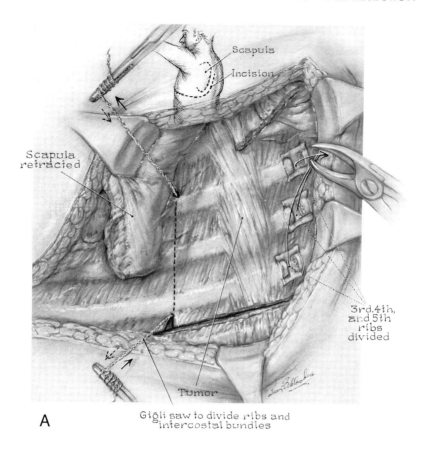

Scapula

Incision

Scapula retracted

3rd, 4th, and 5th ribs divided

Tumor

Gigli saw to divide ribs and intercostal bundles

A

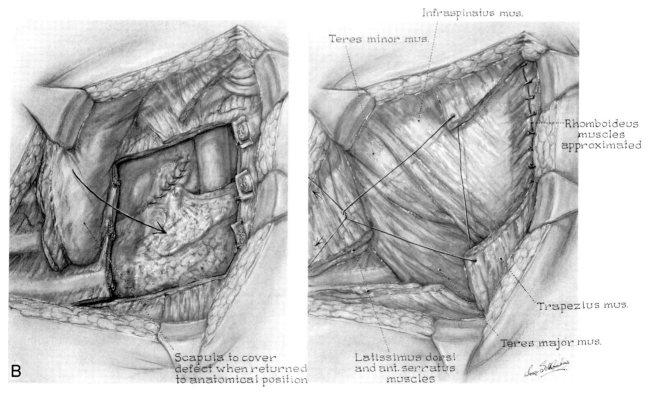

Infraspinatus mus.

Teres minor mus.

Rhomboideus muscles approximated

Scapula to cover defect when returned to anatomical position

Latissimus dorsi and ant. serratus muscles

Trapezius mus.

Teres major mus.

B

263

EXTENDED RESECTION OF SUPERIOR SULCUS TUMOR*

A. The patient is positioned on the side, with the arm suspended. The long parascapular incision begins just above the level of the spine of the scapula and passes down around the tip of the scapula, extending to the anterior axillary line. The trapezius has been divided; usually the upper portion is preserved. The latissimus dorsi has also been divided. Division of the attachments of the serratus anterior muscle to the upper ribs permits good elevation of the scapula. (The large scapula retractor has been omitted for clarity.) The chest is entered through a 3rd interspace incision for evaluation of operability and extent of the tumor. If the 3rd interspace proves to be involved or too close to the tumor, incision is made through the intercostal muscles in the 4th interspace. The anterior and medial scalenus muscles are shown already divided, though in actual practice that is done with the exposure achieved after the ribs have been divided anteriorly and pulled down as shown in B. The intercostal vessels and nerves are serially doubly ligated and divided as the ribs are transected anteriorly.

B. Downward traction on the anterior end of the first rib exposes the structures in the neck and has permitted the division of the scalenus muscles, after the subclavian artery and vein have been identified. The lower trunk of the brachial plexus is identified (not pictured), and the extent of its involvement by the tumor determined. The involved portion of the trunk is transected distal to the point of invasion. The arterial trunks are carefully dissected free in the periadventitial plane. The subclavian artery can almost always be dissected free. Its branches, the internal mammary, thyrocervical, and occasionally the vertebral, may have to be sacrificed because of involvement in the tumor.

---

*Method of D.L. Paulson.

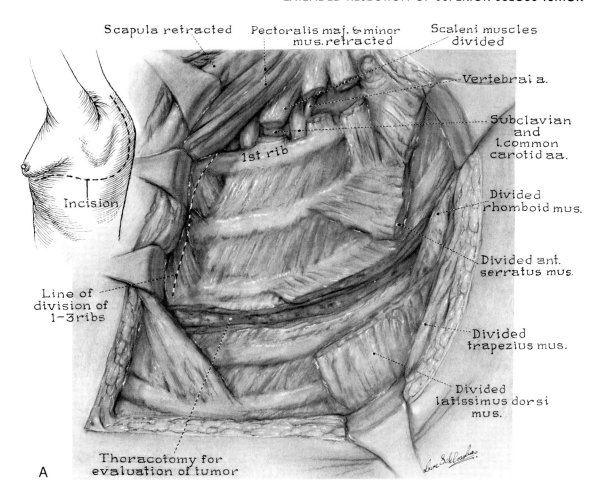

Scapula retracted

Pectoralis maj. & minor mus. retracted

Scaleni muscles divided

Vertebral a.

Subclavian and 1. common carotid aa.

1st rib

Divided rhomboid mus.

Divided ant. serratus mus.

Line of division of 1–3 ribs

Divided trapezius mus.

Divided latissimus dorsi mus.

Thoracotomy for evaluation of tumor

Incision

A

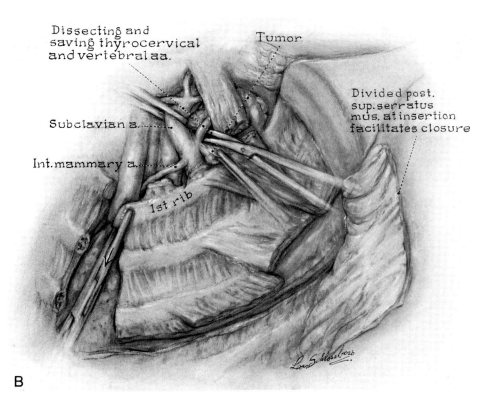

Dissecting and saving thyrocervical and vertebral aa.

Tumor

Divided post. sup. serratus mus. at insertion facilitates closure

Subclavian a.

Int. mammary a.

1st rib

B

C. Posterior phase of the dissection. The intrinsic dorsal musculature has been separated by sharp dissection from the upper ribs and transverse processes to the laminae of the vertebrae. The intrinsic dorsal musculature is retracted, and with bone cutters the transverse processes are divided in sequence, flush with the laminae. The heads of the ribs are levered with the periosteal elevator and the intercostal nerves and vessels are clipped and divided. The dorsal sympathetic chain is divided inferiorly. When the head of the 1st rib is elevated, the large 1st intercostal nerve is seen and divided, and the involved 8th cervical nerve root is also divided, now permitting downward traction on the 1st rib and the underlying tumor mass. In some cases the 8th cervical nerve root is not involved and only the portion of the lower brachial plexus trunk contributing the 1st intercostal nerve needs to be removed. It may be possible to elevate the tumor in its fibrous pseudocapsule from the vertebral body. If not, substantial portions of the involved vertebrae may be chiseled away.

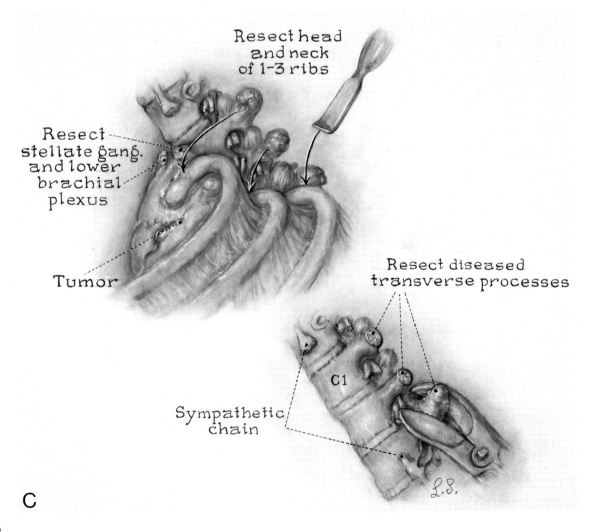

C

D. The specimen has been removed, with the involved portion of lung stapled off and amputated. At times, the involvement may dictate the necessity for upper lobectomy. A hilar and mediastinal node dissection is usually performed. The portion of the serratus posterior preserved as in *B* aids in closing the defect. A posterior and superior defect of this kind can be closed satisfactorily with the remaining shoulder girdle muscles and the scapula. Particularly if it has been necessary to remove the 4th rib as well, Prolene or Marlex mesh reconstruction of the chest wall produces a more satisfactory closure and eliminates paradox.

REFERENCES

1. Shaw, R.R., Paulson, D.L., and Kee, J.L., Jr.: Treatment of the superior sulcus tumor by irradiation followed by resection. Ann. Surg. 154:29–40, 1961
2. Paulson, D.L.: Extended resection of bronchogenic carcinoma in the superior pulmonary sulcus. Surgical Rounds, January 1980, pp. 10–21 and 60

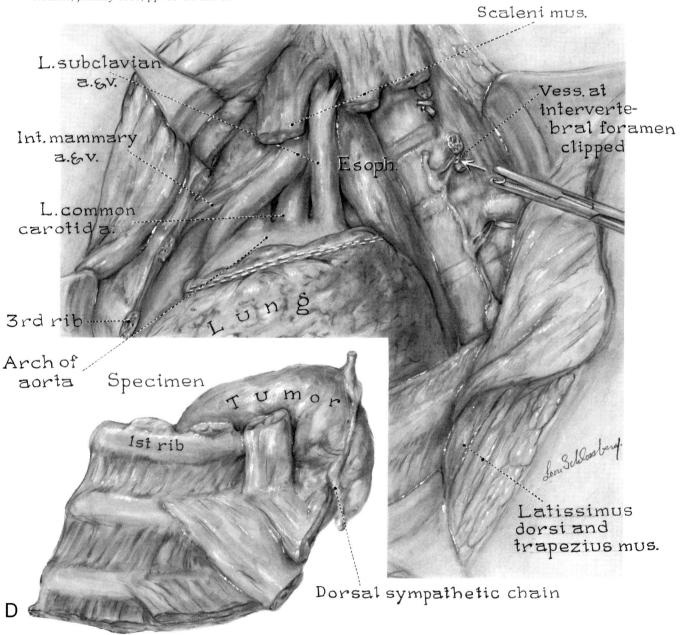

SLEEVE RESECTION—RIGHT UPPER LOBE

Sleeve resection of a major bronchus with lobectomy and reanastomosis of the bronchi of the remaining lobes to the parent bronchus or trachea is specifically applicable to carcinoma of the right upper lobe extending to involve its origin from the right main bronchus.

A. This view of the approach, from behind, shows that the azygos vein has been divided. The lines of division of the main bronchus and the intermediate bronchus are shown. The line of division of the main bronchus is transverse, to provide as much margin as possible, and the line of division of the intermediate bronchus is oblique so as to compensate for the discrepancy in caliber.

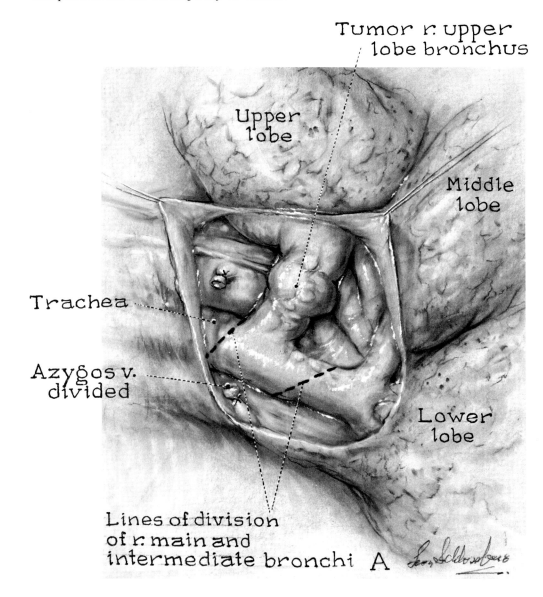

B. The bronchi have been divided, and the vascular supply of the upper lobe is secured and the lobe removed. The main bronchus is necessarily open during the suture, and this has been anticipated by the placement of a Carlens or similar catheter, or the use of a long tube into the left main bronchus for one-lung anesthesia from the start of the operation. Anastomosis is with interrupted through-and-through sutures of nonabsorbable material placed around the cartilage above and below.

C. Depending upon the anatomical situation, it may be necessary to decrease the caliber of the segment of the proximal bronchus by excising a wedge as shown in *D* and *E*.

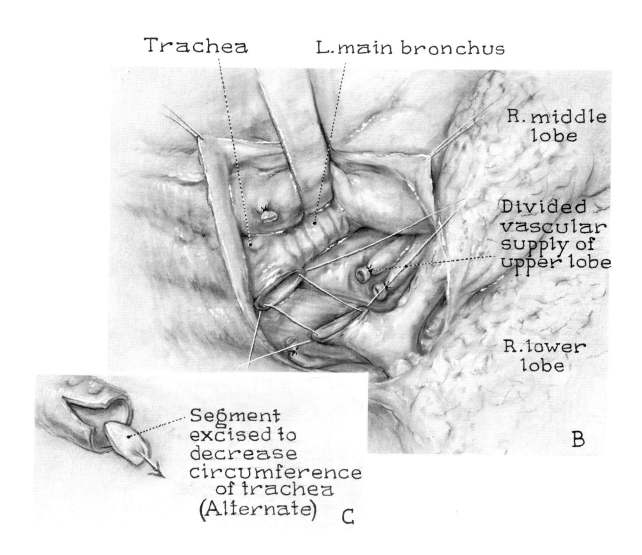

Trachea L.main bronchus

R. middle lobe

Divided vascular supply of upper lobe

R. lower lobe

B

Segment excised to decrease circumference of trachea (Alternate) C

D. The potential margins of bronchus proximal and distal with this type of resection are shown.

E. In spite of the difference in the obliquity of the two bronchial transections, the necessity for taking some trachea has required a wedge excision of the trachea. Closure of the wedge tapers the tracheal opening to the size of the oblique opening of the transected intermediate bronchus.

REFERENCES

1. Crafoord, C.: In discussion of Rabin, C.B., and Neuhof, H.: Adenoma of the bronchus. J. Thorac. Surg. 18:149–163, 1949
2. D'Abreu, A.L., and MacHale, S.J.: Bronchial "adenoma" treated by local resection and reconstruction of the left main bronchus. Br. J. Surg. 39:355–357, 1952
3. Paulson, D.L., and Shaw, R.R.: Preservation of lung tissue by means of bronchoplastic procedures. Am. J. Surg. 89:347–355, 1955
4. Allison, P.R.: Personal communication to C.P. Thomas. In: Thomas, C.P.: Conservative resection of the bronchial tree. J. R. Coll. Surg. Edinb. 1:169–186, 1956
5. Thomas, C.P.: Conservative resection of the bronchial tree. J. R. Coll. Surg. Edinb. 1:169–186, 1956
6. Kittle, C.F.: Atypical resections of the lung. In: Ravitch, M.M., and Steichen, F.M.: *Principles and Practice of Surgical Stapling.* Chicago, Year Book Medical Publishers, 1987

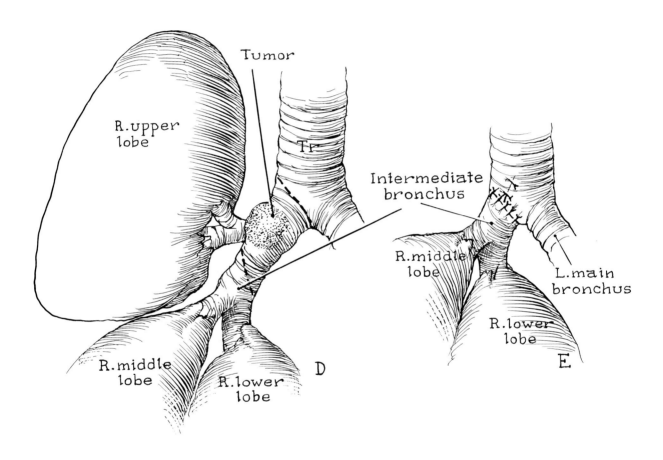

SLEEVE RESECTIONS OF BRONCHI WITH RESECTION OF PULMONARY LOBE OR SEGMENT

In resecting bronchial adenomas and increasingly in the case of favorably situated carcinomas, particularly in patients in whom preservation of pulmonary parenchyma is thought especially important, sleeve resection of the parent bronchus from which the involved bronchus arises, with resection in continuity of one or more lobes or the segment supplied by the involved bronchus, has become increasingly favored. For benign strictures and for strategically located bronchial adenomas, as in the cases of Crafoord and D'Abreu, if the supplied parenchyma is healthy, it becomes possible to perform a localized segmental or partial bronchial resection with reconstruction of the bronchus that avoids any resection of pulmonary parenchyma.

In all of these procedures, anesthesia and ventilation are either through a long tube into the uninvolved lung or with a Carlens or similar tube. Sutures may be made of either monofilament, nonabsorbable (Prolene)), or absorbable (polyglycolic acid) materials.

A. By virtue of the bronchial anatomy, by all odds the most common application of this principle is in resection of the right upper lobe when the tumor involves a portion of the main or the intermediate bronchus (see earlier, *Sleeve Resection—Right Upper Lobe*). Rarely, a portion of the pulmonary artery has also been resected and the artery reconstructed.

At times the required sleeve resection demands resection of the middle lobe as well as the upper. The lower lobe bronchus is then anastomosed to the proximal stump of the main bronchus. The middle lobe has been resected alone by the sleeve technique, and segmental pulmonary resections are possible with sleeve resection of the lobar bronchus.

B. Sleeve resection of left upper lobe.

C. Sleeve resection of left lower lobe.

D. Sleeve resection of superior segment of left lower lobe.

In all sleeve resections for tumor, which are by definition limited, frozen section of the remaining bronchial ends is required, and the operator must be prepared for the necessity of converting to a more extensive extirpation.

After Kittle, C.F.: Atypical resections of the lung. In: Ravitch, M.M., and Steichen, F.M.: *Principles and Practice of Surgical Stapling*. Chicago, Year Book Medical Publishers, 1987.

RIGHT UPPER LOBE
SLEEVE RESECTION

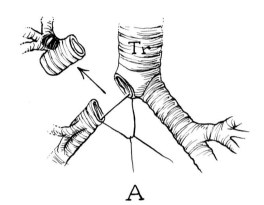

A

LEFT UPPER LOBE SLEEVE
RESECTION

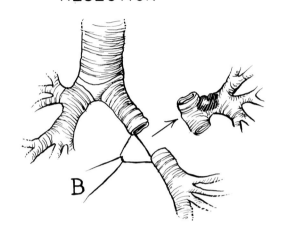

B

LEFT LOWER LOBE SLEEVE
RESECTION

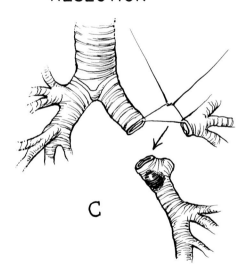

C

SEGMENTAL SLEEVE RESECTION
SUPERIOR SEGMENT
LEFT LOWER LOBE

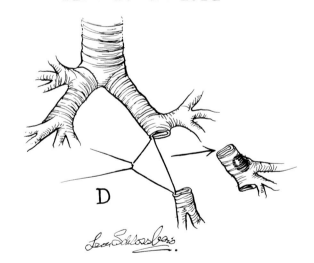

D

273

EXTRAPLEURAL THORACOPLASTY WITH APICOLYSIS
(PRICE-THOMAS)

A. The patient is in the full lateral position with the arm either elevated on a frame or draped free. The vertical limb of the incision begins above the level of the spine of the scapula, rather closer to the vertebrae than to the scapular border. The incision is carried down to well below the scapular angle and then brought forward horizontally. Scratching the skin at the corner of the turn simplifies matching the flaps at the closure.

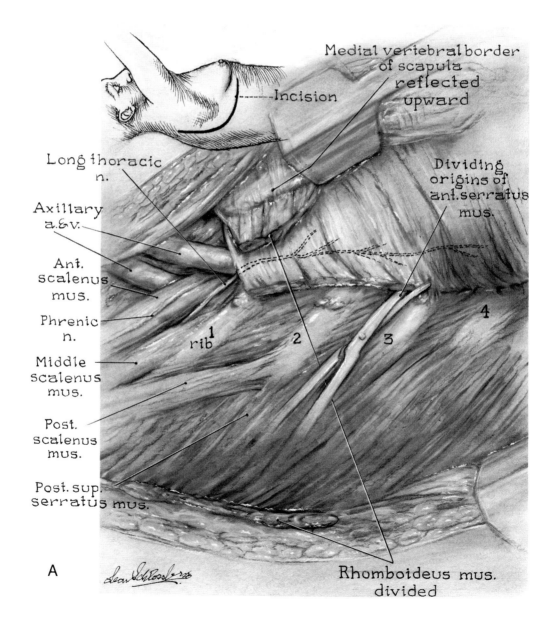

Making the incision well posteriorly permits division of the muscles where they are less fleshy and more tendinous, making for less bleeding and facilitating closure. The trapezius and the rhomboids have been divided. The scapula is held forward and dissection carried anteriorly, close to the ribs with knife, cautery, or scissors. The anterior serratus muscle is shown being divided from its costal attachments. Note the closeness of the long thoracic nerve, which must be protected.

B. It is most convenient simply to excise the posterior serratus muscle next, as shown. *Note:* All muscles are divided or elevated in the line of the skin and subcutaneous incision.

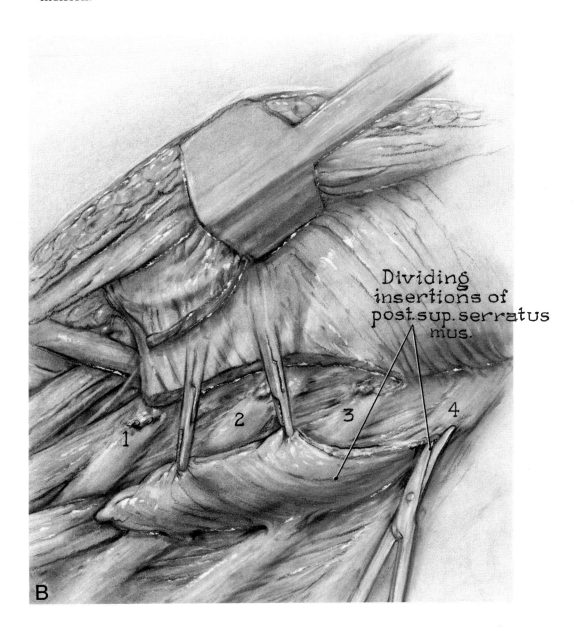

EXTRAPLEURAL THORACOPLASTY WITH APICOLYSIS
(PRICE-THOMAS) *(Continued)*

C. It is a matter of choice and judgment as to how many ribs are to be removed in the first stage; if an essentially total thoracoplasty is planned, usually no more than three or four are involved. In thoracoplasty with apicolysis limited to the first stage, the 2nd, and 1st ribs are excised *in toto*; the 3rd rib is removed back from the anterior axillary line and the 4th rib back from the midaxillary line to the transverse process. The periosteum is incised with the cautery.

D. The periosteum is elevated from the external surface of the ribs, and a tunnel is created under the rib for passing the Doyen raspatory. Note that the Doyen is placed at an angle so as to hold its sharp edge against the rib, minimizing the risk of tearing the posterior periosteum as the rib is denuded.

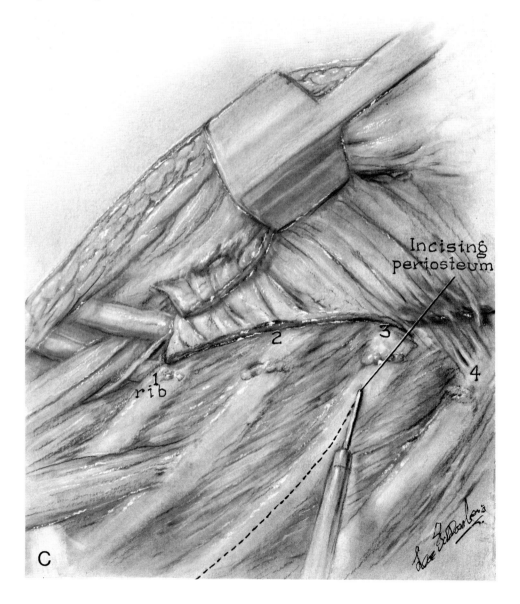

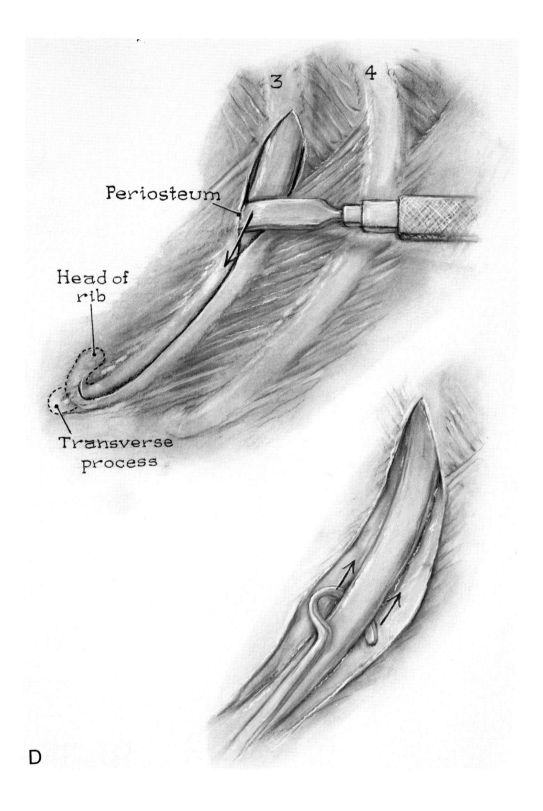

Periosteum

Head of
rib

Transverse
process

3

4

D

EXTRAPLEURAL THORACOPLASTY WITH APICOLYSIS
(PRICE-THOMAS) *(Continued)*

E. Ordinarily, the scaleni are divided before the resection of the ribs is begun. In denuding the ribs posteriorly, the paraspinal muscles are elevated and retracted from the ribs. The rib is stripped of periosteum and the costotransverse joint is opened with the shears to permit division of the rib beyond its shoulder. The rib is then elevated and divided as far anteriorly as required, usually somewhat lateral to the costochondral junction, for total thoracoplasty or, as described under C, for first-stage (limited) thoracoplasty with apicolysis.

The 1st rib requires a special approach if its resection is planned. First, it is denuded, taking care not to injure axillary vessels and brachial plexus. The rib is then divided at its midportion and removed in two portions. By pulling each segment away from its anterior or posterior attachments, it is easier to reach the costotransverse ligament posteriorly and the 1st cartilage behind the clavicle anteriorly.

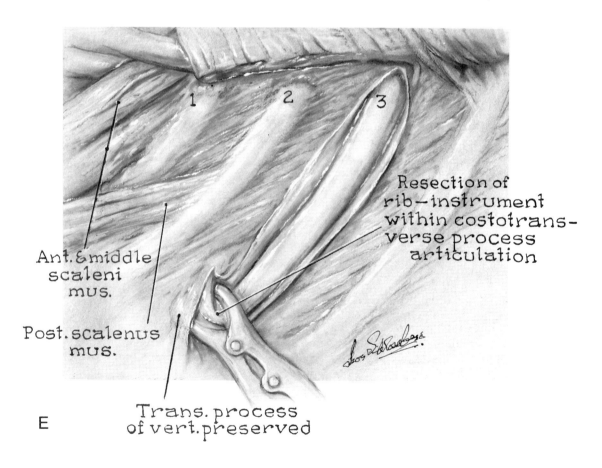

F. The appropriate lengths of the first three ribs have been divided. Once the 1st intercostal muscle is excised, the division of one or two perichondrial beds and intercostal muscles posteriorly is required to provide wide exposure of the extrapleural space. Transverse division of Sibson's fascia, a heavy expansion of the endothoracic fascia over the apex of the lung, provides the readiest access to the space between the inside of the chest wall and the mediastinum on the one hand and the endothoracic fascia on the other. Division of Sibson's fascia clearly and safely exposes the 1st dorsal nerve, the subclavian artery, and the innominate vein.

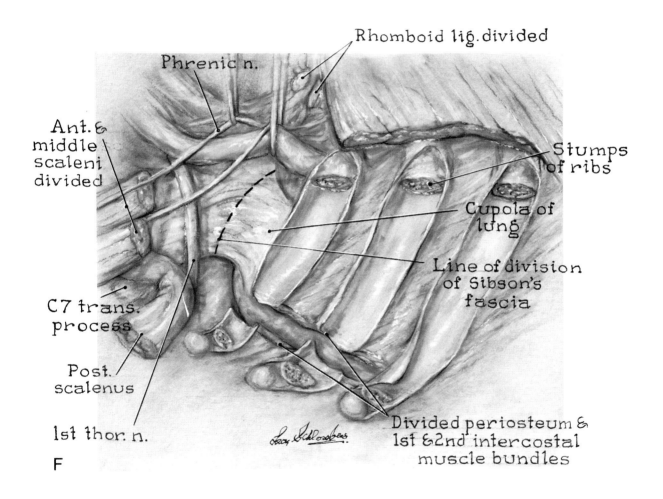

EXTRAPLEURAL THORACOPLASTY WITH APICOLYSIS
(PRICE-THOMAS) *(Continued)*

G. After Sibson's fascia is divided, the lung contained in its pleural sac is stripped from the chest wall by a combination of blunt pressure dissection and cutting with the scissors as the bands of Sebileau (three thickenings of Sibson's fascia) are brought into relief. The first band lies superficial to the nerve, the second between the artery and the nerve, and the third in front of the artery. These bands are isolated and divided, and the intervening less dense, fibrous fascia is also divided.

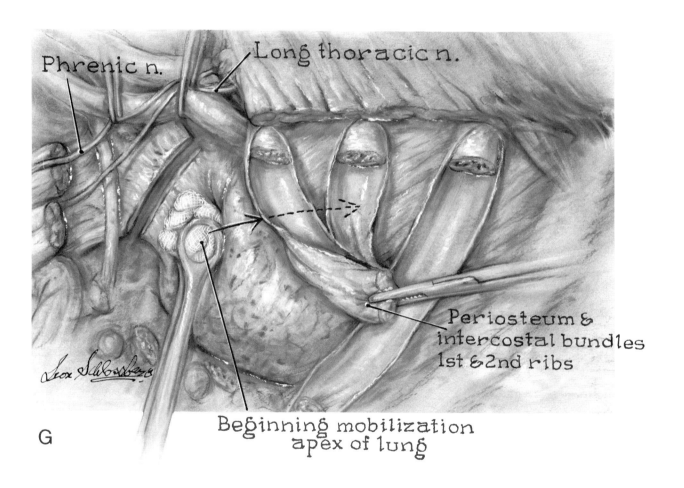

G

H. A very full displacement of the apical portion of the lung is possible. The dissection is with a stick sponge (end shown in dotted lines without its sponge) or with a sponge gently held by the fingers. Fibers of the anterior scalenus that are attached to the pleura may require transection.

In the days when thoracoplasty was the mainstay of the operative collapse therapy of tuberculosis, this operation, which we usually performed under local anesthesia, gave great satisfaction. Innumerable variations were practiced. It is possible, for instance, to strip the 1st rib of periosteum but leave it in place, to provide a better cosmetic result, and still to divide the periosteum and intercostal muscles if apicolysis is indicated. Obviously, if the thoracoplasty is undertaken to collapse an empyema cavity or a space left after lobectomy or pneumonectomy, the apicolysis is superfluous.

REFERENCES

1. Alexander, J.: *The Collapse Therapy of Pulmonary Tuberculosis.* Springfield, Illinois, Charles C Thomas, 1937
2. Thomas, C.P., and Cleland, W.P.: Extrafascial apicolysis with thoracoplasty. Indications, technique and complications. Br. J. Tuberc. 36:109–138, 1942 (Brompton Hospital Reports XII:23–52, 1943)

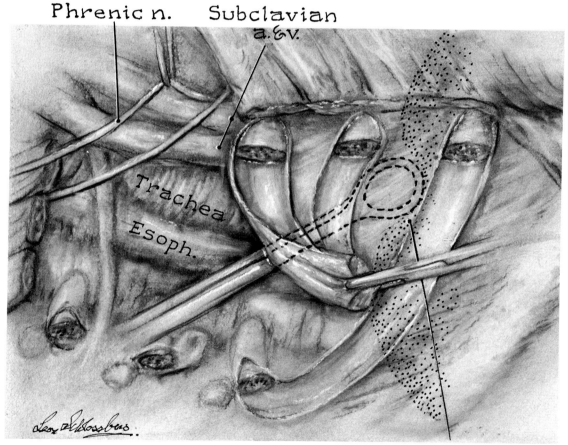

Phrenic n.   Subclavian a. & v.

Trachea

Esoph.

Lung mobilized

H

DECORTICATION

A. The length and site of the incision depends upon the extent of the empyema, but usually a long 6th interspace incision suffices; occasionally the 5th or 7th is used. There is no need to resect the rib. As the pleural cavity is emptied, the clot and pus or coagulum are evacuated (not shown). The incision is gradually enlarged, and the retractors are opened to provide exposure. Incision is made into the fibroblastic peel over the visceral pleura, the edge is grasped, and the anesthetist is asked to expand the lung so it will pout into the incision in the fibrous peel as soon as the visceral pleura has been reached.

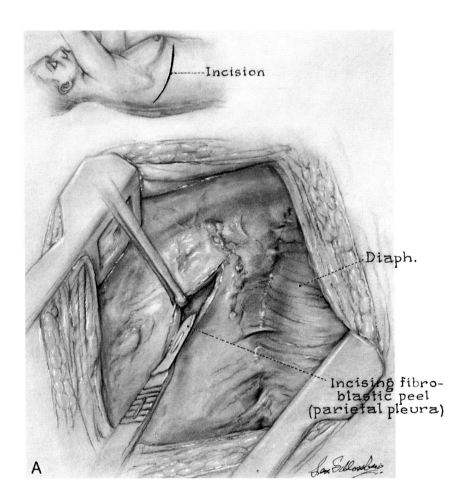

B. At this point, the strong edges of the peel are elevated and the lung displaced from the underside of the peel, by gauze pledget dissection (as shown), by finger dissection, or occasionally by dissection with Metzenbaum scissors. Although injuries to the pleura and bubbling air leaks and oozing here and there are to be expected, the degree to which they occur depends upon the accuracy with which the proper plane is achieved.

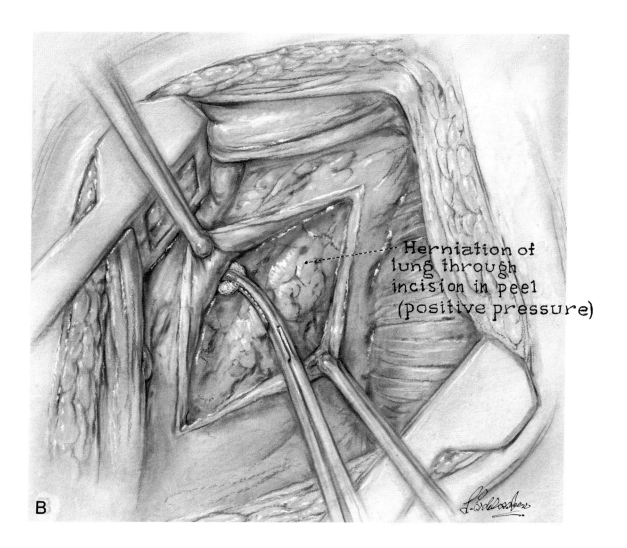

Herniation of lung through incision in peel (positive pressure)

B

C. The borders of the empyema cavity are seen being reached, and the peel is coming around the lung. Every effort should be made to excise the full thickness and the full extent of the visceral peel to allow full expansion of the lung. At the same time, it is usually preferred to excise the parietal peel as well (not shown), including particularly the costal and diaphragmatic surfaces, to permit full respiratory motion.

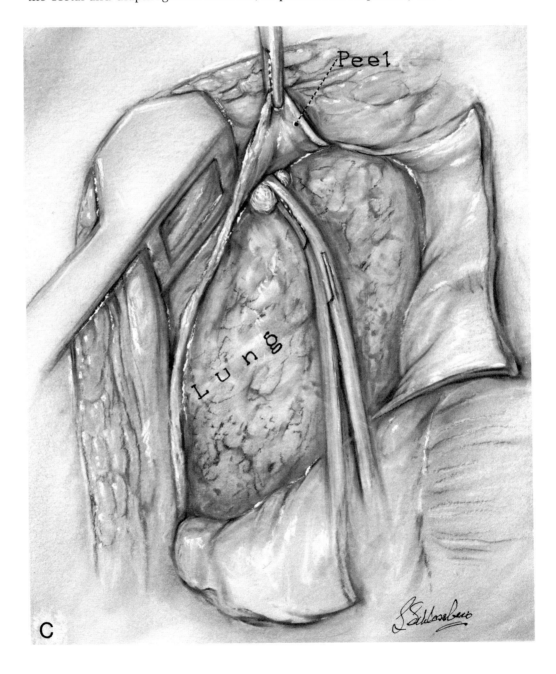

D. The lung is completely expanded and it is seen that the peel has been removed from the fissure as well as from the upper and lower lobes.

Unless injury to the parenchyma has been substantial, it is preferable not to attempt to close the air leaks with sutures but to depend upon suction drainage with at least two tubes, or more if deemed necessary. Bleeding is largely controlled by temporary packing in the course of operation. The tubes should go to the apex of the thorax and have multiple perforations down to the exit from the chest.

REFERENCES

1. Fowler, G.R.: A case of thoracoplasty for the removal of a large cicatricial fibrous growth from the interior of the chest, the result of an old empyema. M. Rec. 44:838–839, 30 Dec. 1893
2. Delorme, E.: Nouveau traitement des empyèmes chroniques. Gaz. d'hop. 67:94–96, 25 Jan. 1894
3. Delorme, E.: Du traitement des empyèmes chroniques par la décortication du poumon—résultats, indications, technique. Assoc. franc. de chir., Paris 10:379–389, 1896
4. Burford, T.H.: Hemothorax and hemothoracic empyema. In: *Medical Department, United States Army. Surgery in World War II. Thoracic Surgery. Volume II.* F.B. Berry (Ed.). Washington, D.C., Office of the Surgeon General, Dept. of the Army, 1965
   The decortications of Fowler, and shortly after of Delorme, were surprisingly modern, but recognition of the importance to respiration of the removal of the parietal peel came later. The modern knowledge and use of decortication dates essentially from the experience in the Mediterranean Theater of Operations during World War II. Burford's description of the gradual development of technique and the accretion of experience and information in the North African Theater of Operations and subsequently in Italy is of surpassing interest and current value.

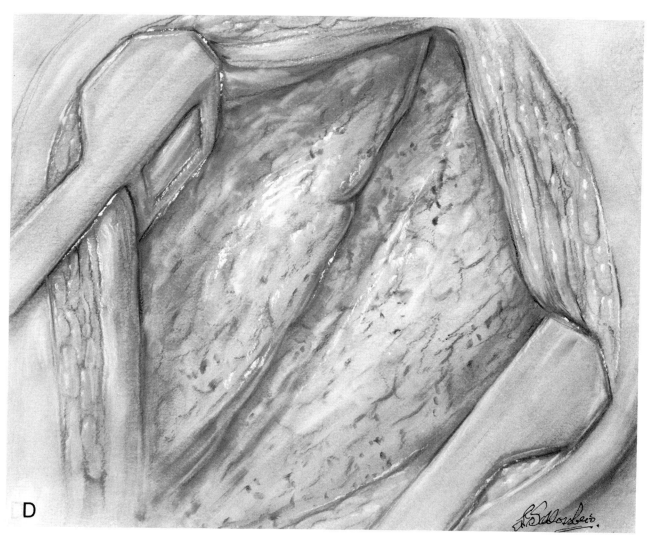

D

EMPYEMECTOMY

At times, the localized nature of an empyema permits one to perform what is essentially a complete decortication without ever entering the empyema cavity. Although wound infection of the thoracotomy incision is surprisingly rare after decortication, there is nevertheless an obvious advantage and appeal to excision of the pus sac *in toto* and without a breach.

A. The empyema cavity is shown. Note in the section of normal chest wall a depiction of the layers involved. Whether the dissection is outside the endothoracic fascia or between it and the parietal pleura will depend upon the circumstances. Ideally and most safely, dissection should be outside the endothoracic fascia, but in fact the inflammatory reaction will often be such as to make it difficult to discern the precise plane of dissection.

B. After the intercostal muscles are opened and the endothoracic fascia, in this case, incised, the fascial edges are held apart while with finger dissection, clamp-held sponges, or the scissors, as variously indicated, the pleural sac is dissected away from the chest wall.

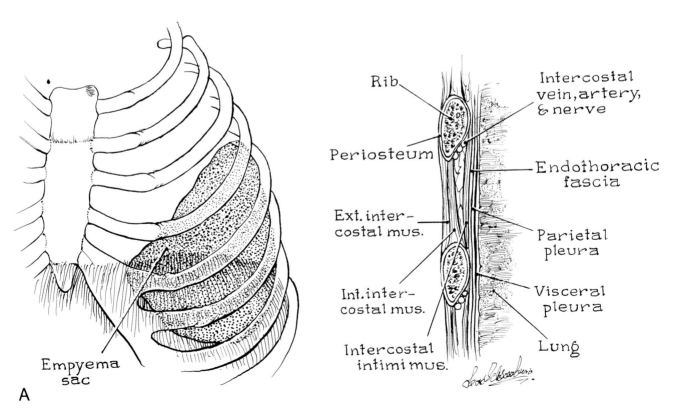

A

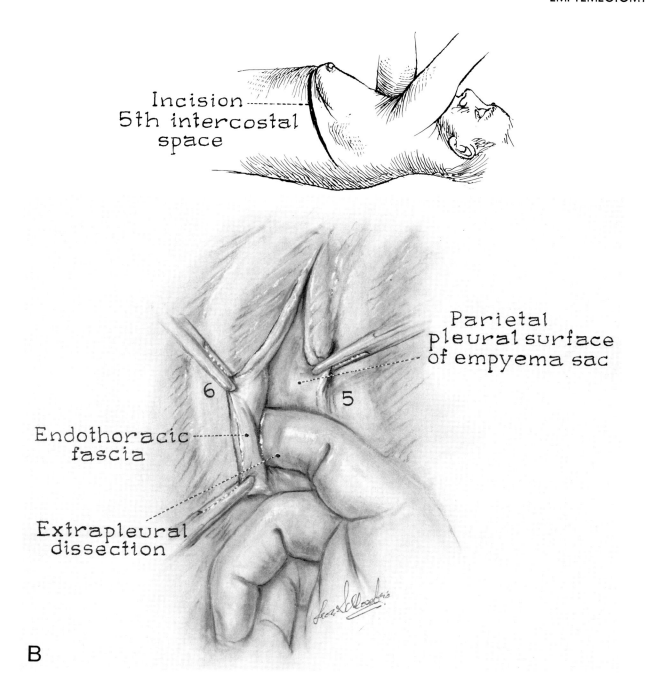

Incision
5th intercostal
space

Parietal
pleural surface
of empyema sac

Endothoracic
fascia

Extrapleural
dissection

6

5

B

EMPYEMECTOMY *(Continued)*

C. One has now come superiorly to the upper border of the empyema sac and is dissecting it away from the visceral pleura of the underlying lung. As in decortication, at times this is readily done by blunt dissection and at other times by sharp dissection.

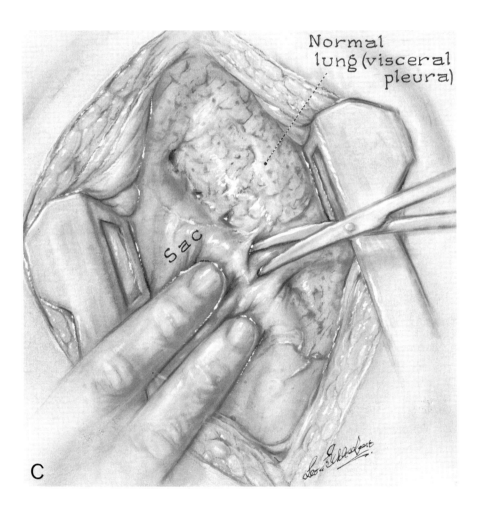

D. The empyema sac has been peeled away from the base of the lung and now is being dissected off the diaphragm. At the completion of the procedure, the empyema sac has been dissected away from the chest wall, the lung, and the diaphragm and its mediastinal attachments; all tissue left behind is uncontaminated and restored to normal mobility. As in decortication, the fibrous peel is often thinnest over the diaphragm, and the dissection there is most taxing.

REFERENCES

1. Dugan, D.J., and Samson, P.C.: Surgical significance of the endothoracic fascia. The anatomic basis for empyemectomy and other extrapleural technics. Am. J. Surg. 130:151–158, 1975
2. le Roux, B.T., Mohlala, M.L., Odell, J.A., and Whitton, I.D.: Suppurative diseases of the lung and the pleural space. Part I: Empyema thoracis and lung abscess. Current Problems in Surgery, January 1986

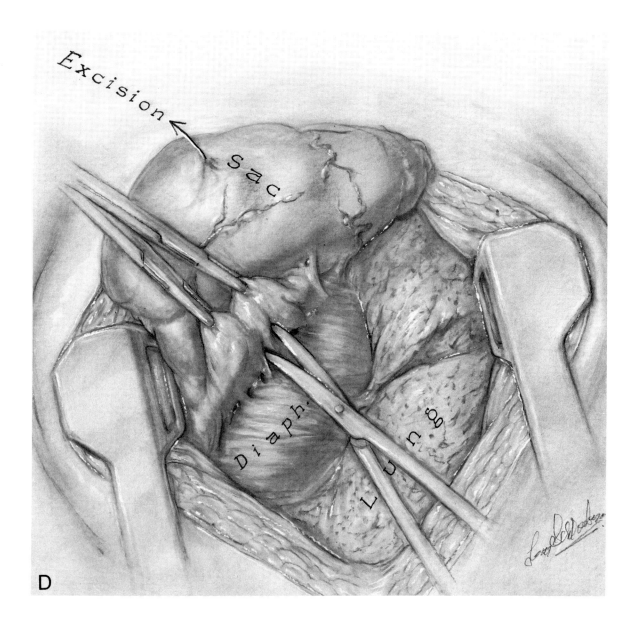

EMPYEMA DRAINAGE—ELOESSER FLAP

In general, early empyema is treated by tube thoracostomy, and empyema discovered late, by decortication or empyemectomy. If the small size of the empyema, or the feeble condition of the patient, or the underlying condition (such as with postpneumonectomy empyema) so indicate, the Eloesser flap is undertaken. This was originally devised by Eloesser for drainage of tuberculous empyema. A U-shaped flap of skin and fat is raised; the flap is made 8 to 10 cm wide or a little wider to nourish its full 6 to 8 cm in length. The base of the flap is at the level of the lowest rib clearly above the bottom of the empyema cavity and at whatever point on the circumferences of the chest the roentgenograms demonstrate to be the lowest point of the cavity. This rib at the base of the flap is resected with its periosteum and intercostal vessels. The intercostal muscles and parietal pleura in the defect are excised. The tip of the flap is now turned up into the chest and tacked to the pleura. A gauze sponge wrapped around a catheter into the chest helps to hold the flap in place until it has become adherent. The edges of the wound are advanced from below to cover over the chest wall below the incision.

REFERENCE

1. Eloesser, L.: An operation for tuberculous empyema. Surg. Gynecol. Obstet. 60:1096, 1935

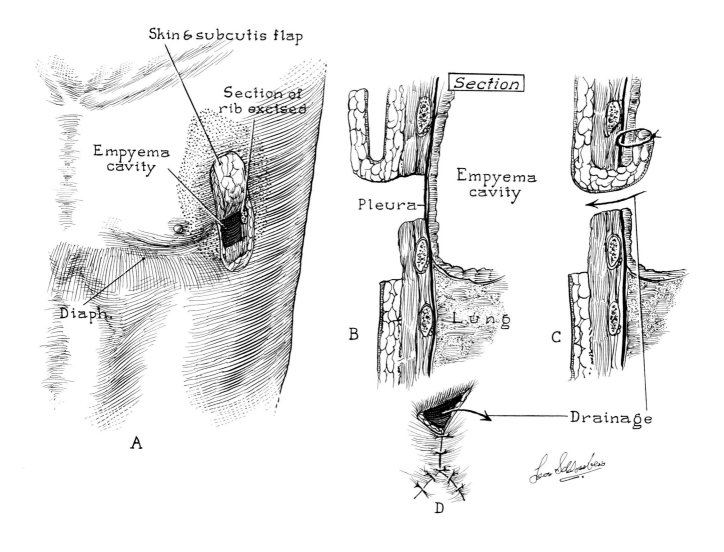

Skin & subcutis flap

Section of rib excised

Empyema cavity

Diaph.

A

Section

Pleura

Empyema cavity

Lung

B

C

Drainage

D

The Trachea

The Trachea

BLOOD SUPPLY OF THE TRACHEA

Upper, left and right: Anterior and left lateral views of vessels supplying the trachea. There is some variation from case to case. Note that the major arterial supply comes in laterally or slightly posterolaterally, essentially from branches of the subclavian artery above and from the bronchial arteries below. The distal trachea is invariably supplied by the bronchial arteries, with contributions coming varyingly from the supreme intercostal artery, directly from the subclavian artery, from the internal mammary artery, and from the innominate artery. The several tracheal arteries branching up and down on the lateral aspect of the trachea interconnect with the tracheal arteries above and below, producing a variable and irregular but usually complete longitudinal vascular anastomosis on the lateral wall of the trachea. The cervical trachea receives its blood supply chiefly from the inferior thyroid artery, the tracheal branches of which pass anterior or posterior to the recurrent laryngeal nerve, or both.

Lower: Trachea showing details of arterial supply. The entire dependence of the trachea upon vessels entering the wall a little posterior to midlateral is clearly demonstrated. The lateral tracheal pedicle of Grillo is an irregular sheet of connective tissue coming from the deep surface of the aorta and the innominate and subclavian arteries. In it are contained branches from the thyrocervical, costocervical, subclavian, and internal thoracic arteries to the trachea and esophagus. The three to seven primary tracheal arteries are found at intervals along the entire length of the trachea in this tissue, and the recurrent laryngeal nerves are involved in its fibers.

Note the tendency for the tracheal blood supply to split off from the tracheoesophageal artery, producing a separation of the tracheal and esophageal arteries.

After Salassa, J.R., Pearson, B.W., and Payne, W.S.: Gross and microscopical blood supply of the trachea. Ann. Thorac. Surg. 24:100–107, 1977.

294

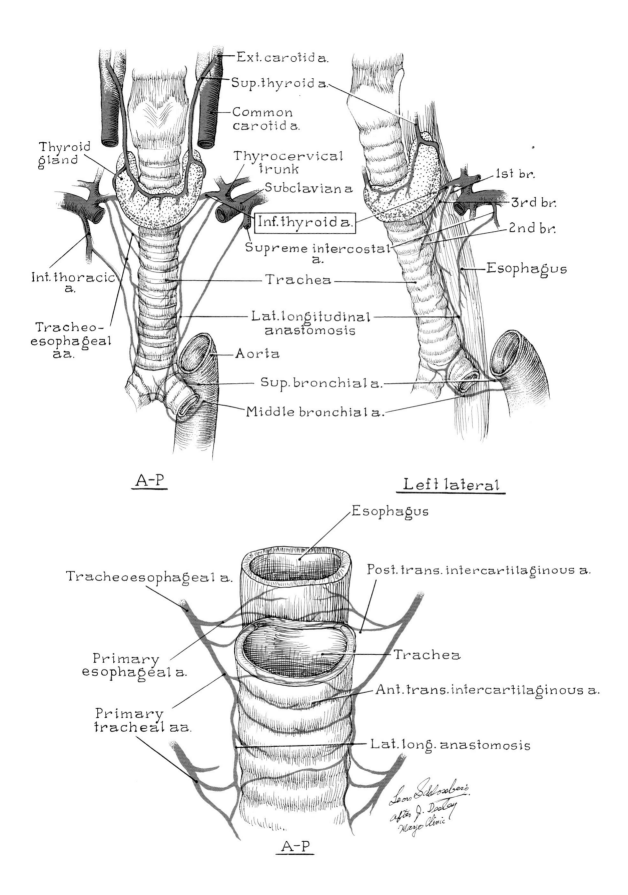

A-P

Left lateral

A-P

TRACHEAL RESECTION—ANTERIOR APPROACH

The cervical or upper cervicomediastinal approach is used for limited tumors of the upper trachea and for almost all benign strictures of the trachea. The patient is usually anesthetized with halothane, and a rigid bronchoscope is passed. A stricture less than 6 mm in diameter is dilated under direct vision with a rigid pediatric bronchoscope. If the stricture is more than 6 mm in diameter, an endotracheal tube may be placed to just above the lesion. If the lesion is subglottic, the stricture must be dilated and a small endotracheal tube passed through it. A small endotracheal tube may be slipped past most tumors, and if jet ventilation is employed, a tube as small as No. 14 French suffices.

A. The trachea is explored through a collar incision, which may circumcise an existing tracheal stoma. If the stoma is too high for that, the incision is made appropriately low, and the stoma is separately excised. Skin flaps are raised to the cricoid cartilage above and the sternal notch below. The strap muscles are elevated on both sides. There may be dense scarring at the site of the stoma. The anterior surface of the trachea is exposed from the cricoid cartilage to the carina. The thyroid isthmus is divided, dissected from the trachea anteriorly, and retracted with sutures. The innominate artery may be densely adherent to the trachea. In inflammatory lesions, it is essential to keep the dissection close against the trachea to avoid the risk of injury to the back wall of the innominate artery. If the lesion extends too far below the sternal notch to be easily accessible through the collar incision, the exposure is increased by making a T incision, the vertical arm extending downward to a point 1 cm below the sternal angle. The sternum is divided to that point only and separated with a small chest spreader. It is better to let the sternum fracture at will on one side or the other, as the retractor is opened, than to cut across the sternum. Nothing is gained by full median sternotomy, since the carina lies at the level of the angle of Louis and the great vessels anterior to it obstruct access from in front.

For an approach to an upper tracheal tumor of uncertain extent, the patient is positioned with support behind the upper back to the right of the midline, the right arm is abducted, and the chest, to the posterior axillary line, is included in the operative field. The midline incision may, if necessary, be extended laterally beneath the breast, entering the right hemithorax through the 4th interspace, beneath the elevated pectoral muscle. The resultant "trapdoor" incision offers exposure of the entire trachea from the cricoid to the carina and provides access to the posterior aspect of the carina.

B. The upper sternum has been divided to provide access to the lower trachea. The innominate vein, lying caudal to the dissection, is not divided. The tissues containing the innominate artery are dissected away from the trachea, *without* exposing the wall of the artery, and are retracted gently. The carina and the right and left tracheobronchial angles can be exposed as necessary.

In cases of inflammatory stenosis, dissection is made meticulously along the lateral sides of the involved trachea and posteriorly approximately 1 cm below the lesion. If there is difficulty in identifying the level of the lesion, as there may be particularly in patients who have cuff-produced stenosis without prior tracheostomy, it may be necessary to bronchoscope the patient intraoperatively. The position of the bronchoscope light is identified at the upper and then the lower end of the lesion, and these levels are marked with fine sutures. For this purpose a flexible bronchoscope may be slipped through the endotracheal tube, or the patient may be extubated, examined with a rigid bronchoscope, and reintubated. Dissection close to the tracheal wall or the scar replacing it avoids injury to the recurrent laryngeal nerves, which lie in the tracheoesophageal groove on either side, often in dense scar but not exposed. This is particularly important if the stenosis lies just below the cricoid cartilage, since the nerves enter the larynx just medial to the inferior cornua of the thyroid cartilages.

The trachea is circumferentially dissected, most often at a level immediately below the distal margin of the lesion, since here the trachea is less likely to be adherent to the esophagus. Care must be taken not to perforate either the esophagus or the membranous wall of the trachea. A tracheal perforation produced immediately below the lesion may be excised with the specimen. A tape is passed beneath the trachea.

Sterile anesthesia equipment is assembled on the field prior to division of the trachea, unless high frequency ventilation is being used, and the corrugated tubing is passed off the table to the anesthetist. Lateral traction sutures are placed on either side of the trachea approximately 1 cm below the anticipated level of transection; they pass vertically through the full thickness of the tracheal wall and around one or more rings. The trachea is opened anteriorly just distal to the lesion, staying close to the lesion if it is benign. If the wall is still diseased at this point, a second incision is made one ring lower, until good tissue is identified, and the trachea is transected. Healthy cartilage should be visible in the cut edge or lie immediately below. Transection is generally just above a ring, but it is acceptable to make the incision in cartilage. Continuous suctioning prevents seepage of blood into the distal trachea. After the transection, an assistant maintains tension on the two lateral traction sutures and holds the flexible armored tube in the distal trachea.

Circumferential dissection of the residual distal trachea is limited to its first 1 to 2 cm to protect the segmental blood supply, which comes in laterally. Devascularization invites necrosis and a possibly irreparable restenosis.

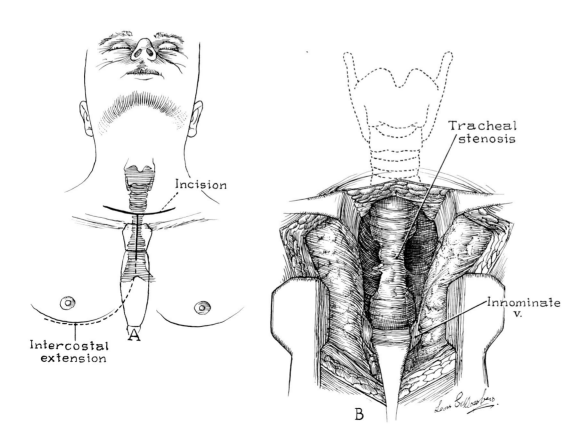

297

C. If the events producing the stenosis are sufficiently far in the past that much of the fibrosis has resolved, it may be possible to dissect out the entire involved segment before transecting the trachea. Ordinarily this is not feasible. In the illustration, the endotracheal tube has already been passed into the distal trachea. The specimen is elevated to permit easier dissection from the esophagus, and the trachea is then transected above. If the lesion is distal or supracarinal, circumferential dissection and transection are first carried out at the upper end of the lesion. For stenotic lesions that lie just above the carina, the traction sutures are placed in the tracheobronchial angles on either side. In such cases, the endotracheal tube is passed into the right or left main bronchus for single lung anesthesia. High frequency ventilation simplifies the process.

In the case of *tumors* of the upper trachea, since there is no peritracheal inflammation, the recurrent laryngeal nerves are usually identified and followed to above the level chosen for tracheal transection. This permits excision of paratracheal lymph nodes immediately adjacent to the tumor-bearing segment. To determine the appropriate level of tracheal transection, the trachea is initially opened through a tumor-free area at the level of the tumor. A lobe of the thyroid may be included if it is thought the tumor has penetrated the tracheal wall. A button of invaded esophageal wall may require excision, attached to the trachea. Unavoidably, the esophagus is narrowed by the two-layer closure that follows.

Lateral traction sutures are placed proximally about a centimeter above the proposed proximal level of transection. Again, no more than at the most 1 cm of trachea is freed circumferentially. If the upper level of transection is at the inferior border of the cricoid cartilage, no attempt is made to dissect more cephalad posteriorly, since this would be into the zone of fusion between the upper esophagus and the cricoid, just below the arytenoids, and posterolaterally might also endanger the recurrent laryngeal nerves.

To test the ease with which the tracheal ends can be brought together, the anesthetist flexes the patient's neck and the operators draw upon the crossed proximal and distal traction sutures, bringing the tracheal ends together. The endotracheal tube may have to be removed to make certain the ends come together satisfactorily. An experienced surgeon can readily judge whether the tension is excessive. The length of trachea that may be safely removed obviously must be determined prior to division. Whether resection is feasible is based on radiologic and endoscopic observations made before operation, and rarely on exploration.

Occasionally, adjunctive measures are necessary to reduce tension. For upper tracheal resections, a suprahyoid laryngeal release according to the technique of Montgomery (see next procedure, *Suprahyoid Laryngeal Release [Montgomery]*) may be utilized to gain an additional 1 or 2 cm. Thyrohyoid release as described by Dedo and Fishman gives similar relaxation but is more likely than the suprahyoid release to lead to aspiration during swallowing.

D. Approximation of the tracheal ends after upper tracheal resection is achieved chiefly by the simple maneuver of cervical flexion. In children or young adults, up to 50% of the trachea rises into the neck on hyperextension, and in them marked flexion alone will permit tracheal anastomosis after resection of up to 50% of the trachea. In older, kyphotic, obese patients, or when there is fibrosis from previous operations, flexion may overcome only a short gap. Freeing its anterior surface helps the trachea to slide a little in the mediastinum. Circumferential dissection of the distal trachea, in the hope of gaining more length, risks devascularizing the trachea.

E. Once it has been demonstrated that the ends will come together without excessive tension, the neck is again hyperextended. The first anastomotic suture (currently 4-0 coated Vicryl) is placed in the posterior midline with the knot to lie outside, and the suture is clipped to the drapes above. The next suture is placed lateral to this and clipped to the drapes just caudad to the previous one. The sutures are thus serially inserted until a point is reached just posterior to the midlateral traction suture. The same placement of sutures is now carried out on the opposite side, from the posterior midline to the midlateral suture. Serial sutures are similarly placed

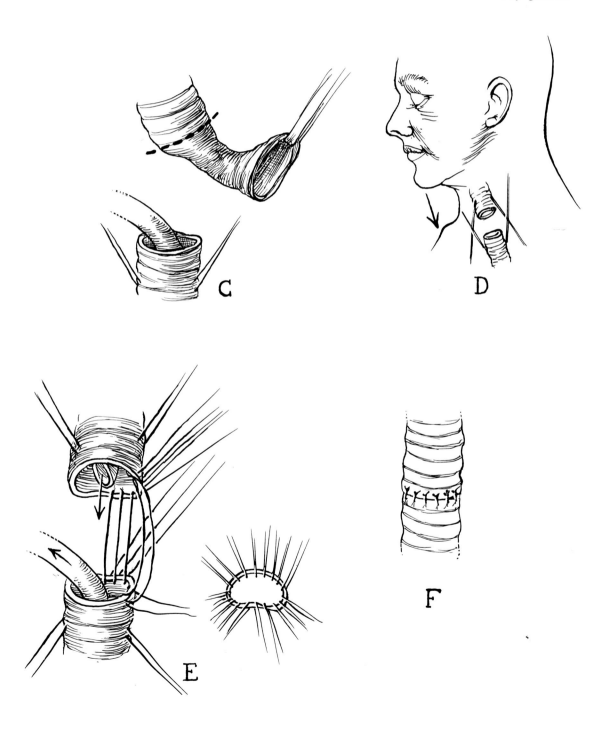

anteriorly, proceeding from the lateral traction sutures to the midline. The endotracheal tube may have to be removed intermittently for the placement of difficult sutures, or drawn to one side as the sutures are inserted.

The sutures, usually through cartilage, are placed approximately 4 mm back from the cut edge of the trachea and 4 mm apart. Particularly in children, it is better not to pass sutures around the cartilage, since their soft cartilages buckle easily, with resultant narrowing of the anastomosis.

F. When all sutures have been placed, the endotracheal tube is advanced from above until the end is visible in the wound. In upper tracheal resections, a catheter is sutured into the tip of the endotracheal tube at the time of initial proximal transection of the trachea. This allows withdrawal of the tube through the vocal cords to get its bulk out of the way of the surgeon but leaves a guide for easy advancement of the tube into the field.

The distal trachea is suctioned, the tube in it is withdrawn, and anesthesia is now taken over by the original endotracheal tube, which is advanced into the distal trachea. The tube is placed just barely into the distal trachea, since approximation of the trachea will push it down further, potentially into the right main bronchus.

The patient's head is firmly supported on blankets in full flexion. The crossed lateral traction sutures are pulled together on either side and tied with surgeon's knots. The tracheal ends are apposed end-to-end, not intussuscepted.

The anterior anastomotic sutures are tied first, without tension, and each is cut as it is tied. The assistant now rotates the trachea by gently drawing on the traction suture on the surgeon's side of the table, and the surgeon ties the suture just behind the lateral traction suture and works posteriorly to the posterior midline, cutting each suture as it is tied. This is repeated on the opposite side. The traction sutures are removed and the integrity of the anastomosis is checked under saline.

Some surgeons prefer to tie the posterior sutures first and then place and tie the anterior ones. While this is feasible in the simpler cases, it becomes much more difficult when a 50% resection has been performed and the patient is in marked flexion during completion of the anastomosis. We find it better to perform all anastomoses in the same fashion so that a dependable routine is established. With experience one can avoid breaking the posterior sutures.

If there is dense calcification of the cricoid or upper trachea, it may be necessary to use a fine dental drill to make holes for sutures. On occasions when the tissues have been very rigid, we have used one or two heavier sutures anteriorly.

The thyroid isthmus is reapproximated. No particular protection is necessary for the innominate artery unless, as a result of a previous tracheal operation, scar involves the arterial wall. A pedicle can be made from a strap muscle, and this may be interposed between the trachea and the innominate artery. Flat suction drains are placed in the pretracheal and substernal spaces, and the strap muscles are approximated in the midline. The sternum is wired with two or three heavy sutures.

After the incision has been closed, a heavy suture (Prolene or Mersilene) is placed through the skin crease beneath the chin and through the presternal skin. Two sutures, one on each side, may be used if there is a midline incision. These sutures are tied with the patient's neck in flexion to guard against sudden hyperextension of the neck in the first week following operation.

The patient is usually extubated as he awakens. An airway not satisfactory at this point is not likely to improve later on unless the problem is one of laryngeal edema, for which a small endotracheal tube is left in position for a few days, preferably with cuff deflated. A tracheostomy is not to be performed since the stoma may lie near the anastomosis and injure it. Tracheostomy also leads to inspissation of secretions. No stent is necessary if the anastomosis has been done properly.

REFERENCES

1. Montgomery, W.W.: The surgical management of supraglottic and subglottic stenosis. Ann. Otol. Rhinol. Laryngol. 77:534–546, 1968
2. Dedo, H.H., and Fishman, N.H.: Laryngeal release and sleeve resection for tracheal stenosis. Ann. Otol. Rhinol. Laryngol. 78:285–296, 1969
3. Grillo, H.C.: Surgery of the trachea. Current Problems in Surgery, July 1970
4. Grillo, H.C.: Surgical treatment of postintubation tracheal injuries. J. Thorac. Cardiovasc. Surg. 78:860–875, 1979
5. Grillo, H.C.: Primary reconstruction of airway after resection of subglottic laryngeal and upper tracheal stenosis. Ann. Thorac. Surg. 33:3–18, 1982

SUPRAHYOID LARYNGEAL RELEASE (MONTGOMERY)

When the gap after resection of an upper tracheal lesion is too great (more than 4 to 4.5 cm) for direct anastomosis, a laryngeal release operation, dropping the larynx down, permits approximation of the two tracheal ends.

A. The lesion in the upper trachea.

B. The "unbridgeable gap," or at least a gap that would require closure under undesirable tension.

C. The effect of laryngeal release.

D. The situation in full front view after excision of a segment of trachea. The gap is bridgeable only under tension. The dotted line shows the beginning division of the mylohyoid, geniohyoid, and genioglossus muscles and of the two horns of the hyoid bone.

E. The downward distraction of the larynx and upper trachea made possible by this maneuver closes the gap in the trachea. Visible above is the anterior pharyngeal wall with the exposed pre-epiglottic space and the ends of the hyoid on either side.

REFERENCE

1. Montgomery, W.W.: *Surgery of the Upper Respiratory System*, Volume 2. Philadelphia, Lea & Febiger, 1973

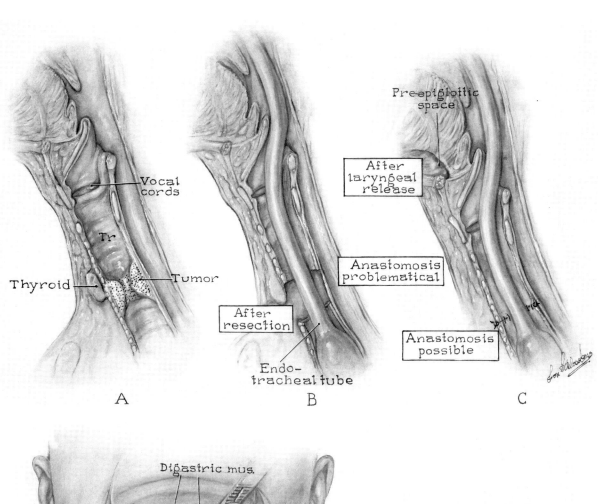

A

B

Pre-epiglottic space

After laryngeal release

Anastomosis problematical

Anastomosis possible

C

After resection

Endo-tracheal tube

Vocal cords

Tr

Thyroid

Tumor

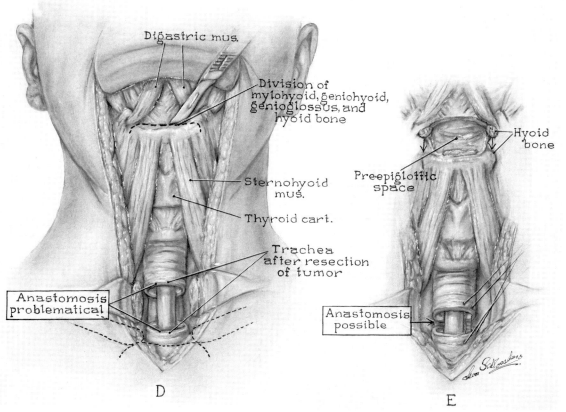

Digastric mus.

Division of mylohyoid, geniohyoid, genioglossus, and hyoid bone

Sternohyoid mus.

Thyroid cart.

Trachea after resection of tumor

Anastomosis problematical

D

Hyoid bone

Pre-epiglottic space

Anastomosis possible

E

303

Combined Subglottic and Upper Tracheal Stenosis

In many patients, an upper tracheal stenosis extends into the subglottic larynx, impinging upon the anterior cricoid cartilage and sometimes extending circumferentially and posteriorly. Such lesions are the result of damage—from endotracheal tubes used for ventilation, from cricothyroidostomy, or from a high stoma that eroded superiorly. If the stenosis reaches to the vocal cords without any free interval in the immediate subglottic larynx, it is difficult to perform a single-stage operation for correction. A bit of uninvolved airway immediately below the vocal cords permits a single-stage repair. Such procedures, very different from a simple segmental tracheal resection, are difficult and require experience and considerable attention to detail. Obviously it is not possible to perform a segmental airway resection at this level, since both recurrent laryngeal nerves would be destroyed. Two situations are considered—anterior and circumferential subglottic stenosis.

ANTERIOR SUBGLOTTIC STENOSIS

A and D. The stenosis is subglottic but involves only the anterior portion of the cricoid cartilage. Although the stenosis is circumferential in the trachea in this example, the posterior cricoid plate is not significantly involved. In some cases, the posterior wall of the trachea is totally uninvolved, as in a stenosis arising from a stomal injury with upward erosion. If the lesion extends only to the lower part of the anterior cricoid, resection may be performed as described in *Tracheal Resection—Anterior Approach*, except that a portion of the anterior cricoid is beveled off with the resection. If the full width of the anterior cricoid has to be resected as well as some distal trachea, a different approach must be used.

B and E. The specimen from resection of an upper tracheal stenosis includes a portion of the subglottic anterior larynx and a segment of the anterior cricoid.

C and F. The distal trachea has been tailored to match the defect above. Over the width of one ring of distal trachea, the line of division swings in a gentle curve from full width of the cartilage anteriorly to its inferior margin posteriorly. The membranous wall is divided transversely. The anastomosis is fashioned as in *Tracheal Resection—Anterior Approach*. The cut in the larynx may be quite sharply oblique. Inferiorly only one ring is divided obliquely, in order not to lead to loss of substance of the trachea by creating a floppy anterior flap. The effect is to arch the trachea slightly forward, widening the anastomosis. Since often there is submucosal thickening of the subglottic larynx up to the conus elasticus, the airway at this level is not fully normal. The arched anterior anastomosis allows full advantage to be taken of the necessarily oblique division at the lower end of the larynx.

G and H. At the conclusion of the tracheal anastomosis, the thyroid isthmus is reapproximated in front of the tracheal suture line. In some instances, when subglottic narrowing and edema suggest that temporary postoperative airway difficulty may develop, provision is made for a possible tracheostomy by suturing strap muscle to the anterior wall of the trachea, above the innominate artery and well below the anastomosis. This provides a triangle of tracheal wall below the resutured thyroid isthmus and above the strap muscle in which a tracheostomy may later be placed for temporary airway management. We no longer routinely employ tracheostomy with these high anastomoses, and if resection of a long tracheal segment leaves little space for the placement of a needed stoma, it is better to use a small endotracheal tube for four or five days. The tube is removed in the operating room and reinserted if the airway is still inadequate, and the tracheostomy is made through the previously marked triangle. By this time, tissue planes have begun to seal and the small tracheostomy tube is less likely to damage the anastomosis.

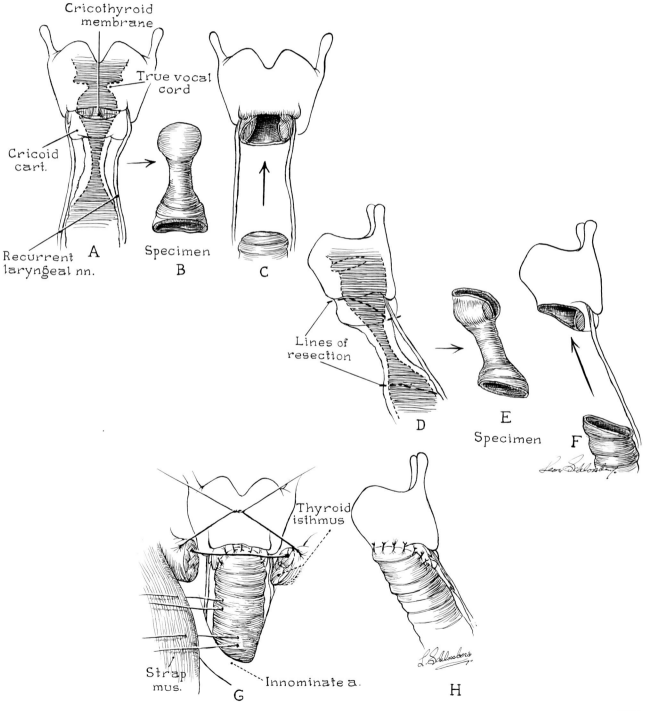

CIRCUMFERENTIAL SUBGLOTTIC STENOSIS

A. In the more difficult case illustrated here, damage in the lower subglottic region is circumferential and includes the mucosa over the cricoid plate.

B and C. The line of resection of the larynx begins as before in the midline, anteriorly, just below the inferior margin of the thyroid cartilage; it sweeps laterally through the cricothyroid membrane and across the posterior portion of the lateral lamina of the cricoid cartilage. The posterior cricoid plate remains intact. The lines of lateral division on both sides are anterior to the points of entry of the recurrent laryngeal nerves. The shelf of stenosis posteriorly is excised by making a transverse cut against the cricoid, inferior to the arytenoid cartilages and above the level of stenosis. The scarred mucosa and ridge of scar are removed from the anterior surface of the cricoid, leaving the denuded cartilage as intact as possible.

The distal tracheal cartilage, cut as in C and F in *Anterior Subglottic Stenosis*, forms a prowlike structure. When the membranous wall is reached posteriorly, instead of being cut transversely, a broad-based, gently rounded flap of membranous wall is shaped. This has excellent blood supply.

D. The anastomosis is performed much as in *Tracheal Resection—Anterior Approach* and *Anterior Subglottic Stenosis*, except that the posterior flap is tacked to the cricoid cartilage and sutured to the mucous membrane below the arytenoids. The anastomosis is somewhat difficult. We preplace four sutures from the base of the outside of the membranous flap to the inferior margin of the posterior plate of the cricoid cartilage. The posterior mucosal sutures are placed next, followed by the first lateral sutures on each side. All sutures (4-0 Vicryl) are placed so that their knots will be outside. The lateral anastomotic sutures are now begun from the back of the cartilage ring initially to what is left of the lateral lamina of the cricoid cartilage, continuing to the cricothyroid membrane up to the lateral traction sutures. The tracheal ends are drawn up by the traction sutures and the anastomotic sutures tied, beginning with the four sutures applying the membranous lower flap to the cricoid cartilage plate posteriorly. The posterior mucosal sutures are tied by placing the finger down into the lumen through the still-gaping anterior wall, and the sutures are cut as each is tied. The balance of the anastomotic sutures, anteriorly, are placed from the tracheal cartilage to the thyroid cartilage, and the anastomosis is completed in the usual manner. These cases are particularly difficult and should not be undertaken without considerable experience in the simpler types of tracheal reconstruction.

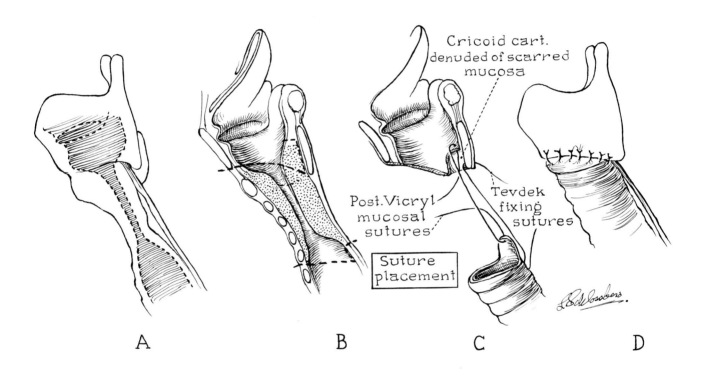

Cricoid cart. denuded of scarred mucosa

Post. Vicryl mucosal sutures

Tevdek fixing sutures

Suture placement

A   B   C   D

TRACHEOESOPHAGEAL FISTULA

A and B. Tracheoesophageal fistula after prolonged ventilatory support usually occurs as a result of pressure on the apposed walls of esophagus and trachea, between an inflated tracheal cuff and an in-lying esophageal feeding tube. The fistula usually lies at the level of the cuff, somewhat below the level of the tracheal stoma. More often than not, the circumferential pressure damage produced by the intratracheal balloon has resulted in tracheal stenosis as well. If the fistula is identified while the patient still requires respiratory support, repair of the fistula is postponed. The esophagus is kept empty, and the lowest pressure high-volume cuff that will provide a gentle seal of the trachea is used for continuation of the ventilation. A gastrostomy tube is inserted to drain the stomach and prevent reflux, and the patient is fed through a jejunostomy. Once the patient has been weaned from the respirator, a single-stage operation is performed.

The collar incision often circumcises the stoma. Rarely is the vertical limb needed. The initial dissection is identical to that described for upper tracheal resection.

C and D. After the trachea has been transected below the distal margin of the stenotic segment, the specimen is elevated and the fistulous connection completely isolated circumferentially and dissected off the esophagus. In many cases the anterior tracheal stoma is so close to the injured segment of trachea as to be conveniently included in the resection. If there is a segment of fairly normal trachea between the stoma and the stenotic segment, the stoma may be left in place. If the fistulous opening is long and the tracheal wall is not destroyed anteriorly as far down as the fistula extends, the margin of the tracheal opening is excised as a V, with the point of the V aimed distally, so that the posterior membranous wall may be reconstructed with a vertical suture line before the tracheal ends are anastomosed, and without any resection (not shown). We have seen a granuloma form at the junction of the T closure in such cases. If necessary, some of the esophageal wall may be left at the sides of the V so that there will be enough tissue for reconstruction of the membranous wall.

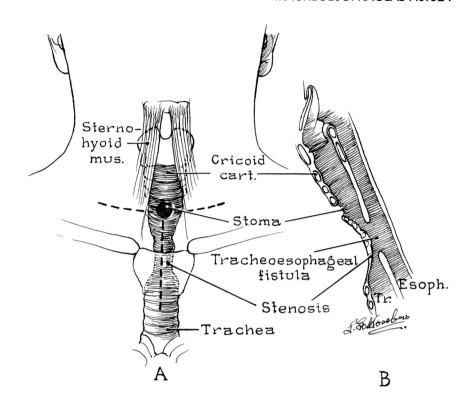

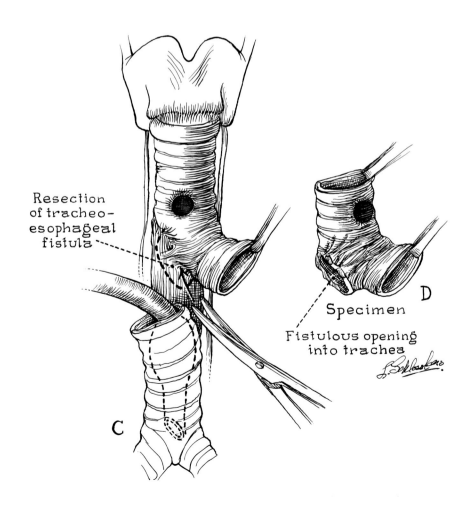

TRACHEOESOPHAGEAL FISTULA *(Continued)*

E. The esophagus is closed longitudinally with two layers of 4-0 silk.

F. The sternohyoid muscle, or sometimes the sternothyroid, is used to create a pedicle and is sutured into place over the esophageal closure, interposing healthy muscle between the vertical suture line in the esophagus and the transverse suture line of the tracheal anastomosis about to be made.

G. The completed anastomosis of the trachea is shown.

In the rare case when direct trauma has produced a tracheoesophageal fistula without circumferential damage to the trachea, repair does not require resection of the trachea. The trachea and esophagus are carefully dissected by keeping close to the trachea and esophagus until the fistula is fully identified. The recurrent laryngeal nerves are not deliberately exposed. In such cases, extra tissue from the anterior esophageal wall is used to provide sufficient tissue for closure of the membranous tracheal wall without tension. The esophagus is first closed in layers, muscle is interposed, and the trachea is repaired longitudinally. Exposure is more difficult because the trachea has not been divided.

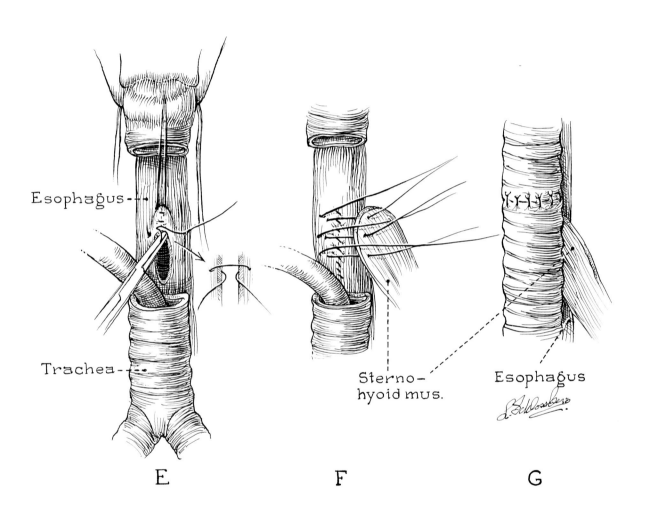

Esophagus

Trachea

Sterno-
hyoid mus.

Esophagus

E   F   G

TRANSTHORACIC TRACHEAL RESECTION

A. The transthoracic approach is used for tumors of the lower trachea and carina and some inflammatory lesions. Occasionally it is made necessary by a previous transthoracic approach for stenosis. When it is necessary to re-explore a stenotic trachea previously operated on inappropriately through the chest, it is generally better to use a trapdoor chest wall incision, which allows exposure of the upper as well as the lower trachea. It is indeed possible to resect the lower trachea and the carina through a median sternotomy, by dividing the pericardium anteriorly and posteriorly between the superior vena cava and the aortic arch and displacing the innominate artery upward and the pulmonary artery inferiorly (see pages 250–253, *Transpericardial Stapling of Bronchus for Postpneumonectomy Bronchial Fistula*). But this exposure is adequate only for small and wholly intratracheal tumors. For more extensive dissection, difficult anastomosis, or excision of parts of other organs, such as the esophagus, the high right posterolateral thoracotomy in the 4th interspace remains the incision of choice. The right arm is draped free, and the neck and anterior chest are included in the field. This allows for alteration of the incision or addition of a cervical component, should laryngeal release or other maneuvers be necessary. The arm may be swung back and forth for access to the chest.

The endotracheal tube used is extra long to reach into a main bronchus and of a diameter to fit in a main bronchus. The end is cut off squarely, so that it may be placed in the right or left main bronchus without obstructing the upper lobe orifice. It also carries a shorter cuff, which seals the main bronchus without herniating. Double-lumen tubes are not useful in this sort of operation. High frequency ventilation with small catheters is an advantage. In general, it is better not to consider using cardiopulmonary bypass, except for the simplest type of resection, and then it is unnecessary.

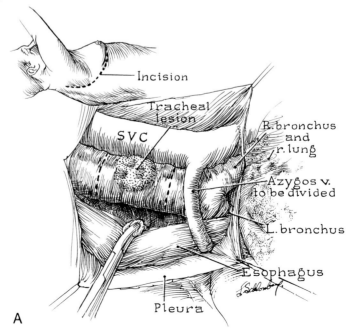

A

312

B. Dissection of the trachea is carried out with gentle compression of the lung. Effort is made to take surrounding tissues with the tumor. Eventually, the trachea is dissected circumferentially below the tumor, and sometimes above it, although the upper portion of the dissection may be completed after division of the trachea below. Traction sutures are placed in the midlateral tracheal wall distal to the tumor. If the transection is close to the carina, the sutures are placed in the lateral walls of the right and left main bronchi. Anesthesia tubing brought across the field is joined to the tube in the distal trachea or, preferably, the left main bronchus, to allow collapse of the right lung for better exposure during the anastomosis. If this results in intrapulmonary shunting, the right pulmonary artery may be gently clamped.

If a significant length of trachea must be resected, the necessary mobilization is preferably carried out before transection of the trachea. In the initial exposure, the azygos vein is divided or, if adherent to tumor, a segment is taken with the specimen; the vagus nerve is similarly approached, well below the takeoff of the right recurrent laryngeal nerve. The specimen is elevated and resection completed. The left recurrent laryngeal nerve lies over the aortic arch, immediately on the left lateral side of the trachea. Extensive mediastinal node dissection is not performed, for fear of devascularizing the trachea. If the tumor invades the esophageal wall, either a plaque of muscularis or a full-thickness disc of esophageal wall may be excised with the trachea. The esophagus is closed in two layers. The sutured segment, though narrowed, will permit the patient to swallow saliva and take liquids. In most cases, the segment will later dilate with use. In occasional cases, instrumental dilatation is required. If there is any question about the security of the esophageal closure, it should be reinforced with a flap of pleura or with a pedicled intercostal muscle flap.

Flexion of the neck, even with the patient in the lateral thoracotomy position, delivers much of the proximal trachea into the chest. This is a key maneuver in getting a tension-free anastomosis. Finger dissection of the anterior tracheal wall does not disturb blood supply and may help to allow the trachea to slide down into the chest. By gentle anterior dissection of the right and left main bronchi, the distal trachea may be mobilized enough to decrease tension.

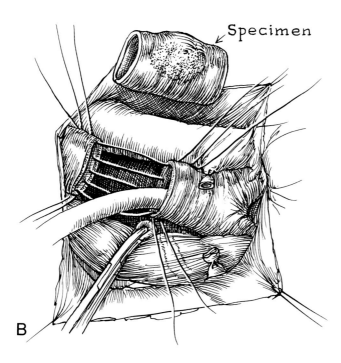

Specimen

B

TRANSTHORACIC TRACHEAL RESECTION *(Continued)*

C. More formal mobilization maneuvers involve dissection of the pulmonary artery and veins (*left*). The inferior pulmonary ligament is divided. The pericardium is opened with a U-shaped incision beneath the inferior vein. The attachment of the pericardium is divided just below the vein. This step alone allows the right hilum to rise up about a centimeter, as shown at right. If necessary, the pericardium may be incised completely around the hilum (*dotted lines*). Posteriorly, we prefer to do this beneath the pedicle of the lymph nodes and bronchial arteries that go to the right main bronchus. These are preserved to avoid lymphatic obstruction in the right lung in the early postoperative days. The subcarinal lymph nodes should not be radically resected. Blunt dissection of the left main bronchus anteriorly, beneath the aortic arch, may be of some help. The technique of anastomosis is similar to that used in the upper trachea.

D. The airtightness of the completed anastomosis is checked under saline after the tip of the endotracheal tube has been withdrawn proximal to the anastomosis. A pedicled pleural flap is wrapped around the anastomosis. If there is any question about the security of the anastomosis, a pedicled intercostal muscle flap is placed around it. From such a flap we prefer to excise the costal periosteum, which in one case formed a circular ring of bone about the esophagus, causing an obstruction that ultimately required operative relief.

If the patient requires postoperative ventilatory support, the cuff should be placed so that it will not rest on the suture line.

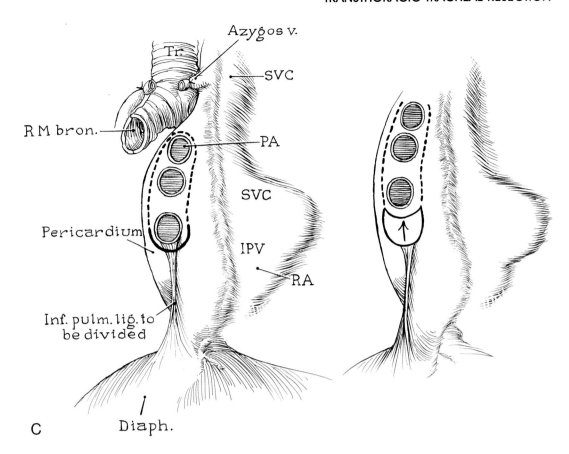

Azygos v.

Tr.

SVC

R M bron.

PA

SVC

Pericardium

IPV

RA

Inf. pulm. lig. to
be divided

Diaph.

C

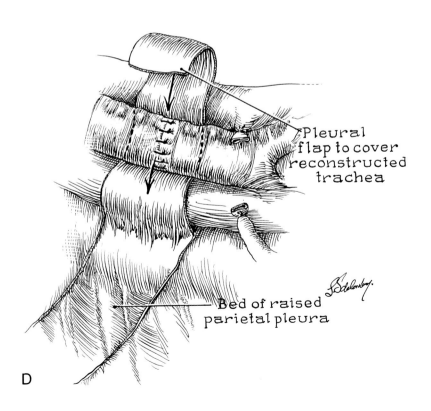

Pleural
flap to cover
reconstructed
trachea

Bed of raised
parietal pleura

D

315

Tracheo-Innominate Artery Fistula

EROSION BY TRACHEOSTOMY TUBE

When the neck is hyperextended for performance of tracheostomy in children or young adults, over half the trachea, and the innominate artery, rise into the neck. It follows that if the tracheal stoma is placed in relation to the sternal notch, rather than in relation to the cricoid cartilage, the stoma will actually be in the mid trachea and lie just above the innominate artery.

A, B, and C. A tube may erode through the artery immediately inferior to the margin of the stoma, producing the lesion shown in B. The premonitory hemorrhage that often occurs should lead to inspection of the tracheal stoma, if necessary by bronchoscopy.

D. In the event of massive hemorrhage, control may be obtained by finger compression down and forward, against the sternum at the site of the bleeding. An endotracheal tube is slipped into the airway and the cuff firmly inflated to prevent blood from running into the lung. The surgeon's finger is held in place while the patient is moved to the operating room.

E. Exposure is best obtained through a collar incision at the level of the stoma and a vertical sternotomy; hemorrhage is controlled with finger pressure during the initial dissection. Dissection is carried distally on the innominate artery to just proximal to its bifurcation, and a gentle vascular clamp or tourniquet is applied. The recurrent laryngeal nerve is to be avoided as it passes around the subclavian artery just beyond this. With bleeding controlled, the best maneuver is usually resection of the damaged segment of the artery and careful oversewing of the proximal and distal ends with double suture lines. Neurological sequelae are rare. An arterial repair would lie in a potentially septic field. Simple ligation is not as secure against secondary hemorrhage as is suture closure. The stumps of the artery proximally and distally are buried under whatever healthy tissue is available—thymus or strap muscles. It is usually best to create a new tracheal stoma at a higher, more appropriate level (2nd or 3rd tracheal ring) by inserting a tube long enough to pass beyond the previous stoma. Strap muscle is sutured over the original stoma.

Such an arterial fistula is best prevented by correct initial placement of the tracheostomy tube.

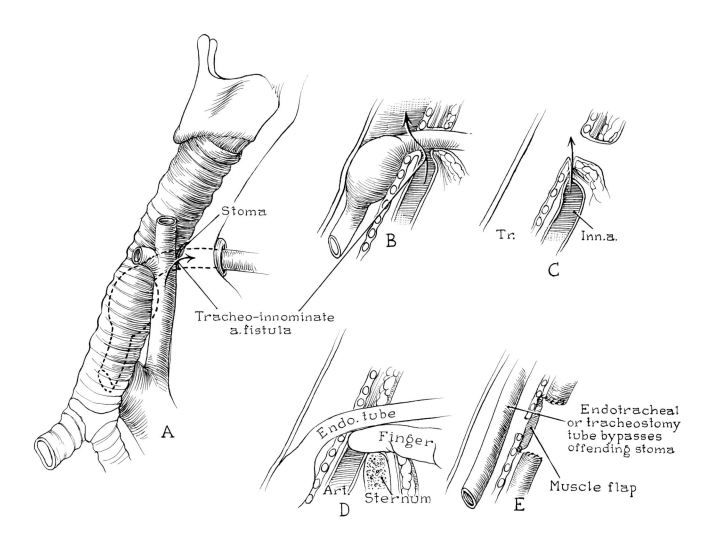

EROSION FROM HIGH PRESSURE TRACHEOSTOMY CUFF

A and B. The high pressure cuff eroded anteriorly through the tracheal wall and into the overlying innominate artery. Occasionally the tip of a tube angulating forward produces a similar erosion.

C. It is impossible to get a finger down to the level of this fistula, which lies entirely within the mediastinum. The immediate hemorrhage is controlled by placement of an endotracheal tube with a high pressure cuff or with a low pressure cuff inflated sufficiently to compress the opening.

D and E. After control of hemorrhage, exposure is achieved as in the circumstance in *Transthoracic Tracheal Resection*. There is usually circumferential damage to the trachea at cuff level. The involved arterial segment is excised, and proximal and distal ends are sutured closed. The circumferential damage produced by the high pressure cuff requires tracheal resection and end-to-end anastomosis (see section on *Combined Subglottic and Upper Tracheal Stenosis*). Such patients obviously will continue to require the ventilation that they were receiving just prior to the hemorrhage. The tube cuff must be positioned either well above or well below the anastomotic line to avoid pressure on the tracheal anastomosis.

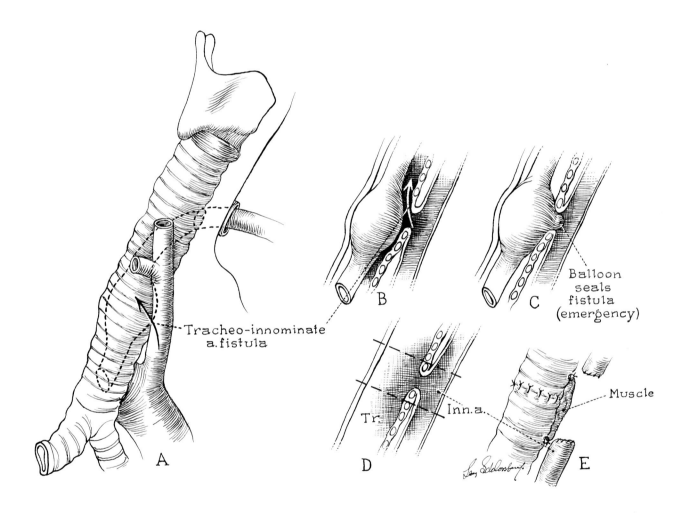

Tracheo-innominate
a.fistula

Balloon
seals
fistula
(emergency)

B

C

Tr.

Inn.a.

Muscle

D

E

A

Carinal Resection and Reconstruction

There is no one technique for reconstruction of the carina. The type of resection varies with the size and location of the tumor. The principal decision to be made by the surgeon is whether in fact the tumor is amenable to resection and primary reconstruction, without complicated skin flaps or use of prosthetic materials. In the present state of evolution of surgical technique and prostheses, we consider it preferable to use primary radiotherapy if a direct anastomosis will not be possible. Judgment as to resectability is based on personal evaluation rather than upon arbitrary criteria. The approach is from the right chest.

REFERENCES

1. Grillo, H.C.: Tracheal tumors: Surgical management. Ann. Thorac. Surg. 26:112–125, 1978
2. Grillo, H.C.: Carinal reconstruction. Ann. Thorac. Surg. 34:356–373, 1982

SMALL CARCINOMA CONFINED TO THE CARINA

In this situation, only a little of the trachea and of the right and left main bronchi must be removed. Reconstruction is by suturing the medial edges of the right and left main bronchi together, then fitting the trachea into the V thus made to create a new carina. Sewing the right and left bronchi together tethers them at a level beneath the aortic arch. Any length to be gained must thus be obtained by cervical flexion, which produces a downward movement of the trachea. This method of reconstruction is therefore applicable in only a few patients.

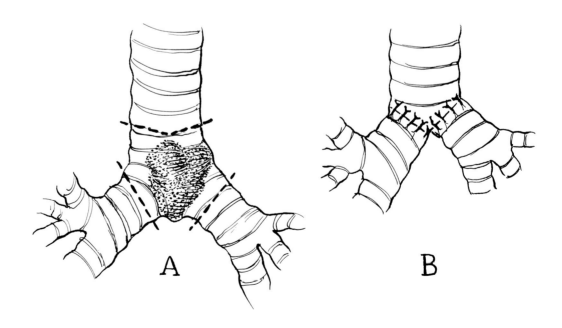

A   B

A. When the tumor is larger and more trachea must be resected, the reconstruction shown previously in *Small Carcinoma Confined to the Carina* is impossible. One must determine whether, without tension, the trachea will more easily reach the right or the left main bronchus.

B. If the trachea will reach the left main bronchus, the situation is technically simpler. Anastomosis is made from the end of the trachea to the end of the left main bronchus. It is not necessary to taper the tracheal end by any plastic or constricting technique. If all sutures are placed symmetrically from the larger tracheal end to the smaller bronchial end, a symmetrical and airtight anastomosis will be achieved. The endotracheal tube from above is passed downward into the left main bronchus, and ventilation is continued with the right lung collapsed. An ovoid right lateral opening is made in the trachea, 1 cm proximal to the anastomosis (to maintain blood supply in the isthmus between the two anastomoses). The opening is kept entirely in the lateral wall, with cartilage on all sides of it, and is not extended into the membranous wall. The right lung, which has been partly mobilized by division of the pulmonary ligament and often by an incision in the pericardium below the inferior vein (see page 315, *Transthoracic Tracheal Resection, C*), is elevated and the bronchus sutured to the aperture in the trachea. Both anastomoses are covered with pleural flaps. The anesthesia tube is pulled above the anastomoses and the right lung is allowed to expand.

C. In a rarely used alternative, the trachea is anastomosed to the right main bronchus, and the left main bronchus is anastomosed to the trachea through a lateral oval opening. Ventilation in the left lung must be continued during the second anastomosis so that the inflated left lung will keep its bronchial stump within easy reach.

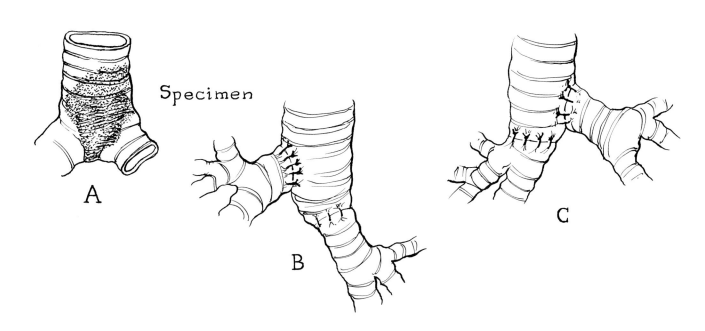

Specimen

A

B

C

EXTENDED RESECTION OF CARINA

For extensive resections, the techniques in *Small Carcinoma Confined to the Carina* and *Larger Carinal Tumor* will not be adequate, since the left main bronchus, tethered by the aortic arch, will not reach the stump of the trachea without excessive tension. The right lung is mobilized as described in *Larger Carinal Tumor*, and the right main bronchus is approximated to the end of the trachea. As first described by Barclay, McSwan, and Welsh, the left main bronchus is brought across the mediastinum and sutured into the medial wall of the bronchus intermedius a little farther from the tracheal anastomosis than shown.

REFERENCE

1. Barclay, R.S., McSwan, N., and Welsh, T.M.: Tracheal reconstruction without the use of grafts. Thorax 12:177–180, 1957

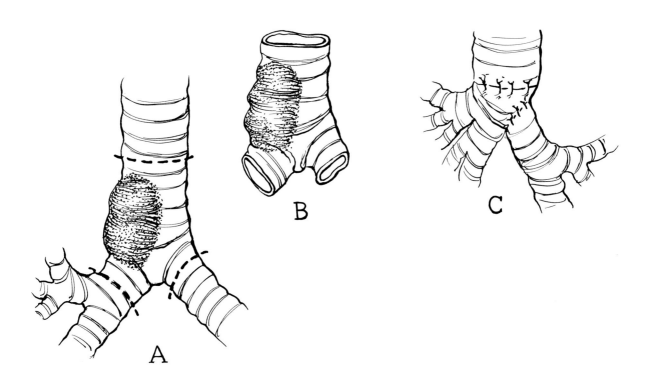

A and B. The carina and right main bronchus are resected with the right upper lobe attached, saving the middle and lower lobes, or at least the lower lobe.

C. The trachea and left main bronchus are anastomosed end-to-end, and the bronchus intermedius is elevated to be sutured into an oval window in the lateral wall of the trachea, sufficiently above the anastomosis of the trachea with the left main bronchus to ensure the viability of the intervening portion of tracheal wall.

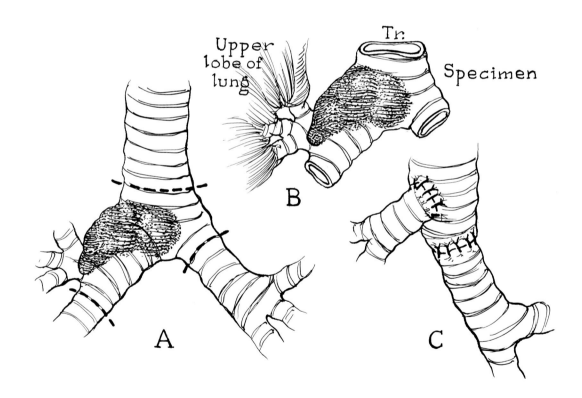

CARINAL RESECTION AND RIGHT PNEUMONECTOMY

A and B. This is applied more often for patients with bronchogenic carcinoma involving the main bronchus and carina than for those with primary tracheal tumors. If the tumor does not extend very far up the trachea, the operation is conceptually and mechanically quite simple to perform. Physiologically, the operation is the equivalent of a right pneumonectomy, but it has been the general experience that mortality is much higher than for simple pneumonectomy, in part perhaps due to pulmonary lymphatic obstruction in the early postoperative days if extensive lymph node dissection is done.

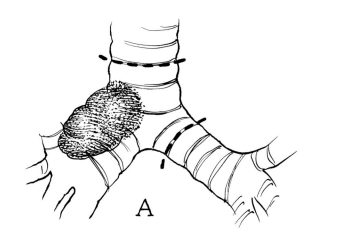

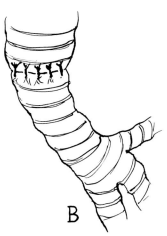

CARINAL RESECTION FOR LESION INVOLVING
LEFT MAIN BRONCHUS

A, B, and C. There is no good solution for the lesion that involves a considerable segment of trachea and enough of the left main bronchus so that the left lung cannot be salvaged. It must first be determined that the right lung can be elevated sufficiently and the trachea brought down sufficiently so that the right lung can be safely connected to the trachea. If it is considered that this is feasible, there are a number of approaches. Perelman resects the tracheobronchial specimen and transects the left main bronchus—from the right chest—by stapling it off distally and leaving the lung *in situ*. We had difficulty with such a patient who developed a persistent vascular shunt through the residual lung and eventually required left pneumonectomy. Another option is to remove the left lung concurrently, but through a left thoracotomy. A median sternotomy could be used in this difficult situation but presents obvious technical problems. Another approach employed has been transverse bilateral thoracotomy through the 4th interspaces, across the sternum. This provides adequate exposure, but the physiological burden imposed on the patient recommends that this approach be reserved for young patients with excellent respiratory reserve.

REFERENCE

1. Perelman, M., and Koreleva, N.: Surgery of the trachea. World J. Surg. 4:583–593, 1980

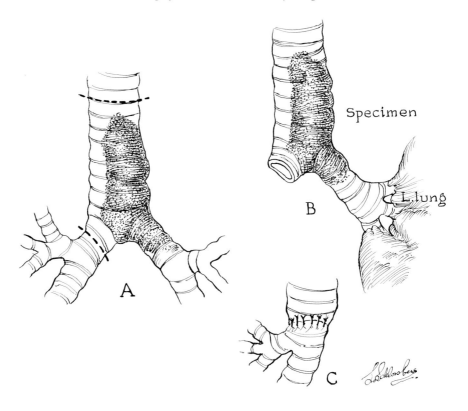

A and B. Residual tumor found microscopically in the line of resection after left pneumonectomy, or recurrence in the main bronchial stump of a tumor such as a carcinoid, has been approached through the right chest by gently displacing the lung forward but keeping it inflated throughout the operation. High frequency ventilation has a clear role here. The specimen is resected, and end-to-end anastomosis is performed.

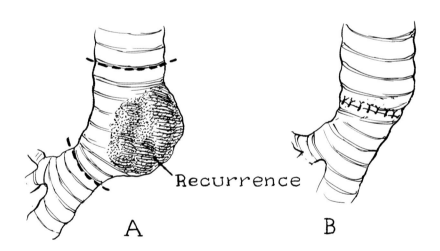

327

TRACHEOSTOMY

A. With the patient supine, a folded or rolled towel 3 to 4 inches in thickness is placed below the shoulders to allow for hyperextension of the head.

    The procedure is best performed in the operating room and with a transoral endotracheal tube in place. The various anatomical landmarks of importance during the operation are shown. If local anesthesia is used (1% lidocaine), care should be taken to anesthetize all of the soft tissues down to the pretracheal fascia.

    The anatomical landmarks are shown from the lateral view. The transverse incision, made some 2 to 3 cm above the suprasternal notch, is carried through the platysma muscle down to the strap muscles, which are separated in the midline, and down to the pretracheal fascia.

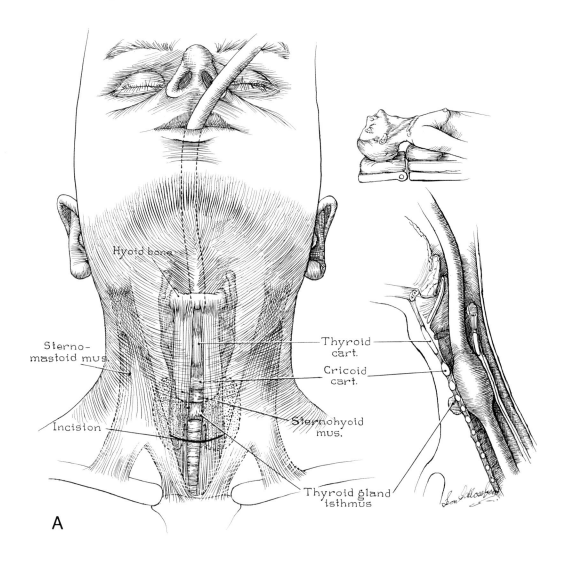

A

B. *1, 2, and 3:* The thyroid isthmus is retracted superiorly in most instances. Occasionally in a low-lying thyroid, it may be easier to push the isthmus downward. Rarely, if ever, is it necessary to transect the thyroid isthmus. The trachea is cleared of all adventitial tissue and elevated with a hook placed into the 1st tracheal or the cricoid cartilage. The transoral endotracheal tube is withdrawn to just below the vocal cords, and the 3rd and 4th tracheal rings are incised vertically.

 4: A tracheal spreader holds the tracheal incision open, and a tracheostomy cannula of size appropriate for the given patient is inserted into the trachea. The tracheal balloon, tested before insertion, is then inflated to the point of preventing air leak, and the tracheostomy tube is tied in place.

 The technical and anatomical pitfalls of this operation include injury to the anterior cervical veins, left innominate vein, innominate artery, internal jugular vein, and carotid artery, as well as the creation of a pneumothorax, especially in children, and the placement of the stoma too low, which may ultimately result in erosion of the innominate artery. Tracheostomy is often considered a "minor" procedure, delegated to a less experienced surgeon who often has to work in far from ideal circumstances, when in fact this operation should be performed under the guidance of the most competent surgeon and ideally in an operating room or at least a well-equipped procedure room or intensive care unit.

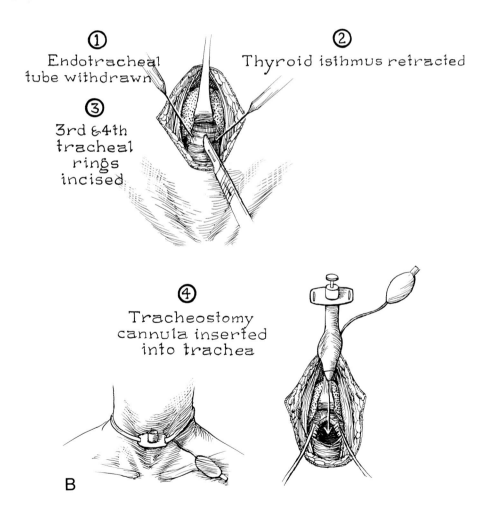

① Endotracheal tube withdrawn

② Thyroid isthmus retracted

③ 3rd & 4th tracheal rings incised

④ Tracheostomy cannula inserted into trachea

B

CLOSURE OF A PERSISTENT TRACHEAL STOMA

Persistent tracheal stomas are usually found to have a mucocutaneous union of trachea and skin. Often the patient has had the tracheostomy for a long time, with extended periods of ventilation, and is old or debilitated. Simply drawing a strap muscle over the aperture creates the potential for formation of a granuloma from the raw tissue presented to the interior of the trachea; this is particularly likely to occur with a large stoma. We prefer to cover the stomal orifice with a circular flap developed from the peristomal skin.

A. A circular incision is made around the stoma to define the skin that will be used for closure. Triangles of skin are excised on either side in the classic technique for permitting linear closure of a circular defect.

B and C. The collar of skin is carefully elevated, leaving sufficient attachment to the trachea to preserve its blood supply.

D and E. The skin is now inverted on itself by a subcuticular suture that effectively closes the stoma with an epithelial, (skin)-lined surface.

F and G. Margins of the skin defect are elevated. The strap muscles are dissected free on either side and approximated in the midline in layers. The platysma and skin are closed transversely.

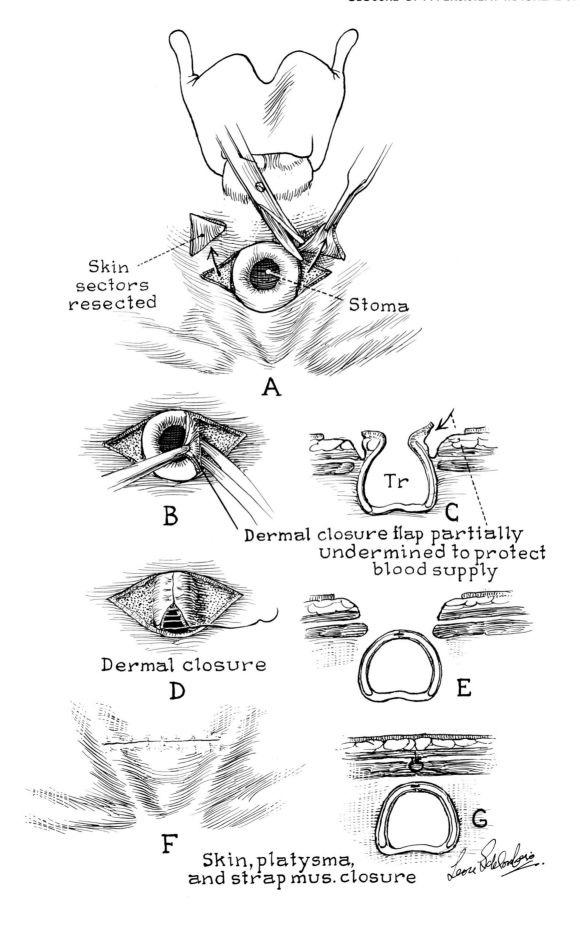

Skin sectors resected

Stoma

A

B

Tr

C

Dermal closure flap partially undermined to protect blood supply

Dermal closure

D

E

F

G

Skin, platysma, and strap mus. closure

The
Esophagus

The Esophagus

ANATOMY OF THE ESOPHAGUS

A. Arteries and nerves.
B. Lymphatics of esophagus and stomach.

Of particular importance in esophagectomy is the somewhat variable arrangement of the esophageal arteries arising from the bronchial and intercostal arteries and the thyrocervical trunk. The procedure for laryngo-pharyngo-esophagectomy without thoracotomy (trans-hiatal esophagectomy) and pharyngogastrostomy (pages 141–142) shows the way in which these may be secured in the procedure of esophagectomy

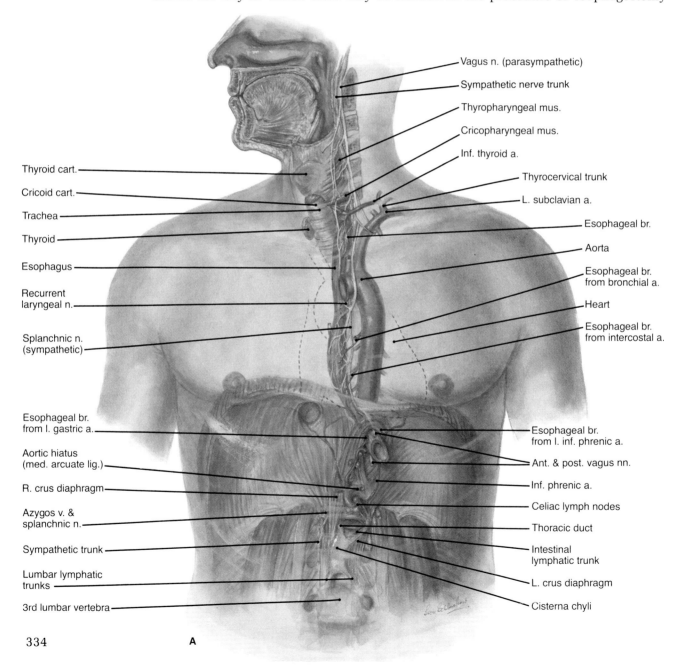

Vagus n. (parasympathetic)
Sympathetic nerve trunk
Thyropharyngeal mus.
Cricopharyngeal mus.
Inf. thyroid a.
Thyrocervical trunk
L. subclavian a.
Esophageal br.
Aorta
Esophageal br. from bronchial a.
Heart
Esophageal br. from intercostal a.

Thyroid cart.
Cricoid cart.
Trachea
Thyroid
Esophagus
Recurrent laryngeal n.
Splanchnic n. (sympathetic)

Esophageal br. from l. gastric a.
Aortic hiatus (med. arcuate lig.)
R. crus diaphragm
Azygos v. & splanchnic n.
Sympathetic trunk
Lumbar lymphatic trunks
3rd lumbar vertebra

Esophageal br. from l. inf. phrenic a.
Ant. & post. vagus nn.
Inf. phrenic a.
Celiac lymph nodes
Thoracic duct
Intestinal lymphatic trunk
L. crus diaphragm
Cisterna chyli

A

without thoracotomy. The distribution of the lymphatics is such that most surgeons, while giving an individual cancer as wide a margin of resection as is reasonably possible, have abandoned the idea of a "super-radical cancer operation" as impractical and unfeasible so far as the soft tissues of the mediastinum are concerned. However, it is increasingly common practice to remove the entire esophagus for a carcinoma at any level and, for cancers of the lower esophagus and the esophagogastric junction, to include in the resection proximal stomach, lesser curvature, spleen, omentum, and lymph nodes about the celiac axis.

From Zuidema, G.D. (Ed.) and Schlossberg, L. (Illustrator): *Atlas of Human Functional Anatomy*, 3rd Edition. Baltimore, Johns Hopkins University Press, 1985, with permission.

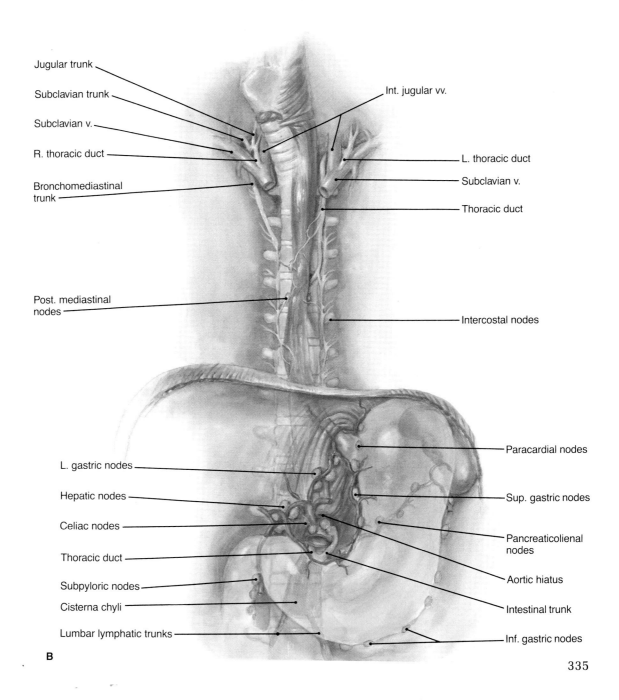

B

335

ZENKER'S DIVERTICULUM OF THE PHARYNX

A, B, and C. The diverticulum arises from the posterior midline of the pharynx between the oblique and transverse fibers of the inferior constrictor of the pharynx and above the cricopharyngeal muscle, ordinarily then presenting somewhat to the left as shown. The diverticulum descends along the esophagus, to which it is attached by loose areolar tissue.

D. The approach is by incision along the anterior border of the sternocleidomastoid muscle, allowing for freedom in exposing both the origin and the lower end of the diverticulum. The only structure of significance to be divided is the middle thyroid vein. The thyroid gland is retracted medially and the carotid sheath retracted laterally, providing access to the esophagus. The recurrent laryngeal nerve, shown on the drawing, need not be dissected out. The diverticulum, having been identified at its distal end and lifted up in the wound, is followed down to its neck, while the esophagus is displaced medially.

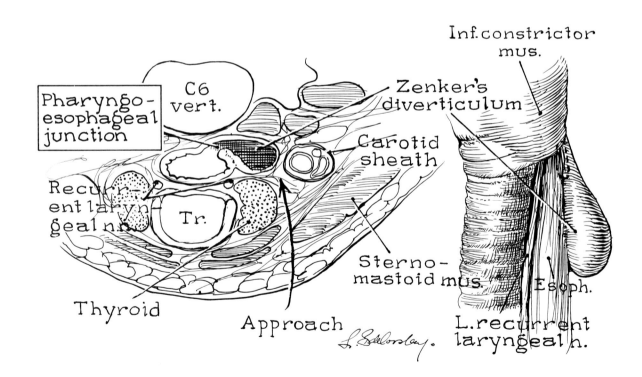

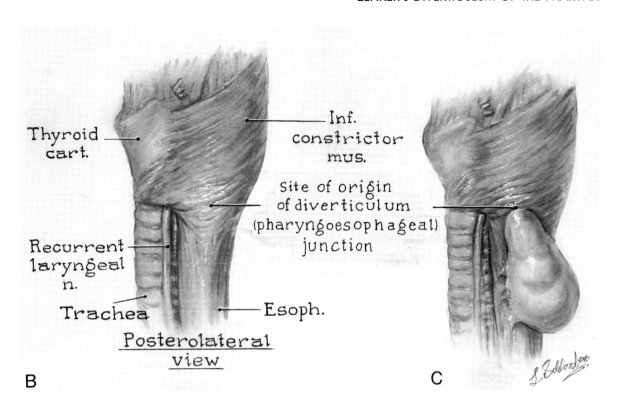

Thyroid cart.

Inf. constrictor mus.

Site of origin of diverticulum (pharyngoesophageal) junction

Recurrent laryngeal n.

Trachea

Esoph.

Posterolateral view

B

C

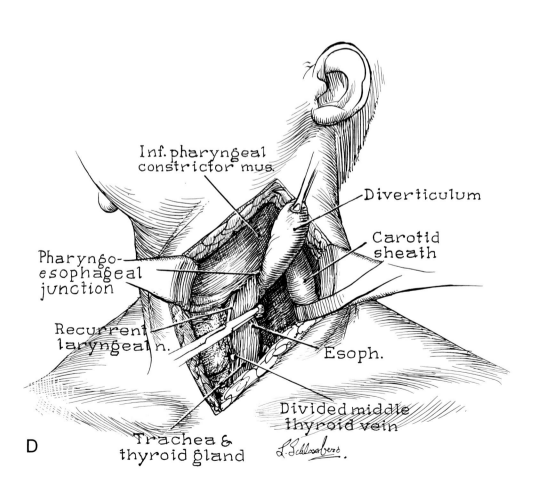

Inf. pharyngeal constrictor mus.

Diverticulum

Carotid sheath

Pharyngo-esophageal junction

Recurrent laryngeal n.

Esoph.

Trachea & thyroid gland

Divided middle thyroid vein

D

E. The muscular fibers—inferior constrictor and cricopharyngeal—below the orifice of the diverticulum are elevated and divided to prevent recurrence of the diverticulum. There are some who, at least for the smaller diverticula, rely on this myotomy alone, with resection of the diverticulum.

F. A single application of the linear stapler, here the TA 30 instrument, suffices to close off the neck of the diverticulum. The closure need not be oversewn. A tube in the esophagus, from the beginning of the operation, helps with initial identification of the esophagus and prevents tenting of the esophagus as the neck of the diverticulum is stapled.

G. The submucosa bulges forward as the myotomy, 2 to 3 cm long, is extended down from the stapled neck of the diverticulum.

REFERENCE

1. Payne, W.W.: The role of stapling devices in the treatment of pharyngoesophageal (Zenker's) diverticulum. In: M.M. Ravitch and F.M. Steichen (Eds.). *Principles and Practice of Surgical Stapling.* Chicago, Year Book Medical Publishers, 1987

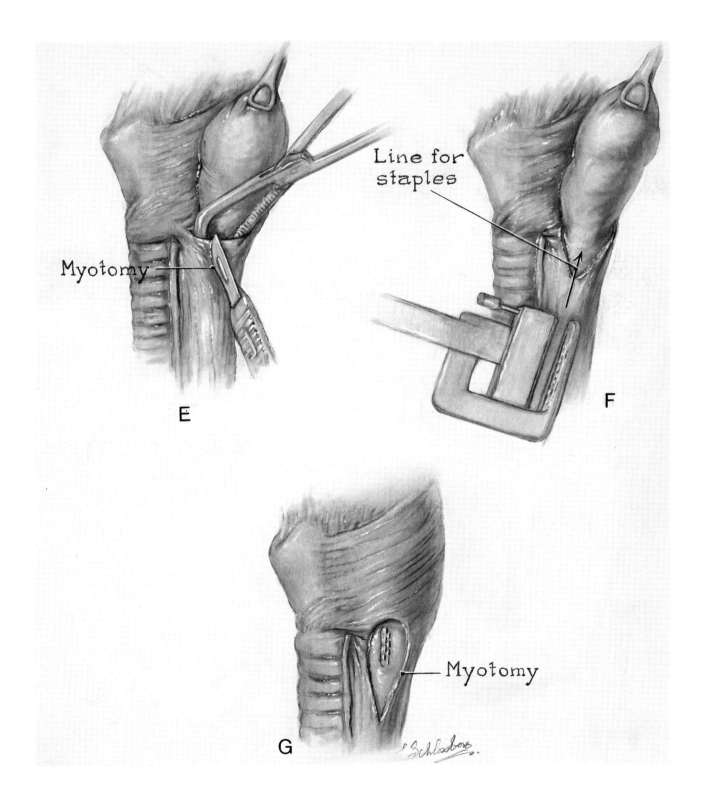

Line for staples

Myotomy

E

F

Myotomy

G

LARYNGO-PHARYNGO-ESOPHAGECTOMY WITHOUT THORACOTOMY (TRANSHIATAL ESOPHAGECTOMY) AND PHARYNGOGASTROSTOMY

A. The operation is performed by two teams, coordinating efforts in neck and abdomen as shown in the two sketches on the right side of the plate. For carcinoma of the cervical esophagus, the concomitant laryngectomy and—for disease metastatic in the lymph nodes—a radical neck dissection (here on the right) are performed by a second team of surgeons. The approach to the neck is through a single, or double transverse, or Y incision, at the surgeon's discretion. A complete right radical neck dissection precedes the elevation of the cervical esophagus; the specimen is left atttached medially to the trachea and esophagus. The trachea is transected at the level appropriate for a secure permanent tracheostomy, and the peroral endotracheal tube is replaced by one inserted into the open end of the distal trachea, connected to tubing passed off the table to the anesthetist. At this point, the hypopharynx may be divided, as shown, anteriorly above the larynx as for laryngectomy and proceeding circumferentially, transecting posteriorly down to the prevertebral fascia. (Alternatively, after the radical neck dissection and transection of the trachea distally, the esophagus may be delivered into the neck following the mobilization illustrated in B and C, and the entire specimen—of esophagus, larynx and nodes, sternocleidomastoid muscle, and jugular vein on the side of the radical neck dissection—may be all delivered, with the specimen now attached only at the level of the hypopharynx. The transection of the hypopharynx can be performed at this moment, immediately before the anastomosis with the stomach shown in D.)

Upper Left: Transection superiorly has freed the larynx and hypopharynx, which are shown wrapped in a sponge. Anesthesia is given through the tube transferred to the distal trachea. A right radical neck dissection has been performed for lymph nodal disease. Mobilization of the stomach is now accomplished by ligating the short gastric, the left gastroepiploic, and the left gastric vessels (*bottom left*) while preserving the right gastric and right gastroepiploic vessels as well as the gastroepiploic arcade.

With retractors or an "upper hand" retractor elevating the rib cage (not shown), the phrenoesophageal ligament is opened. The upper edge of the diaphragmatic hiatus is elevated by traction with the curved small end of a Deaver retractor, the hiatal rim is incised if necessary, and the lower esophagus is brought into view by sharp and blunt dissection. A tape passed around the gastroesophageal junction to make traction permits identification and ligation or clipping of the lower esophageal vessels under direct vision or with palpation. The hiatus is progressively enlarged until the whole hand can be introduced around the esophagus into the posterior mediastinum. With a little care, major blood loss can be avoided.

Simultaneously, blunt finger dissection through the lower neck into the thoracic inlet develops the plane around the upper esophagus and identifies upper esophageal vessels by finger palpation.

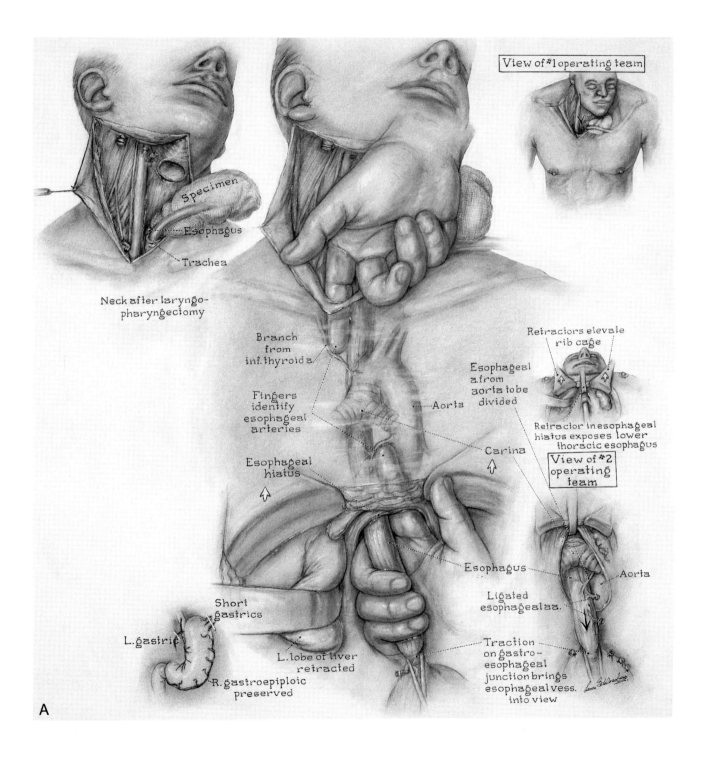

View of #1 operating team

Neck after laryngo-
pharyngectomy

Specimen

Esophagus

Trachea

Branch
from
inf. thyroid a.

Fingers
identify
esophageal
arteries

Esophageal
hiatus

Aorta

Carina

Retractors elevate
rib cage

Esophageal
a. from
aorta to be
divided

Retractor in esophageal
hiatus exposes lower
thoracic esophagus

View of #2
operating
team

Esophagus

Aorta

Short
gastrics

L. gastric

R. gastroepiploic
preserved

L. lobe of liver
retracted

Ligated
esophageal aa.

Traction
on gastro-
esophageal
junction brings
esophageal vess.
into view

A

B. With alternate traction on the stomach from below, and on the specimen from above, the esophageal arteries seen or palpated in the mediastinum are controlled with surgical clips and divided. The palpating finger guiding the tip of the surgical clip carrier is not illustrated, so as to render a clearer illustration. Lower esophageal arteries from the left gastric artery have already been divided.

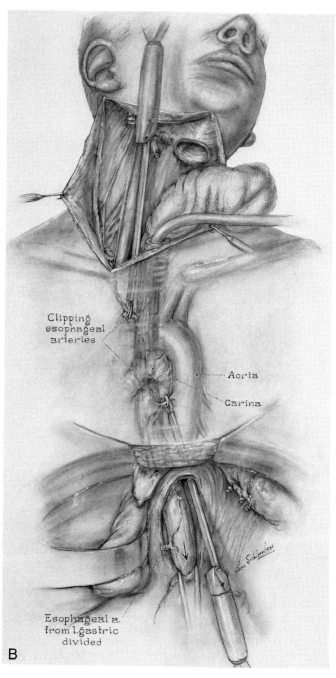

C. Following complete liberation of the entire, uninvolved, thoracic esophagus by sharp and blunt dissection and ligation of all visible and palpable esophageal vessels, the esophagus is drawn up through the thoracic inlet, followed by the stomach with intact right gastric and right gastroepiploic vessels. This upward displacement is facilitated by an extensive Kocher mobilization of the duodenum, which comes to occupy the former course of the stomach. The gastroesophageal junction, now in the neck, is divided and stapled with the GIA instrument. The gastric side of this GIA staple closure is reinforced with manual sutures. The pharyngogastrostomy will be into the apex of the gastric fundus. Pyloroplasty is optional.

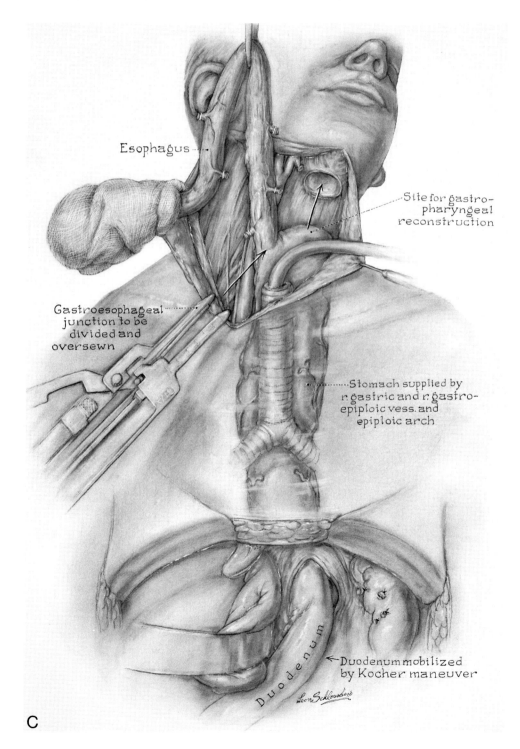

Esophagus

Site for gastro-
pharyngeal
reconstruction

Gastroesophageal
junction to be
divided and
oversewn

Stomach supplied by
r. gastric and r. gastro-
epiploic vess. and
epiploic arch

Duodenum

←Duodenum mobilized
by Kocher maneuver

C

343

D. Pharyngogastrostomy. Joining the lower oropharynx to an incision made into the apex of the gastric fundus is accomplished with one or two layers of manual interrupted nonabsorbable sutures. The posterior rows of the classical two-layer anastomosis are shown in the small insets. The tracheostomy will be brought through the incision or through an opening in the lower flap, depending upon the circumstance.

REFERENCES

1. Denk, W.: Zur Radikaloperation des Ösophaguskarzinoms. (Vorläufige Mitteilung.) Zentralbl. Chir. 27:1065–1068, 1913
   Early (earliest?) suggestion for transhiatal esophagectomy—cadaver operation only
2. Turner, G.G.: Some experiences in the surgery of the oesophagus. N. Engl. J. Med. 205:657–674, 1931
3. Ong, G.B., and Lee, T.C.: Pharyngogastric anastomosis after oesophago-pharyngectomy for carcinoma of the hypopharynx and cervical oesophagus. Br. J. Surg. 48:193–200, 1960
4. Ong, G.B.: Resection and reconstruction of the esophagus. Current Problems in Surgery, September 1971
   Transhiatal esophagectomy, historical review of resection of esophagus
5. Orringer, M.B., and Sloan, H.: Esophagectomy without thoracotomy. J. Thorac. Cardiovasc. Surg. 76:643–654, 1978
6. Orringer, M.B.: Transhiatal esophagectomy without thoracotomy for carcinoma of the thoracic esophagus. Ann. Surg. 200:282–288, 1984

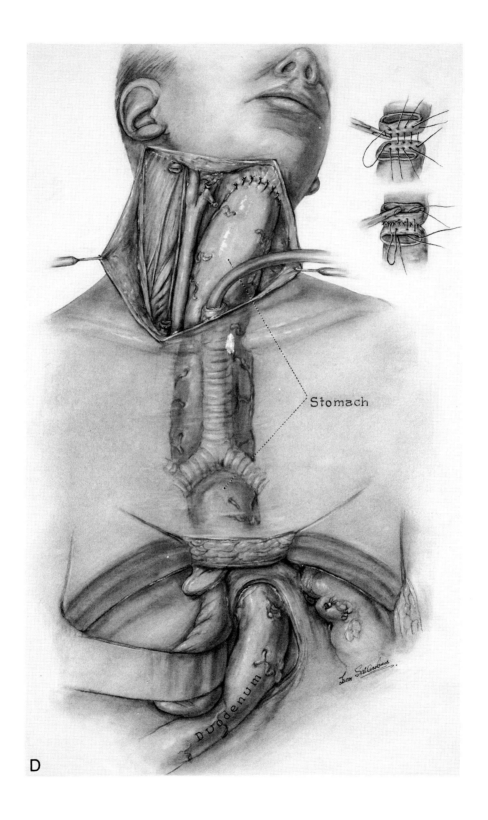

Stomach

Duodenum

D

TRANSHIATAL ESOPHAGECTOMY AND CERVICAL ESOPHAGOGASTROSTOMY

A. The abdominal incision is through the upper midline, and the cervical incision is oblique, upward from the sternal notch along the anterior border of the sternocleidomastoid muscle.

B. The stomach is mobilized by division of the left gastric artery and the coronary veins on the lesser curvature side and the short gastric vessels and the omentum, peripheral to the gastroepiploic vessels, on the greater curvature side. Mediastinal dissection and securing of the esophageal vessels are as in the illustrations for the previous procedure. The esophagus in the neck is approached between the right lobe of the thyroid and the carotid sheath, by dividing the middle thyroid vein. Dissection is immediately upon the esophagus to spare the recurrent laryngeal nerves.

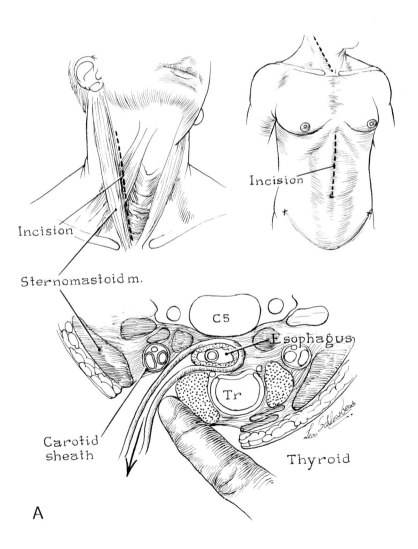

A

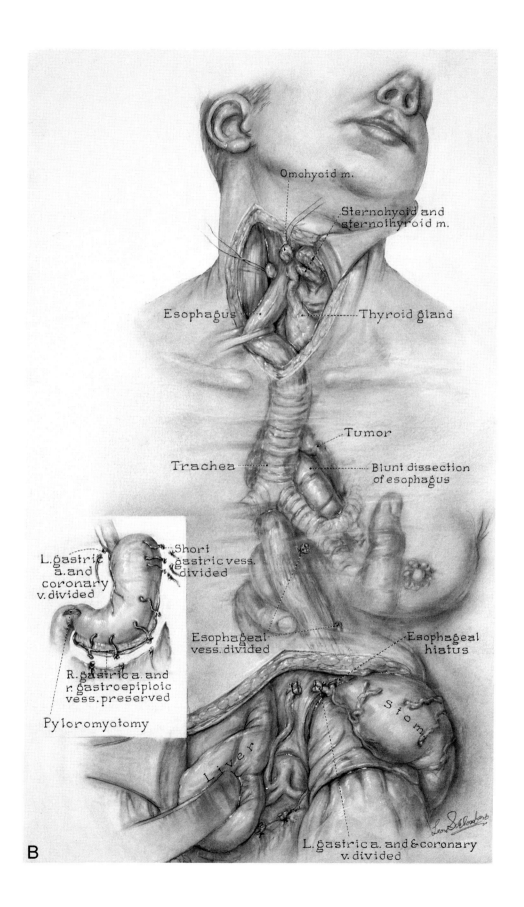

Omohyoid m.

Sternohyoid and sternothyroid m.

Esophagus

Thyroid gland

Tumor

Trachea

Blunt dissection of esophagus

L. gastric a. and coronary v. divided

Short gastric vess. divided

R. gastric a. and r. gastroepiploic vess. preserved

Pyloromyotomy

Esophageal vess. divided

Esophageal hiatus

Stom

Liver

L. gastric a. and coronary v. divided

B

C. Traction on the esophagus delivers the entire thoracic esophagus and the gastric cardia into the cervical wound. The cervical esophagus is transected, and the gastric cardia is amputated with the stapler. Anastomosis can be made with the traditional two-layer technique to the anterior wall of the stomach, as shown in the inset, or with the EEA end-to-end anastomotic stapler passed through the mouth, if the proximal esophagus is of sufficient size. If the extensive Kocher maneuver has sufficiently mobilized the stomach so that enough of it can be delivered into the neck, the esophagogastrostomy may be performed with the GIA-TA technique (see pages 358–361, *Palliative Esophagogastrostomy in Continuity, for Inoperable Carcinoma of the Gastroesophageal Junction*); the specimen is divided after completion of the anastomosis. Traction on the stomach from below then reduces the anastomosis into the chest.

From Stewart, J.R., Sarr, M.G., Sharp, K.W., Efron, G., Juanteguy, J., and Gadacz, T.R.: Transhiatal (blunt) esophagectomy for malignant and benign esophageal disease: Clinical experience and technique. Ann. Thorac. Surg. 40:343–348, 1985, with permission.

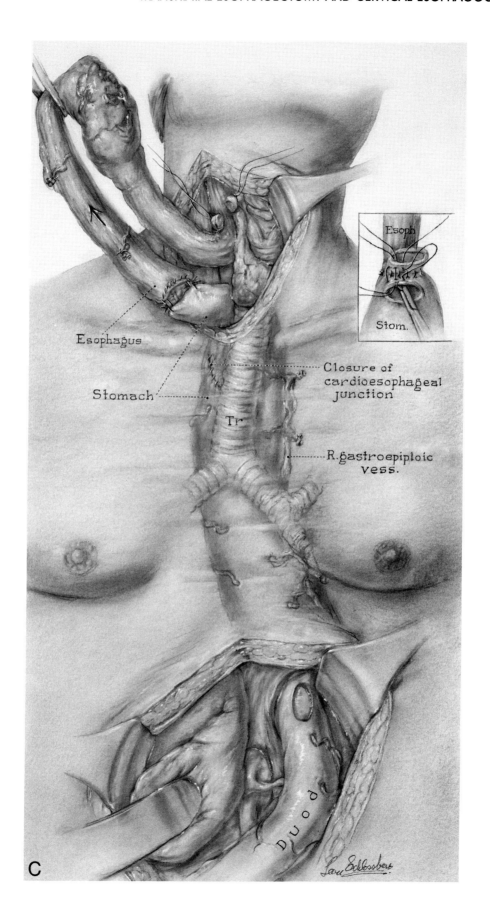

Esophagus

Stomach

Closure of
cardioesophageal
junction

R. gastroepiploic
vess.

Esoph.

Stom.

Tr

Duodn

C

COMBINED LAPAROTOMY AND RIGHT ANTEROLATERAL THORACOTOMY FOR CARCINOMA OF THE ESOPHAGUS— INTRATHORACIC ESOPHAGOGASTROSTOMY

Most surgeons, whether operating with one team or two, prefer to explore the abdomen through a midline laparotomy, proceeding to thoracotomy if the situation is favorable. Fisher, Brawley, and Kieffer, whose technique is illustrated, prefer a simultaneous thoracotomy by a second team. With the steadily decreasing mortality and morbidity of the resection and the reconstruction, it is generally agreed that the presence of involved nodes in the abdomen or mediastinum need not contravene resection and anastomosis, which is, in general, the best palliation.

A. The abdomen is entered through a midline incision. In providing exposure, the upward extension to the left of the xiphoid is more important than any extension below the umbilicus. Depending upon the case, the triangular ligament may be incised to free up the left lobe of the liver, or the left lobe may be held out of the way by a large retractor. The vasa brevia are ligated or clipped, and divided, and the omentum is divided from the stomach, preserving intact the gastroepiploic arcade. The gastrohepatic ligament is divided. The coronary vein and the fatty tissue surrounding it are ligated and divided, and the left gastric artery is exposed, cleaned of any fat and lymph nodes, secured, and divided. The phrenoesophageal ligament is incised and the vagi divided, liberating the stomach and esophagus. Although to bring the stomach into the neck (see *Laryngo-Pharyngo-Esophagectomy without Thoracotomy*) it may be necessary to carry on the division of the gastrohepatic ligament to the pylorus and then to mobilize the duodenum, the additional length so provided may not be required for an intrathoracic esophagogastrostomy. We usually do perform a pyloroplasty (not shown), generally the Heineke-Mikulicz, with the stapler; at times, we perform a pyloromyotomy. Other divulse the pylorus by a variation of the Loreta procedure through the invaginated stomach (without gastrotomy), and others find no need for any pyloroplasty or divulsion.

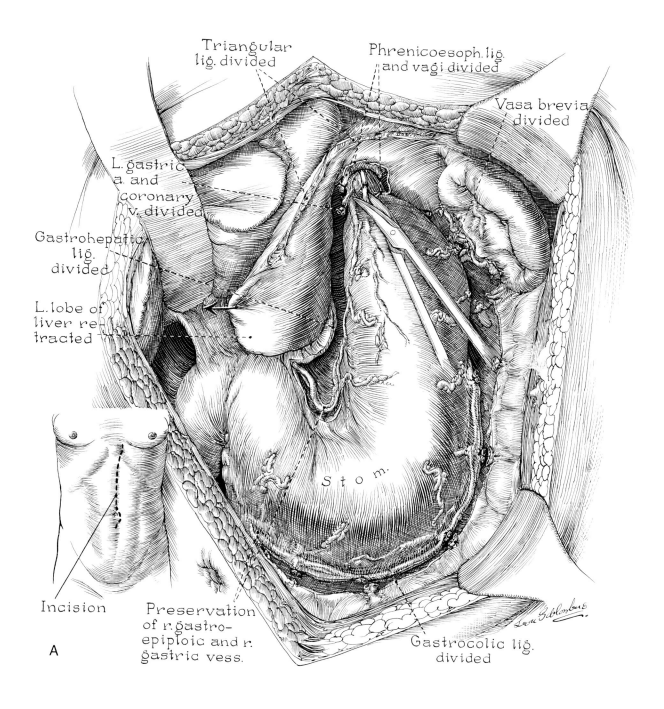

Triangular lig. divided

Phrenicoesoph. lig. and vagi divided

Vasa brevia divided

L. gastric a. and coronary v. divided

Gastrohepatic lig. divided

L. lobe of liver retracted

Sto m.

Incision

A

Preservation of r. gastroepiploic and r. gastric vess.

Gastrocolic lig. divided

COMBINED LAPAROTOMY AND RIGHT ANTEROLATERAL
THORACOTOMY *(Continued)*

B. The chest is entered through an anterolateral 4th interspace incision (see *Anterior (Anterolateral) Thoracotomy*); the patient is positioned with the right arm supported on a frame and the right half of the thorax tilted forward by a pad underneath the right shoulder. Maximal exposure is obtained by carrying the incision to the sternum anteriorly, securing and dividing the internal mammary vessels, and, laterally, splitting the intercostal muscles far posteriorly, to the necks of the ribs if necessary. Infrequently is it necessary to divide a rib by resecting a 1-cm segment posteriorly in order to provide easier access above or below. Alternatively, and preferably, the 3rd or 4th cartilage anteriorly can be divided obliquely for the same purpose. Displacing the lung anteriorly permits direct exposure of the lower-third esophageal tumor shown and determination whether it is resectable or not. Tapes are passed around the esophagus, which is dissected free of the mediastinal structures. Although every attempt is made not to violate the tumor and to take the pleura, involved mediastinal lymph nodes, and other tissue with it, we do not subscribe to the doctrine of super-radical mediastinal dissection. If, with an advanced tumor, the esophagus can be safely mobilized only by dissecting through a tumor bed attached to the posterior wall or the trachea, the main bronchus or aorta, or the pulmonary vein, the resection is carried out in that fashion, accepting the unavoidability of leaving tumor behind and accommodating to the reality of a palliative operation to restore deglutition.

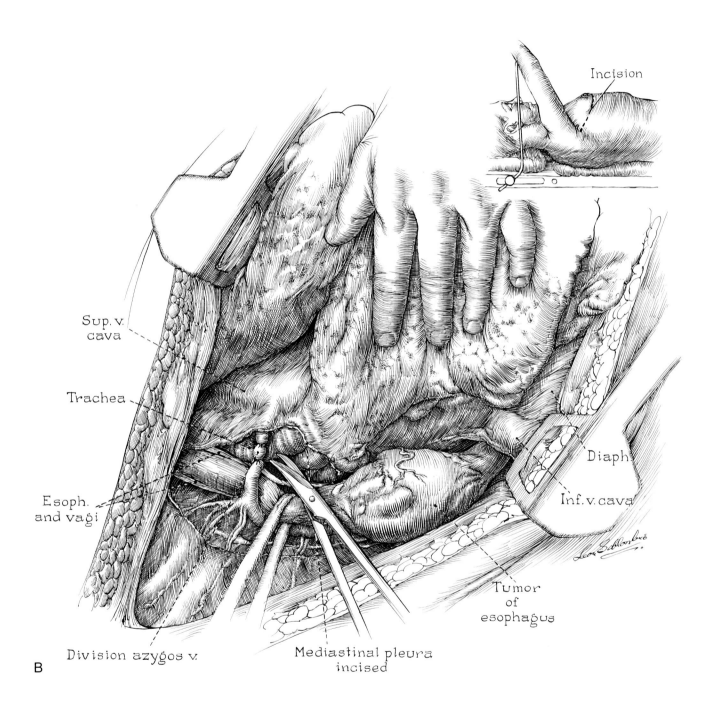

Incision

Sup. v. cava

Trachea

Esoph. and vagi

Diaph.

Inf. v. cava

Tumor of esophagus

Division azygos v.

Mediastinal pleura incised

B

COMBINED LAPAROTOMY AND RIGHT ANTEROLATERAL THORACOTOMY *(Continued)*

C. If exposure of the mediastinum is difficult because of the inflated lung, the anesthetist may be asked to deflate the lung, and the bronchus then may be temporarily occluded with a noncrushing clamp, as shown. This is an unattractive-appearing maneuver but one that is safe and may have to be resorted to if the original intubation was with a single-lumen rather than a double-lumen tube. The stomach is now readily drawn up through the hiatus and into the right chest, the esophagogastric junction is divided, and the gastric closure is inverted. We would today ordinarily employ the stapler and, in this situation, at the upper end of the partially devascularized stomach, do invert the stapled gastric closure. The stomach is drawn up to the apex of the pleural cavity, with the lesser curvature lying against the mediastinum. The gastric fundus is anchored by sutures fixing it posteriorly to the prevertebral fascia. With the stomach now secured in its new position, the abdominal team closes the esophageal hiatus about the distal stomach with interrupted sutures and closes the midline incision.

The esophagus is laid down on the anterior surface of the gastric fundus and doubled back on itself. The anastomosis will be made between the esophagus at the point at which it is folded back and the fundus at some 3 cm below its upper end. A row of Lembert sutures (*inset*) forms the posterior row of the two-layer anastomosis. Transverse incisions are made in stomach and esophagus half a centimeter or so beyond the Lembert sutures, providing cuffs to be sutured through-and-through.

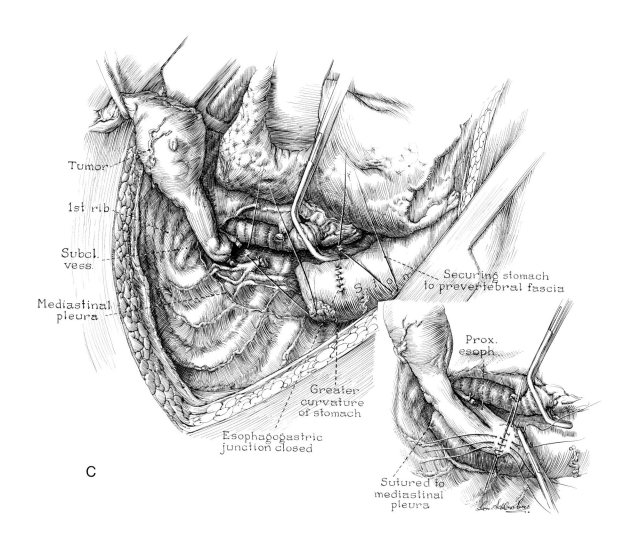

Tumor

1st rib

Subcl.
vess.

Mediastinal
pleura

Securing stomach
to prevertebral fascia

Greater
curvature
of stomach

Esophagogastric
junction closed

C

Prox.
esoph

Sutured to
mediastinal
pleura

D. The esophagus is now amputated by dividing its anterior wall at a level somewhat distal to the incision in the posterior wall so as to form a somewhat longer anterior flap. The anterior closure is again two-layer—inner through-and-through, outer Lembert. Shown in the lower figure is an additional row of Lembert sutures, covering over much of the suture line with stomach and anchoring the distal esophagus to the gastric bed on which it lies. The EEA stapler lends itself ideally to an anastomosis at this level (see *Techniques of Stapled Esophagogastric Anastomosis*).

From Fisher, R.D., Brawley, R.K., and Kieffer, R.F.: Esophagogastrostomy in the treatment of carcinoma of the distal two-thirds of the esophagus. Ann. Thorac. Surg. 14:658–670, 1972, with permission.

REFERENCES

1. Lewis, I.: The surgical treatment of carcinoma of the oesophagus. With special reference to a new operation for growth of the middle third. Br. J. Surg. 34:18–31, 1946
   Read has given an account of the contribution of Ivor Lewis (Weiss, G.D., and Read, R.D.: The Ivor Lewis procedure. Surgical Rounds 7 (5):41–48, 1984). In fact, although the adoption of the laparotomy plus right thoracotomy technique for esophagectomy and esophagogastrostomy is largely attributable to Ivor Lewis' teachings in Britain and the support from Kent and Harbison in the United States, as detailed by Meade (Meade, R.H.: A History of Thoracic Surgery. Springfield, Illinois, Charles C Thomas, 1961), J.L. Faure of Paris, Alton Ochsner, and others had preceded them.
2. Kent, E.M., and Harbison, S.P.: The combined abdominal and right thoracic approach to lesions of the middle and upper thirds of the esophagus. J. Thorac. Surg. 19:559–571, 1950

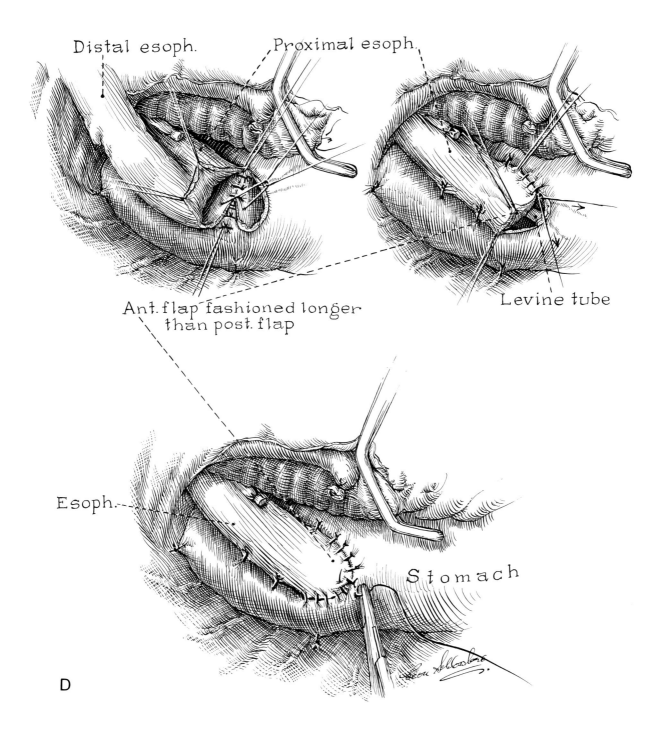

Distal esoph.

Proximal esoph.

Ant. flap fashioned longer
than post. flap

Levine tube

Esoph.

Stomach

D

PALLIATIVE ESOPHAGOGASTROSTOMY IN CONTINUITY, FOR INOPERABLE CARCINOMA OF THE GASTROESOPHAGEAL JUNCTION

A. Through a left posterolateral thoracotomy in the periosteal bed of the 6th rib, left in place with the periosteum attached inferiorly, the mediastinum is opened and the esophagus exposed above the tumor. The diaphragm is incised lateral to the hiatus, leaving the gastroesophageal junction and tumor undisturbed. Three to four vasa brevia are ligated and divided, as well as the gastroepiploic vessels proximally. The mobilized fundus of the stomach is drawn into the chest through the diaphragmatic incision and brought along the uninvolved esophagus proximal to the tumor. Stab wounds for introduction of the anastomosing instrument (GIA) are made in the esophagus, 6 to 7 cm proximal to the tumor and in the apex of the gastric fundus.

B. One limb of the GIA instrument is advanced distally into the esophagus, and the matching limb is inserted down from the apex of the gastric fundus. The instrument halves are locked and the instrument is activated, creating a side-to-side esophago-gastrostomy proximal to the obstructing tumor.

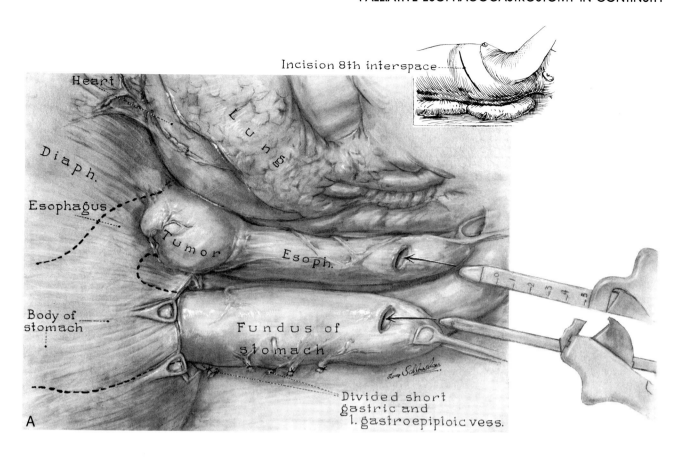

Incision 8th interspace

Heart

Lung

Diaph.

Esophagus

Tumor

Esoph.

Body of
stomach

Fundus of
stomach

Divided short
gastric and
l. gastroepiploic vess.

Leon Schlossberg

A

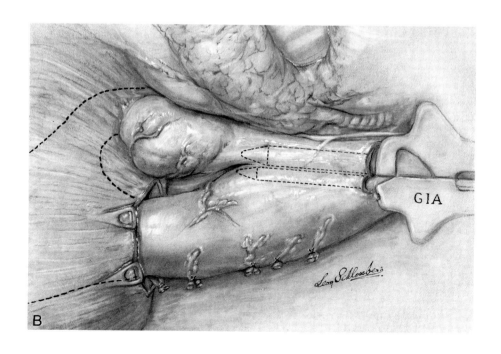

GIA

Leon Schlossberg

B

C. Following removal of the GIA stapler, the now common stab wound has been closed transversely with the TA 55 stapler; it can also be closed manually. The diaphragmatic opening is closed, as indicated, leaving a comfortable aperture for the stomach which is anchored to the edge of the incision in the diaphragm. To avoid any tension on the staple lines, the stomach is attached to the esophagus by single sutures, proximal and distal to the GIA anastomosis. This procedure is substantially simpler than the alternatives, such as a bypassing Roux-Y esophagojejunostomy. In either case, an attractive modification is to staple and transect the esophagus above the tumor, implanting the proximal end into the stomach or the Roux limb.

Method of P. A. Kirschner, Kwun, K.-B., and Kirschner, P.A.: Palliative side-to-side oesophagogastrostomy for unresectable carcinoma of the oesophagus and cardia. Thorax 36:441–445, 1981.

Martin Kirschner of Königsberg, in 1920, presented almost precisely this technique, with the addition that he employed what we now call a Nissen wrap, which he called a "Witzel canal."

REFERENCE

1. Kirschner, M.: Ein neues Verfahren der Oesophagoplastik. Archiv für klin. Chirurgie 114:606–663, 1920

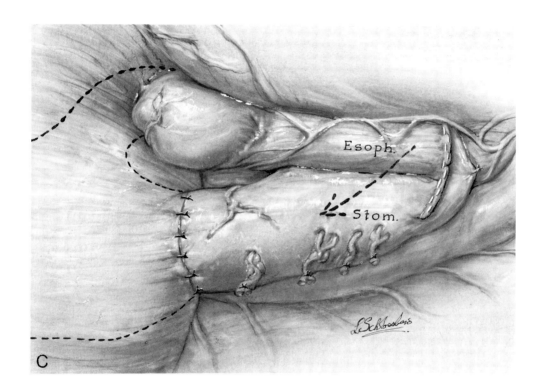

Esoph.

Stom.

C

GREATER CURVATURE GASTRIC TUBES FOR REPLACEMENT OF THE ESOPHAGUS

Beck-Jianu-Gavriliu Greater Curvature Tube

A. It is usually well to perform a splenectomy, although this is not invariably necessary. The short gastric and the splenic vessels should be secured close to the hilum to be sure of preserving the left gastroepiploic vessels, on which the circulation of the gastric tube will depend.

B. The omentum is divided along the greater curvature of the stomach, sufficiently far from the gastroepiploic vessels to avoid any injury to them. The level at which the tube will be begun is indicated. The right gastroepiploic vessels have necessarily been divided and secured.

C. A large rubber tube has been inserted through a stab wound or pursestring suture to outline the greater curvature of the stomach. The tube is created by serial applications of the GIA instrument, each application providing a 5-cm cleft doubly stapled on each side.

D. The tube having been completed, the GIA instrument closure of the stomach is being reinforced here by inversion. It is important not to run this continuous suture to the very end of the tube but to use interrupted sutures there for 2 or 3 cm, so that if the tube is overlong and requires amputation, the continuous suture will not be disrupted. The tube can now be brought up retrosternally or through the thorax. If the esophagus has been dissected out transmediastinally, without thoracotomy, as in *Laryngo-Pharyngo-Esophagectomy Without Thoracotomy* and *Transhiatal Esophagectomy and Cervical Esophagogastrostomy*, the gastric tube may be tied to the stapled distal end of the esophagus and pulled through into the neck as the esophagus is withdrawn from above. The anastomosis in the neck is made by hand.

REFERENCES

1. Beck, C., and Carrell, A.: Demonstration of specimens illustrating a method of formation of a prethoracic esophagus. Illinois Medical Journal 7:463–467, 1905
2. Jianu, A.: Gastrostomie und Ösophagoplastik. Dtsch. Ztsch. f. Chir. 118:383–390, 1912
3. Gavriliu, D.: Gastrostomia minima cu guler peritoneal. Procedeu personal. Chirurgia 51, 1952
4. Gavriliu, D., Cohn, A., Albu, E., Dumitriu, C., and Popa, I.: Gastrostomie ou jejunostomie dans les obstructions digestives supérieures. Ann. Chir. 16:337–340, 1962
5. Gavriliu, D.: Aspects of esophageal surgery. Current Problems in Surgery, October 1975
6. Steichen, F.M., and Ravitch, M.M.: *Stapling in Surgery.* Chicago, Year Book Medical Publishers 1984

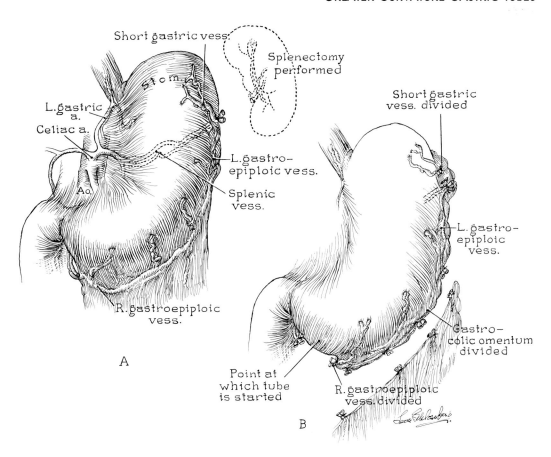

Short gastric vess.

Splenectomy performed

Stom.

L. gastric a.

Celiac a.

Ao.

L. gastro-epiploic vess.

Splenic vess.

R. gastroepiploic vess.

A

Short gastric vess. divided

L. gastro-epiploic vess.

Gastro-colic omentum divided

Point at which tube is started

R. gastroepiploic vess. divided

B

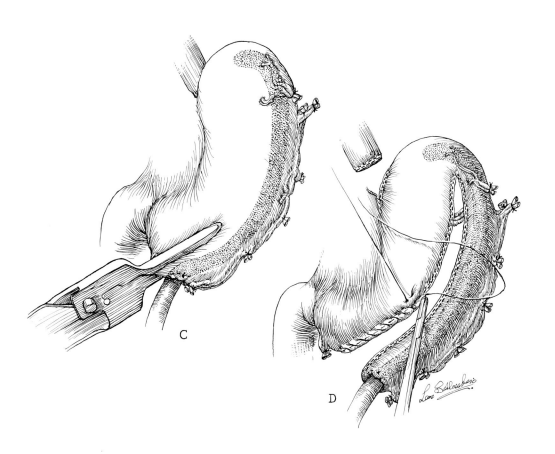

C

D

GREATER CURVATURE GASTRIC TUBES *(Continued)*

Extended Gavriliu Technique

A. The duodenum has been divided with the GIA stapler. The dotted line indicates the line of division of the stomach providing a long greater curvature tube which includes the distal antrum and the proximal duodenum.

B. Serial application of the GIA stapling instrument along the line shown in *A* has constructed the extended greater curvature tube. The gastroduodenostomy has been made by manual suture after excision of the stapled closure of the duodenum and a corresponding portion of the gastric staple line near the lesser curvature. Stapled edges of the stomach and of the gastric tube are covered over with a continuous suture, a measure regularly employed when the stomach has been divided with the GIA instrument. The esophagus is shown having been amputated with the GIA, or with two applications of the TA, at the gastroesophageal junction. The spleen has been resected.

   This procedure, providing 5 or 6 cm of additional length, the tube being nourished by the left gastroepiploic vessels, has the additional advantage of interposing a pyloric sphincter in the line to decrease the likelihood of regurgitation into the cervical esophagus or pharynx.

REFERENCES

1. Gavriliu, D.: Gastrostomia minima cu guler peritoneal. Procedeu personal. Chirurgia 51, 1952
2. Gavriliu, D., Cohn, A., Albu, E., Dumitriu, C., and Popa, I.: Gastrostomie ou jejunostomie dans les obstructions digestives supérieures. Ann. Chir. 16:337–340, 1962
3. Gavriliu, D.: Aspects of esophageal surgery. Current Problems in Surgery, October 1975
4. Steichen, F.M., and Ravitch, M.M.: *Stapling in Surgery*. Chicago, Year Book Medical Publishers, 1984

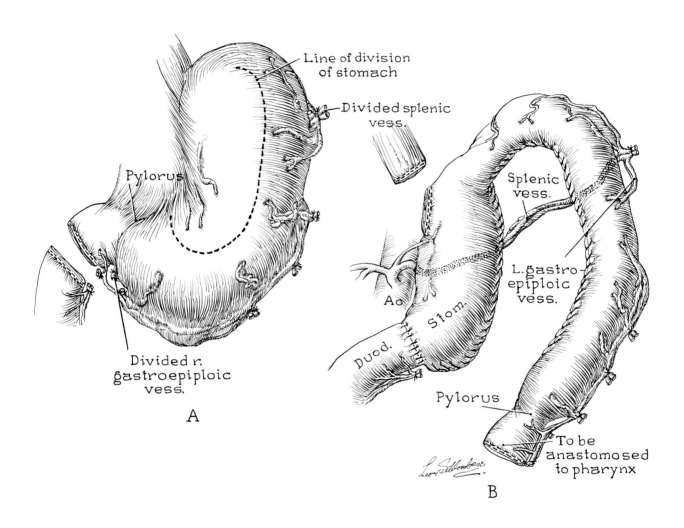

Line of division of stomach

Divided splenic vess.

Pylorus

Divided r. gastroepiloic vess.

A

Splenic vess.

L. gastro-epiploic vess.

Ao.

Stom.

Duod.

Pylorus

To be anastomosed to pharynx

B

"Isoperistaltic" Greater Curvature Gastric Tube (Postlethwait)

A. The omentum has been removed from the stomach, with preservation of the right gastroepiploic vessels that will nourish the tube and division of the left gastroepiploic vessels superiorly. The short gastric vessels are divided and ligated, and the spleen is preserved. Indicated is the point on the stomach at which the spindle of the EEA instrument, having been introduced through an anterior stab wound, will be pressed until it stretches the posterior wall, at which point it is cut down upon through the posterior wall and allowed to push through, and the anvil-carrying nose cone is reapplied.

B. The EEA instrument has produced a circular opening with a double row of staples around it. The GIA instrument is shown about to be inserted, one limb anteriorly and one limb posteriorly, to start construction of the tube.

C. The GIA stapler is closed *in situ.* The inset shows a cross section with the GIA instrument in place. A double row of staples is applied on either side as the knife cuts down the center to within one and one half staples of the end of the staple line, leaving the anterior and posterior walls stapled together with two rows of staples on either side.

D. This view of the completed tube, after several applications of the GIA instrument, now shows the covering over of the staple line. A whipstitch of fine catgut superficial to the staple line, or behind it, is also effective and uses less of the tube. The tube readily reaches the neck through a substernal tunnel for manual anastomosis to the cervical esophagus.

REFERENCES

1. Mes, G.M.: New method of esophagoplasty. J. Int'l Coll. Surgeons 11:270–277, 1948
   We had thought the "buttonhole" technique original with us but, sutured by hand, it was clearly illustrated by Mes of South Africa 50 years ago!
2. Yamagishi, M., Noritsugu, I., and Yonemoto, T.: An isoperistaltic gastric tube. New method of esophageal replacement. Arch. Surg. 100:689–692, 1970
3. Postlethwait, R.W.: Technique for isoperistaltic gastric tube for esophageal bypass. Ann. Surg. 189:673–676, 1979

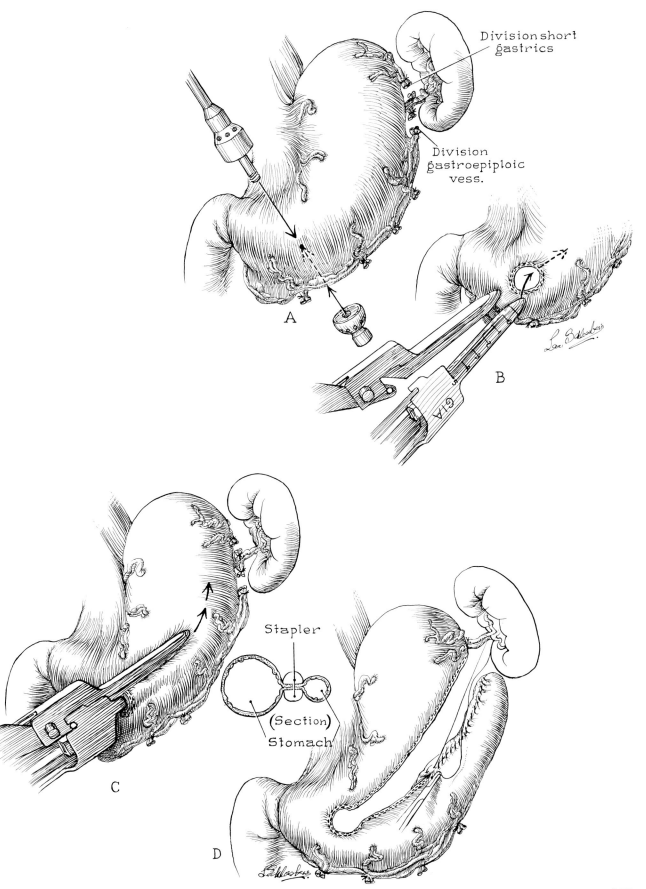

Division short gastrics

Division gastroepiploic vess.

A

B

Stapler

(Section)

Stomach

C

D

TECHNIQUES OF STAPLED ESOPHAGOGASTRIC ANASTOMOSIS

GIA Stapled Anastomosis on the Anterior Surface of the Intact Stomach

Whether in the chest or in the neck, a variety of anastomotic techniques are available, performed manually or with the staplers.

A. The stomach is shown with the gastroesophageal junction divided with the TA instrument, a closure that is usually not reinforced. The end of the esophagus is brought down over the anterior surface of the stomach, and the limbs of the GIA stapler are inserted into the stomach through a stab wound and into the esophagus through its open end or through the cut-away corner of the stapled esophagus.

B. The GIA instrument has been operated and withdrawn. The stippled shading indicates the extent of the V-shaped opening between the esophagus and the stomach.

C. The open lips of the anastomosis, esophagus in front and stomach behind, are held up with clamps (not shown here to avoid busying the field), and the TA linear stapler is slipped behind the three clamps, insuring that the stapler engages the full thickness of esophagus and stomach around the entire circumference of the anastomosis.

D. The finished anastomosis is shown after any tissue projecting beyond the stapler has been cut away and the stapler has been removed.

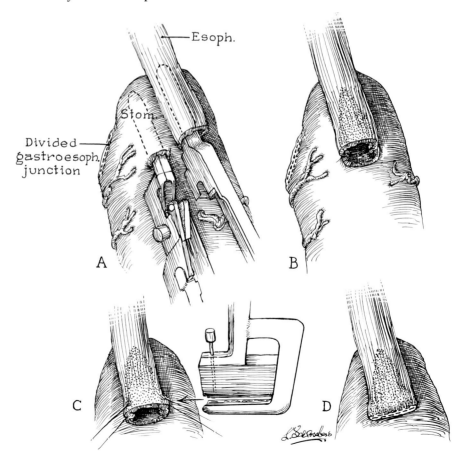

The GIA Stapled Esophagogastrostomy Performed within the Chest (Bayonet Anastomosis)

The stomach is brought up behind the esophagus, the limbs of the GIA are inserted into the stomach through a gastrotomy and into the esophagus through its open end, and the anastomosis is thereafter performed as in the previous drawings. The now-combined orifices of insertion of the GIA instrument will be closed mucosa-to-mucosa with the TA instrument or by inversion with manual sutures. This provides a long and very satisfactory anastomosis. Since with the GIA instrument the upper part of the anastomosis may be made at a level almost out of reach of convenient manual suturing, this technique lends itself to performance of unexpectedly high anastomoses.

REFERENCE

1. Steichen, F.M., and Ravitch, M.M.: *Stapling in Surgery*. Chicago, Year Book Medical Publishers, 1984

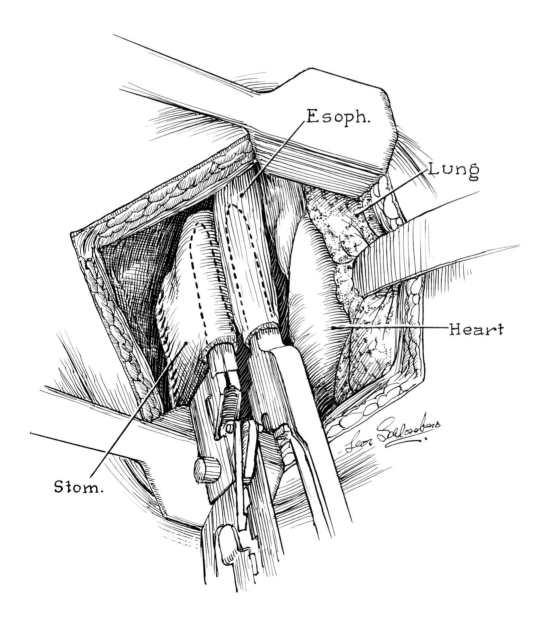

TECHNIQUES OF STAPLED ESOPHAGOGASTRIC
ANASTOMOSIS *(Continued)*

EEA Stapled Anastomosis to the Anterior Gastric Wall— Lesser Curvature Resected

The lesser curvature has been resected by the application of the GIA instrument (hence the oversewing) from a point on the left of the esophagogastric junction to about the position of the "crow's foot" on the lesser curvature, and the vessels on the lesser curvature of the stomach have been appropriately divided and secured.

A. The EEA stapler without its anvil-containing nose cone is inserted through a gastrotomy in the antrum, and the stapler spindle is brought out high up on the anterior wall of the stomach. If the spindle has emerged through a very small incision, so that the stomach fits tightly around the spindle, no pursestring suture is necessary. The nose cone is then reattached and inserted into the esophagus through the pursestring suture.

B. Operation of the EEA instrument has completed the minimally inverting anastomosis. No reinforcing sutures are required. The instrument has been withdrawn and the gastrotomy is about to be closed by application of the TA 55 instrument for mucosa-to-mucosa closure. Depending upon the position of the esophagus on the anterior wall of the stomach and the width of the stomach at that point, it may be possible to cover the anastomosis by a gastric wrap, providing further security as well as an antireflux mechanism.

C. Alternatively, the EEA instrument may be placed in the same manner but with its spindle emerging through the corner of the stapled gastric closure, this portion of which was not oversewn.

REFERENCES

1. Boerema, I.: Oesophagus resection with restoration of continuity by a gastric tube. Arch. Chir. Neerl. 4:120–130, 1952
   Detailed presentation of resection of lesser curvature for tubularization of stomach.
2. Wangensteen, O.H.: In discussion of Neville, W.E., and Clowes, G.H.A., Jr.: Reconstruction of the esophagus with segments of the colon. J. Thorac. Surg. 35:2–22, 1958
   Wangensteen points out the added length given to the stomach if it is straightened out by cutting away the lesser curvature.
3. Steichen, F.M., and Ravitch, M.M.: *Stapling in Surgery.* Chicago, Year Book Medical Publishers, 1984
4. Ravitch, M.M.: Intersecting staple lines in intestinal anastomoses. Surgery 97:8–14, 1985

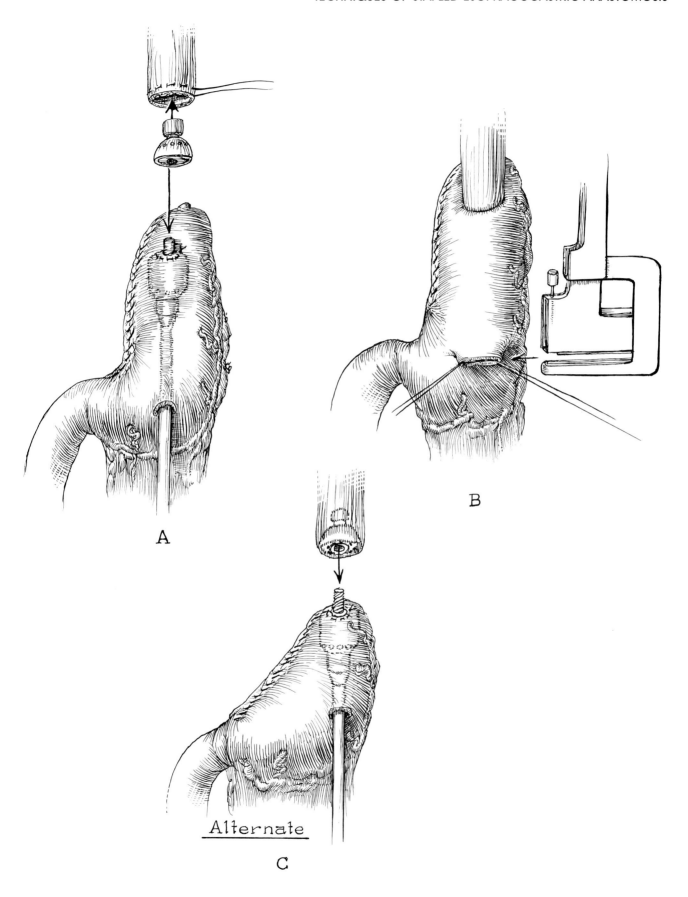

A

B

Alternate

C

EEA Anastomosis to (Tubularized) Stomach

A. The gland-bearing tissue on the lesser curvature is resected, the celiac axis is stripped clean, and the left gastric artery is secured at its origin (not shown). The lesser curvature is resected as shown by stepwise application of the GIA instrument, each cut providing several centimeters of tube, until the greater curvature is reached; a splenectomy is performed as well. The right gastroepiploic vessels are preserved.

B. The EEA instrument, inserted much as in the lesser curvature resection (previous page), reaches sufficiently far superiorly for an anastomosis in the apex of the chest.

C. This anastomosis is made by the same technique, but lower down and in the upper right chest.

D. If sufficient stomach is available in the chest, the curved EEA instrument can be introduced into an anterior gastrotomy through the thoracotomy incision and the anastomosis performed as in C [shown here] or even as in A of the lesser curvature resection (page 371).

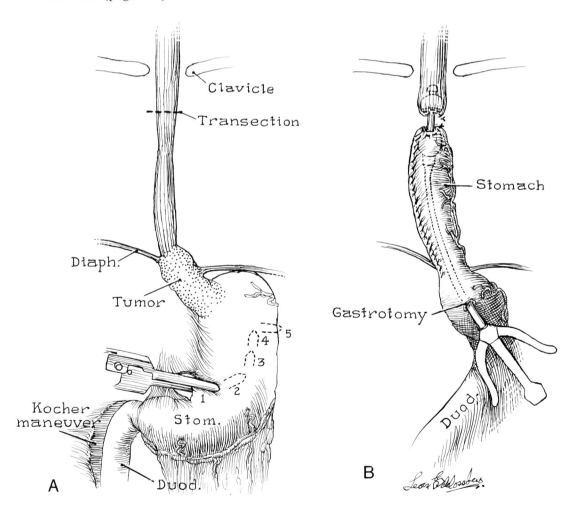

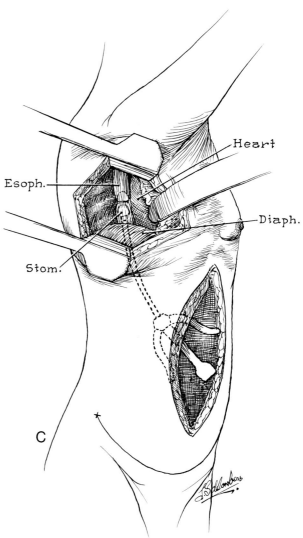

Esoph.

Heart

Diaph.

Stom.

C

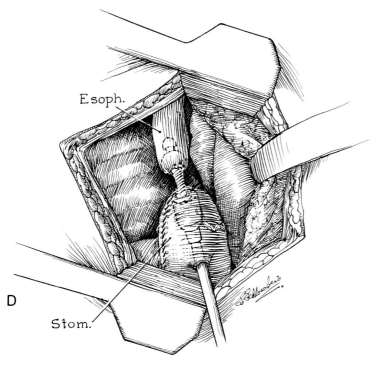

Esoph.

D

Stom.

TECHNIQUES OF REPLACEMENT OF THE ESOPHAGUS WITH COLON

From time to time, particularly for benign lesions, so short a segment of distal esophagus is resected that the gap is most easily filled by interpolating a loop of bowel. A segment of the transverse colon supported by the middle colic vessels is best suited for this purpose. An extrapolated loop of jejunum can be used as well, but preparation of the loop is more tedious. The principle is also applicable to the creation of a bypass in cases of inoperable malignancy in the same location. Exposure is gained by separate laparotomy—midline or left subcostal—and thoracotomy in the 6th or 7th interspace posterolateral on the left, with the patient's left side tilted up some 45°. The thoracoabdominal incision, cutting across the intercostal arch, has been for the most part abandoned because of inviting problems of healing and pain. In any case, the disabling radial division of the diaphragm, which is part of that procedure, is in fact unnecessary. What is needed is exposure *above* the diaphragm and exposure *below* the diaphragm, which is only minimally aided by radial division of the diaphragm. If it is desired to perform the entire operation from above, the simplest technique is to detach the diaphragm by making an incision in it parallel to and 1.5 cm from the chest wall; this avoids injury to the phrenic nerves and paralysis of the diaphragm and gives magnificent exposure through the wide opening created (see page 382).

The replacement of the distal esophagus by colon requires no incision in the diaphragm. The colon may be passed up through the hiatus in the esophageal bed. If inoperable carcinoma is being bypassed, the bowel is passed through a separate opening made at a little distance from the hiatus and the tumor. For curative resections of tumors at the level of the hiatus, a considerable margin of muscle of the diaphragm is resected with the esophagus.

A. For benign disease, the stomach may be stapled with the TA 55 instrument and amputated from above the left gastric vessels, taking only branches of the left gastric artery on the lesser curvature.

B. The required segment of transverse colon has been isolated with applications of the GIA instrument at either end, and the mesocolon has been incised at a little distance from the colon and on either side of the middle colic vessels.

C. The colon has been reanastomosed and the mesenteric defect closed.

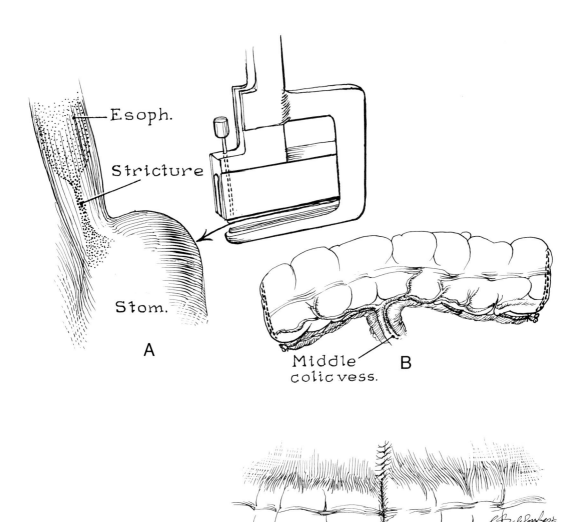

Esoph.

Stricture

Stom.

A

Middle
colic vess.

B

C

D. After the colon is brought up in the chest alongside the esophagus, the limbs of the GIA instrument are inserted upward through stab wounds in colon and esophagus. The point of the GIA instrument reaches the upper limit of colon on its antimesenteric border.

E. Once the instrument is mated, locked, and fired, a long anastomosis has been completed. Thus far, the specimen has not been amputated, an example of the "anastomosis first, resection second" technique.

F. The lower jaw of the TA 55 stapler is now passed behind the esophagus and in front of the colon, so that when it has been closed it will staple off the esophagus and the GIA stapler opening. It is usually placed a little more obliquely, down to the left, than shown. Division of the esophagus and the bit of colon protruding through the TA instrument by cutting on the edge of the instrument completes the procedure.

G. The result is a bayonet-type esophagocolic anastomosis.

H. The EEA instrument can be inserted through the opened distal end of the colonic segment; the bare spindle is pushed through the upper end of the colon, either through a stab wound or through the cutaway antimesenteric corner of the staple line. If the opening fits tightly around the spindle, the pursestring suture shown may not be required. The nose cone, having been screwed onto the spindle, is inserted into the esophagus, the pursestring is tied, and the usual EEA instrument anastomosis is completed. The EEA instrument may be introduced into the colon from below the diaphragm, and the colonic segment is then brought upward as the instrument is advanced.

I. The cologastrostomy. The GIA instrument is inserted into the colon through the cutaway antimesenteric corner and into the stomach through a stab wound.

J. The completed cologastrostomy, after TA instrument closure of the openings for the GIA instrument.

The spleen has not been pictured, but there is no need to remove it for this procedure. *Note* in *I* and *J* that the colon has been passed up behind the gastric antrum, which may otherwise be obstructed by the vascular pedicle.

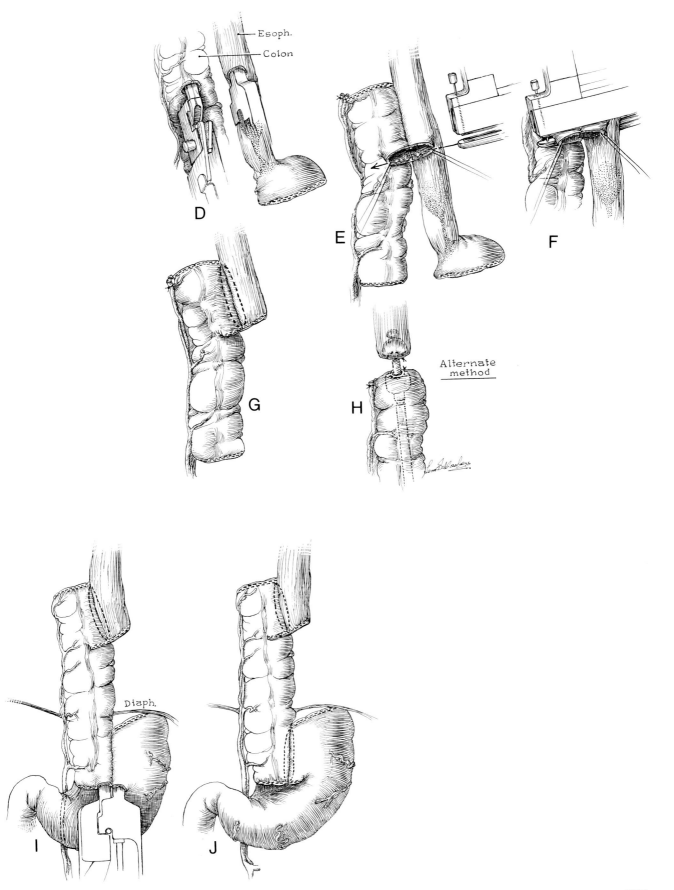

ESOPHAGEAL REPLACEMENT BY RETROSTERNAL ESOPHAGOCOLOPLASTY

Esophagocoloplasty with Stapled Bayonet Anastomosis in the Neck (GIA and TA Instruments)

A. The terminal ileum has been divided with the GIA stapler, the appendix amputated, and the transverse colon divided and stapled, so that the isolated section of cecum, ascending colon, and right transverse colon is nourished by the middle colic artery or its right branch.

B. The bowel has been reconstructed by functional end-to-end anastomosis. After the esophagus has been resected, the isolated section of right colon is brought up in the anterior mediastinum and the proximal end is anastomosed to the esophagus by the GIA–TA technique, creating a bayonet anastomosis (see previous procedure, *Techniques of Replacement of the Esophagus with Colon, D through J*). The anastomosis is shown performed on the right side of the neck. It is frequently more convenient to perform it on the left side. An end-to-side anastomosis with the GIA–TA technique is performed between the distal end of the colon and the stomach (see previous procedure, *I* and *J*). A through-and-through incision in the pylorus has been closed transversely with the TA stapler in the Heineke-Mikulicz fashion.

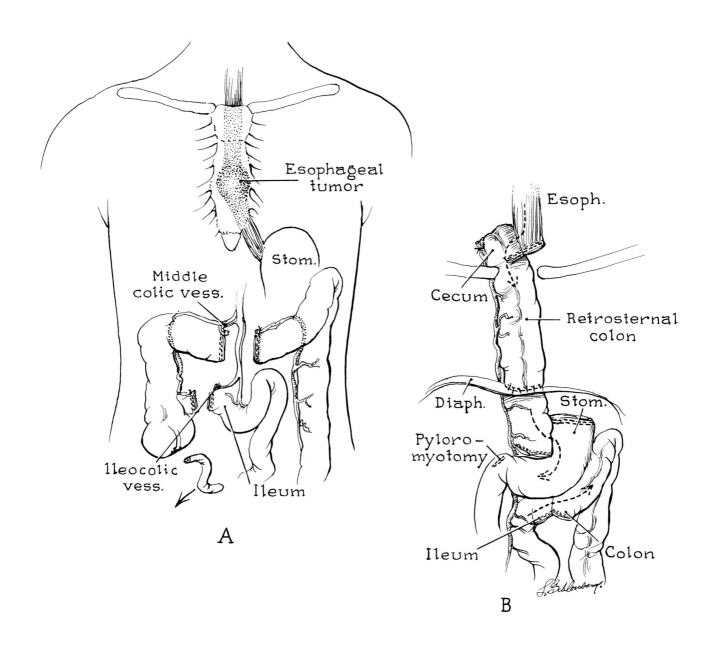

Esophageal tumor

Stom.

Middle colic vess.

Ileocolic vess.

Ileum

A

Esoph.

Cecum

Retrosternal colon

Diaph.

Stom.

Pyloro-myotomy

Ileum

Colon

B

379

Alternate Technique of Stapled Proximal Esophagocoloplasty (EEA Instrument)

A. The cecum and the terminal ileum are brought up in the neck; the EEA stapler, without the anvil-bearing nose cone, is inserted into the terminal ileum through its open end; and the spindle passed through a stab wound in the cecum.

B. The anvil-bearing nose cone has been reapplied and passed up into the proximal esophagus to be secured by a pursestring suture. The pursestring suture shown in the cecum may or may not be necessary, depending upon whether or not the stab wound has been significantly stretched by the manipulation.

C. The EEA stapler, having been used to create the end-to-end anastomosis, has been withdrawn, and the stump of terminal ileum has been amputated with the TA instrument.

Alternate Proximal Esophagocolostomy

Two-layer manual esophagocolostomy in the neck is shown. The inner suture is continuous catgut and the outer is interrupted silk.

REFERENCE

1. Steichen, F.M., and Ravitch, M.M.: *Stapling in Surgery.* Chicago, Year Book Medical Publishers, Inc., 1984

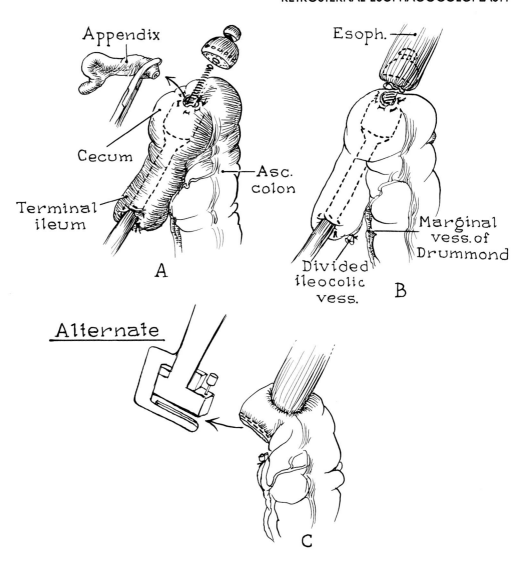

Appendix

Cecum

Terminal ileum

Asc. colon

A

Esoph.

Marginal vess. of Drummond

Divided ileocolic vess.

B

Alternate

C

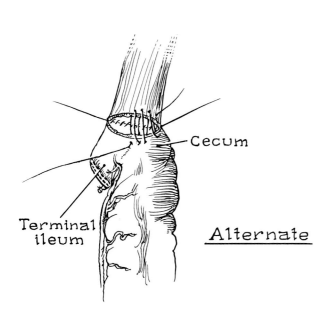

Cecum

Terminal ileum

Alternate

ESOPHAGEAL REPLACEMENT, COLON INTERPOSITION— TRANSTHORACIC, TRANSDIAPHRAGMATIC APPROACH

A. Incision through the periosteal bed of the 7th rib exposes the lower thorax and the long and dense esophageal stricture. The diaphragm is divided peripherally with the cautery about 1 cm from the chest wall, eliminating the necessity for a laparotomy.
B. The colon is delivered into the chest, and the omentum is dissected from it.
C. A segment of transverse colon of requisite length is transected at both ends with the GIA stapling instrument, which at each end simultaneously divides the bowel and staples both ends. The marginal vessels require separate division and ligation.

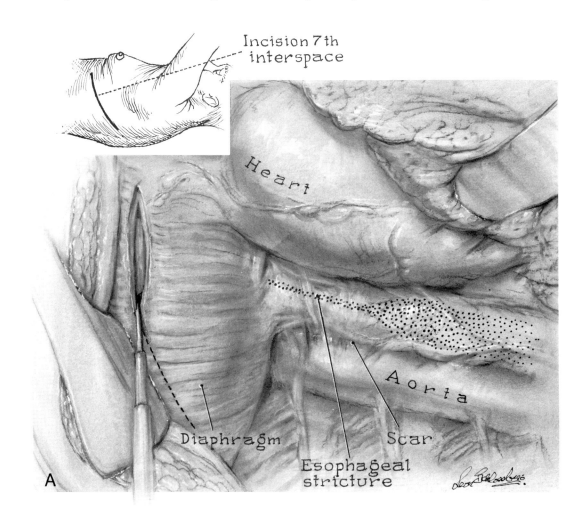

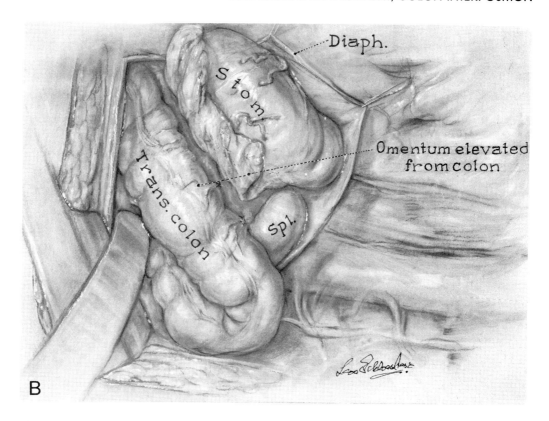

B

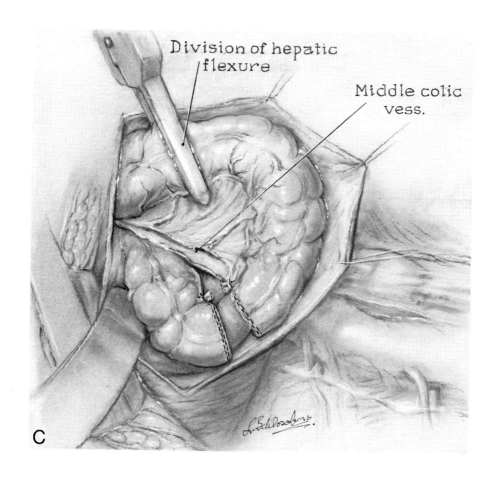

C

D. The esophagus has been dissected out of its scarred bed to above the area of inflammation and scarring. The dashed line indicates the line of proposed transection of the esophagus. The gastroesophageal junction has been stapled and divided, and the proximal end of the colonic segment is shown brought through the esophageal hiatus. The colon has been reconstructed.

E. The colon now lies within the chest. Through a colotomy the curved EEA end-to-end anastomotic stapler is inserted, and the anvil-bearing distal end is passed into the proximal esophagus and secured with a pursestring suture. This is facilitated by drawing the distal end of the colon up into the chest and out toward the wound so that the curved EEA instrument can be passed readily. For both steps F and G, the staple-closed colonic ends are resected and the usual pursestring sutures inserted. Alternatively, the spindle of the stapler can be passed through the end of the segment of colon at or near the staple line, and the anvil-bearing nose cone can then be attached for insertion into the pursestring-sutured esophagus, above, and stomach, below.

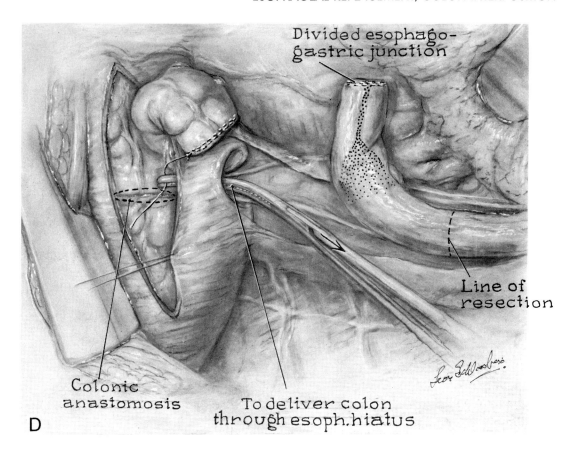

Divided esophago-
gastric junction

Line of
resection

Colonic
anastomosis

To deliver colon
through esoph. hiatus

D

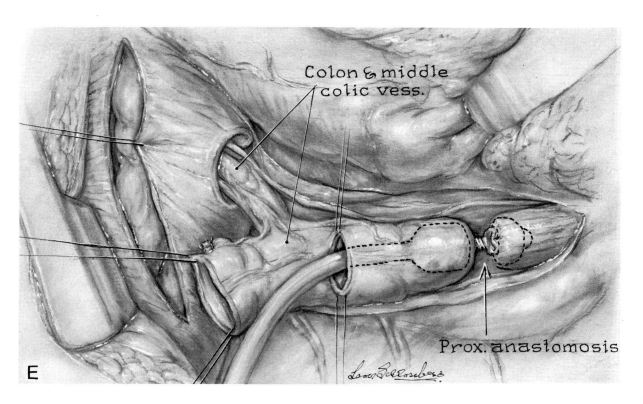

Colon & middle
colic vess.

Prox. anastomosis

E

ESOPHAGEAL REPLACEMENT, COLON
INTERPOSITION *(Continued)*

    F. After the upper anastomosis has been completed, the colon is dropped back into the chest and passed down through the hiatus; the EEA stapler is now passed distally through the same colotomy, and a cologastrostomy is performed with the EEA stapler.

    G. Once the anastomosis is completed, the colon is tacked to the esophageal hiatus. The diaphragm is closed with mattress sutures overlapping the cut edges, which will be reinforced by a series of interrupted sutures tacking the peripheral edge down to the main body of the diaphragm.

        (See also pages 406–409, *Esophageal Atresia Without Fistula.*)

REFERENCES

1. Hopkins, W.: In: Abbott, Osler discussion of Ravitch, M.M., Bahnson, H.T., and Johns, T.N.P.: Carcinoma of the esophagus. J. Thorac. Surg. 24:256–270, 1952
   Peripheral incision of diaphragm.
2. Waterston, D.J.: In D. Gairdner (Ed.): *Recent Advances in Paediatrics.* London, J. & A. Churchill, Ltd., 1954
3. Waterston, D.J.: Replacement of oesophagus with transverse colon. Thoraxchirurgie 11:73–74, 1963
4. Waterston, D.J.: Colonic replacement of esophagus (intrathoracic). Surg. Clin. North Am. 44:1441–1447, 1964
5. Waterston, D.J.: Reconstruction of the esophagus. In: *Pediatric Surgery*, 2nd Edition, W.T. Mustard, M.M. Ravitch, W.H. Snyder, Jr., et al. (Eds.). Chicago, Year Book Medical Publishers, 1969

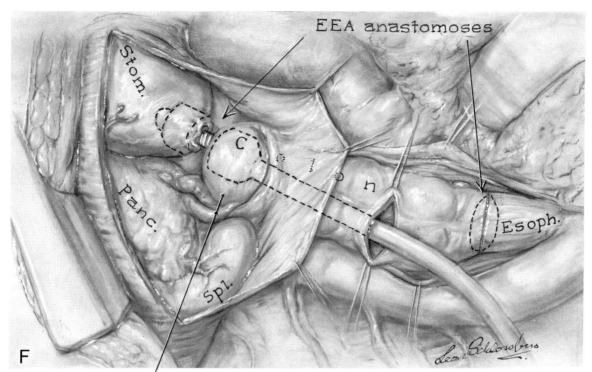

Colon & vascular pedicle through
esoph. hiatus

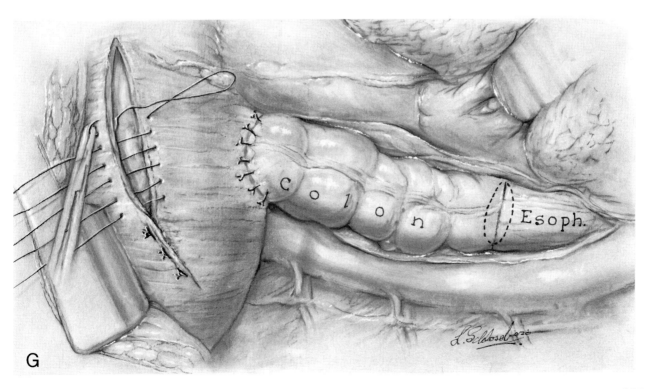

Operation for Esophageal Reflux

THE NISSEN FUNDOPLICATION

The approach is usually through an upper midline abdominal incision, extended superiorly to the left of the xiphoid process. In adults with a broad costal arch, and particularly in children, with their flexible and easily elevated costal margins, we prefer a subcostal incision.

A. Division of the triangular ligament permits retraction of the left lobe of the liver but is often not necessary. A large, heavy retractor will serve to hold the left lobe out of the way and avoids the occasional annoying bleeding from the ligament. The gastric fundus is freed by serial division and ligation of some or all of the short gastric vessels and, occasionally, by dividing upper branches of the left gastric on the lesser curvature in the course of dividing the upper portion of the gastrohepatic ligament. The spleen is depressed out of the way with a laparotomy pad (not shown). The areolar tissues around the crura are dissected free. The aorta and the celiac axis are here shown clearly for reference but are not laid bare in the dissection. The phrenoesophageal ligament is divided and the esophagus liberated from within the mediastinum as required, to provide an adequate length of intraabdominal esophagus. The stomach and esophagus are held to the left by a narrow retractor (not shown), and heavy, nonabsorbable sutures are placed in the crura by taking generous bites from side-to-side, closing the hiatus behind the esophagus.

B. With the esophagus fully liberated from the lower mediastinum and surrounded by a tape or Penrose drain on which a gentle downward traction is maintained, a Babcock clamp is passed behind the esophagus, seizing the right wall of the fundus, which is brought under the esophagus to the right. After the left side of the fundus is seized by another Babcock, the two clamps are approximated anteriorly to be sure of the appropriate placement of the sutures.

C. The collar of gastric fundus is now closed anteriorly with three or four interrupted sutures engaging gastric submucosa. Placement of the sutures in the esophagus as shown—our practice—decreases the likelihood of slippage of the Nissen wrap, but esophageal leaks have been reported to result. Alternatively, the stitches shown may avoid the esophagus and an additional lower stitch may be taken to suture the gastric wrap to the stomach wall just below the gastroesophageal junction.

D. Further to prevent the "slipped Nissen" and to maintain the acute angle of His, an anchoring suture is placed from the apex of the gastric collar to the left leaf of the diaphragmatic crus. The fundic collar should be sufficiently relaxed to admit a No. 34 bougie passed down the esophagus alongside the nasogastric tube, in addition to the surgeon's 5th finger, placed alongside the esophagus within the fundic collar.

For specific reasons, such as in patients with previous left upper quadrant infections or multiple operations, or patients with esophageal strictures in whom the nature of the operation to be performed will be determined intraoperatively, a direct transthoracic approach is undertaken.

REFERENCES

1. Nissen, R.: Chirurgische Erkrankungen der Speiseröhre. Langenbeck's Arch. Klin. Chir. 276:344–356, 1953
2. Ravitch, M.M., Rowe, M.I., and Halperin, D.C.: Hernia of the esophageal hiatus in infants. Illinois Medical Journal 134:269–273, 1968

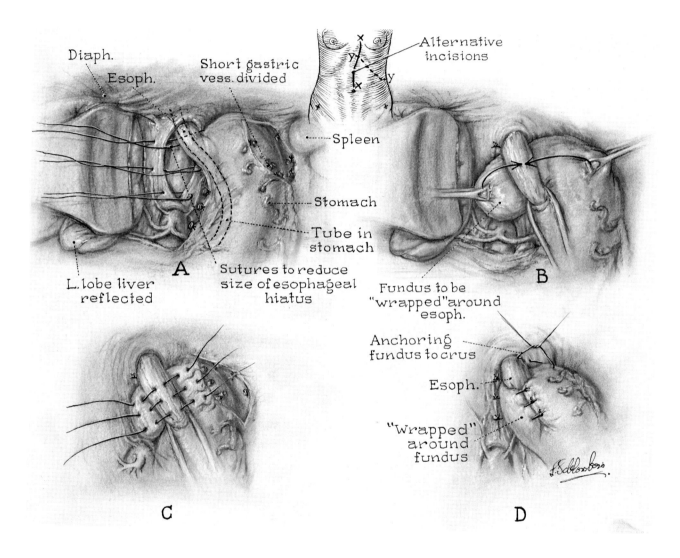

Diaph.

Esoph.

Short gastric
vess. divided

Alternative
incisions

Spleen

Stomach

Tube in
stomach

L. lobe liver
reflected

Sutures to reduce
size of esophageal
hiatus

A

B

Fundus to be
"wrapped" around
esoph.

Anchoring
fundus to crus

Esoph.

"Wrapped"
around
fundus

C

D

THE BELSEY FUNDOPLICATION

A. Mobilization of the distal esophagus and cardia is through a left 6th interspace lateral thoracotomy. The esophagus, with vagus nerves attached, is completely freed up to the lung root. The hernia sac is entered anteriorly, and the entire circumference of the cardia is separated from its attachments. This requires division of branches from the left inferior phrenic artery laterally (illustrated) and left gastric artery posteriorly (not shown).

B. At the start of the repair, sutures are placed in the crura, across the hiatus posteriorly, but are not tied until the completion of the reconstruction. Tension on a Babcock clamp applied to the diaphragm anteriorly makes it easier to identify the strong tendinous tissue in the crus where the sutures should be placed.

C. After complete mobilization of the esophagogastric junction, the pad of fibrofatty tissue at the cardia is excised anteriorly and laterally. The vagus nerves, which tend to be elevated off the esophagus during this dissection, are carefully preserved.

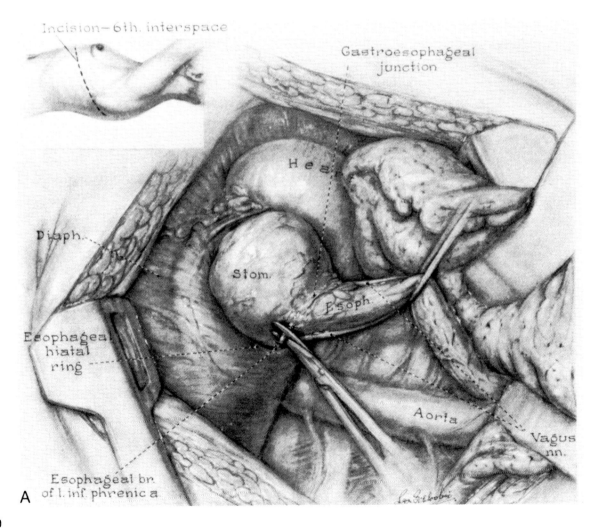

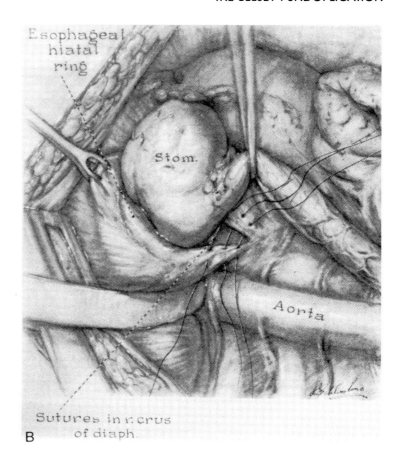

Esophageal
hiatal
ring

Stom.

Aorta

Sutures in r. crus
of diaph.

B

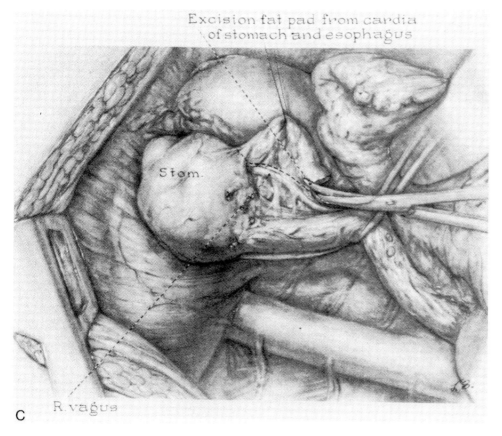

Excision fat pad from cardia
of stomach and esophagus

Stom.

R. vagus

C

THE BELSEY FUNDOPLICATION (Continued)

D. *Top*: The reconstruction is started by placing the first of three mattress sutures between the fundus of the stomach and the esophagus 2 cm above the junction. The spacing of these sutures around the circumference of the esophagus is shown in the cross-sectional inset. *Bottom*: After completion of the first row of sutures, a second row of three mattress sutures is placed through the diaphragm, fundus, and esophagus. In the illustration, the first suture is in place, and the second is being passed through the diaphragm in the bowl of a spoon retractor, which is used to protect structures beneath the diaphragm. The posterior sutures in the crus have still not been tied.

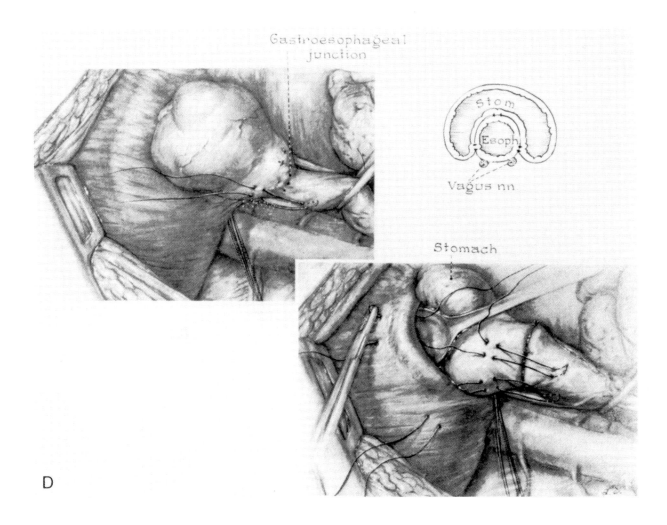

D

392

E. Sagittal sections of the repair. *Left*: The sutures in the crura posteriorly have been placed but not yet tied. The first row of mattress sutures between stomach and esophagus have been tied. One of the mattress sutures in the second row is illustrated. *Right*: The completed repair. The posterior sutures in the crura and second row of mattress sutures joining the diaphragm, stomach, and esophagus are tied after the reconstruction has been placed beneath the diaphragm.

From Skinner, D.B.: Hiatal hernia and esophageal reflux. In: *Davis-Christopher Textbook of Surgery*, 12th Edition, D.C. Sabiston, Jr. (Ed.). Philadelphia, W.B. Saunders Company, 1981, with permission.

REFERENCE

1. Belsey, R.H.R., and Skinner, D.B.: Surgical treatment: Thoracic approach. In: *Gastroesophageal Reflux and Hiatal Hernia*, D.B. Skinner, R.H.R. Belsey, T.R. Hendrix, and G.D. Zuidema (Eds.). Boston, Little, Brown, & Co., 1972

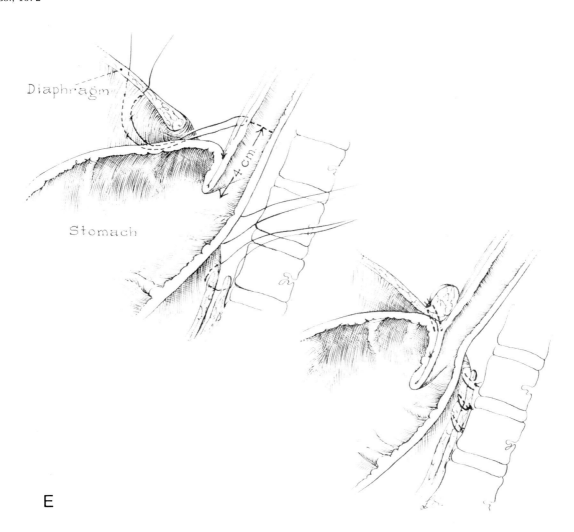

E

THE HILL PROCEDURE

A. The esophagus has been dissected out of the hiatus and the stomach retracted to the left. The vessels and the celiac plexus are here shown to indicate their anatomical location, but they are not operatively dissected out in this clarity. The diaphragmatic crura are reapposed by mattress sutures behind the esophagus.

B. The stomach is sutured by a series of interrupted sutures to the crus of the diaphragm, at the medial arcuate ligament over the midpoint of the aorta and immediately above the trunk of the celiac axis. The edge of the medial arcuate ligament is defined by carefully elevating the preaortic fascia, using blunt-tipped scissors, as shown, or a right-angled clamp. On the left side is shown a suture elevating the fundus of the stomach to the border of the esophageal hiatus, recreating the angle of His.

REFERENCES

1. Hill, L.D., Chapman, K.W., and Morgan, E.H.: Objective evaluation of surgery for hiatus hernia and esophagitis. J. Thorac. Cardiovasc. Surg. 41:60–74, 1961
2. Russell, C.O.H., and Hill, L.D.: Gastroesophageal reflux. Current Problems in Surgery, April 1983

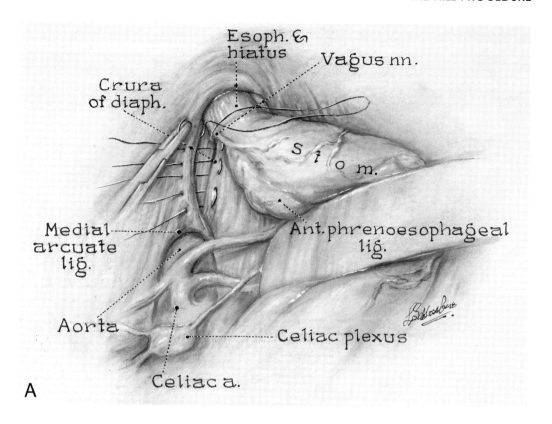

A

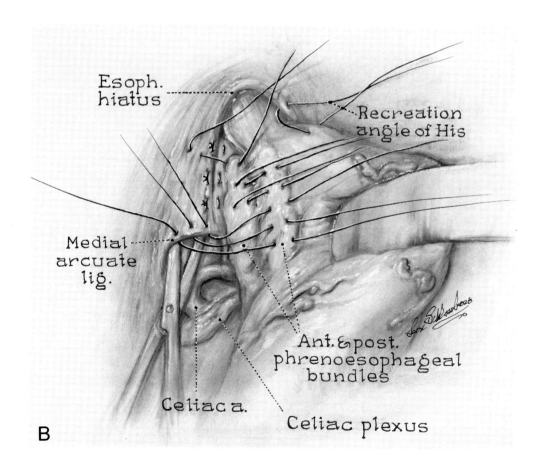

B

THE COMBINED COLLIS GASTROESOPHAGOPLASTY AND NISSEN FUNDOPLICATION

The approach is through a low left posterolateral incision and the bed of the unremoved 6th rib.

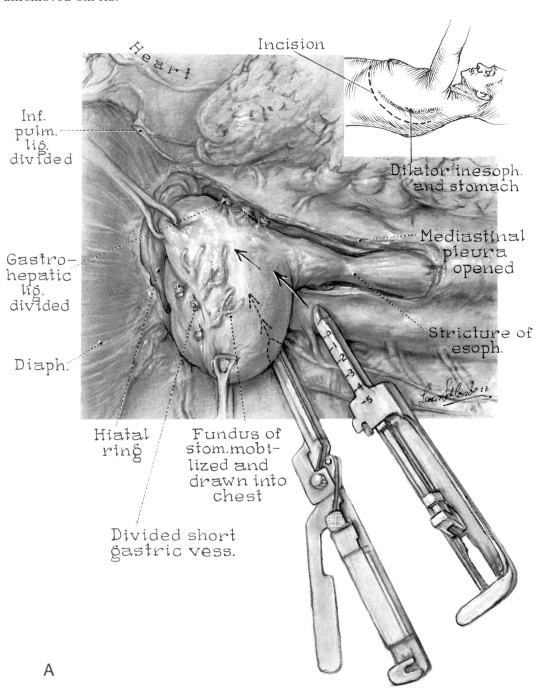

A

A. The mediastinal pleura overlying the lower esophagus is opened, and the shortened, strictured esophagus is dissected out. Through the enlarged hiatus, the fundus of the stomach is mobilized and drawn into the chest. This maneuver is facilitated by dividing three or four short gastric vessels along the greater curvature and, often, the left gastric vessels along the lesser curvature. The arrows indicate the direction in which the GIA stapler is to be passed.

B. The GIA instrument has been applied, compressing the anterior and posterior walls of the fundus between the anterior staple-carrying and posterior anvil-carrying arms of the instrument, in a vertical direction that creates a prolongation of the esophagus onto the lesser curvature of the stomach, making the gastric tube wide enough to allow for the placement of reinforcing sutures without producing too narrow a tube. As the instrument is activated by advancing the stapler pusher-knife assembly, two rows of staples are placed on either side of the dividing knife blade.

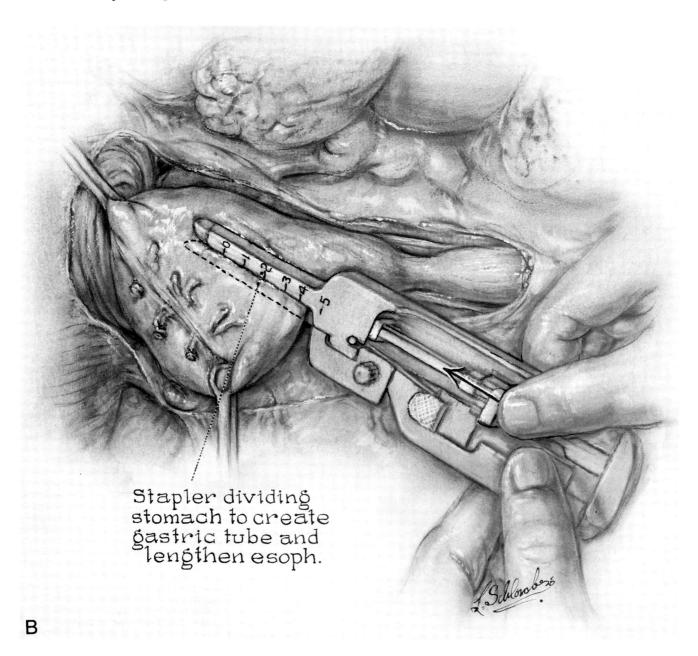

Stapler dividing
stomach to create
gastric tube and
lengthen esoph.

B

THE COMBINED COLLIS GASTROESOPHAGOPLASTY
(Continued)

C. *Top left*: The gastric tube, created as a prolongation of the esophagus, has now been separated from the remainder of the fundus with a double row of staples on both sides. The GIA staple lines are reinforced with a simple over-and-over manual suture, our recommendation when the GIA instrument is employed to suture together two thicknesses of stomach wall. *Top right*: The posteromedial aspect of the fully mobilized fundus is now passed behind the gastric tube (neoesophagus). Three sutures are placed to effect the fundic wrap, which creates a collar of fundus around the gastric tube. Since the tube, or neoesophagus, is formed by muscular gastric wall, the sutures can safely take bites in the tube wall. Before the sutures are tied, the stricture is dilated under direct vision up to a No. 32–34 with a mercury bougie, which is left in place during the tying. The wrap should be sufficiently relaxed to allow for the introduction of the 5th finger between neoesophagus and fundic collar. *Bottom left*: The stomach is sutured to the arcuate ligament (preaortic fascia) to fix it in the abdomen. *Bottom right*: The enlarged esophageal hiatus is then appropriately narrowed with sutures taken in the crura, behind the esophagus (as indicated by the dotted lines).

D. The gastric "wrap around," a Nissen procedure modified by the anatomical effect of the Collis gastroplasty, has been anchored either posteriorly to the arcuate ligament, as shown, or to the diaphragmatic crus with a suture through the upper margin of the gastric collar. Orringer and others employ a simpler modified Nissen wrap. Pearson and Henderson prefer the Belsey vertical inversion of the neoesophagus.

REFERENCES

1. Collis, J.L., Kelly, T.D., and Wiley, A.M.: Anatomy of the crura of the diaphragm and the surgery of hiatus hernia. Thorax 9:175–189, 1954
   Collis's original description of his procedure.
2. Collis, J.L.: An operation for hiatus hernia with short esophagus. J. Thorac. Surg. 34:768–777, 1957
   Collis's presentation before the American Association for Thoracic Surgery with discussions by Richard Sweet, Conrad Lam, Thomas Burford, Stuart Harrington, and others. The comments were complimentary, but enthusiasm was qualified.
3. Pearson, F.G., Langer, B., and Henderson, R.D.: Gastroplasty and Belsey hiatus hernia repair. J. Thorac. Cardiovasc. Surg. 61:50–63, 1971
4. Pearson, F.G., and Henderson, R.D.: Experimental and clinical studies of gastroplasty in the management of acquired short esophagus. Surg. Gynecol. Obstet. 136:737–744, 1973
5. Orringer, M.B., and Sloan, H.: An improved technique for the combined Collis-Belsey approach to dilatable esophageal strictures. J. Thorac. Cardiovasc. Surg. 68:298–302, 1974
6. Orringer, M.B., and Sloan, H.: Collis-Belsey reconstruction of the esophagogastric junction. Indications, physiology and technical considerations. J. Thorac. Cardiovasc. Surg. 71:295–303, 1976
7. Pearson, F.G.: Surgical management of acquired short esophagus with dilatable peptic stricture. World J. Surg. 1:463–473, 1977
   Pearson's experience since 1964 with the addition of a Belsey fundoplication to the Collis gastroplasty.
8. Orringer, M.B.: Combined Collis gastroplasty—Nissen fundoplication operation for reflux esophagitis. Surgical Rounds, August 1978, pp. 10–19
9. Steichen, F.M., and Ravitch, M.M.: *Stapling in Surgery.* Chicago, Year Book Medical Publishers, 1984

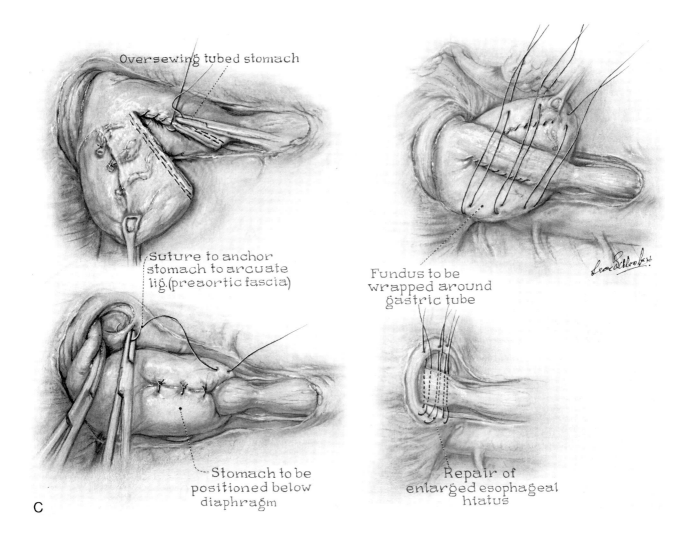

Oversewing tubed stomach

Suture to anchor stomach to arcuate lig.(preaortic fascia)

Stomach to be positioned below diaphragm

Fundus to be wrapped around gastric tube

Repair of enlarged esophageal hiatus

C

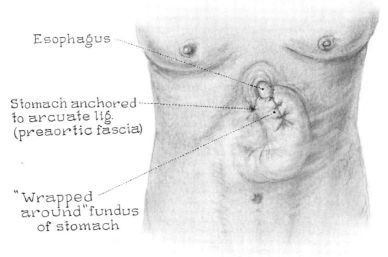

Esophagus

Stomach anchored to arcuate lig. (preaortic fascia)

"Wrapped around"fundus of stomach

D

Operation for Achalasia

HELLER OPERATION FOR ACHALASIA OF THE ESOPHAGUS

Although Heller's esophagomyotomy can be performed through the abdomen or through the chest, it is substantially easier to make the long esophageal myotomy, currently preferred, through the chest than through the abdomen.

A. Incision through the 7th interspace or rib bed exposes the esophagus. A bit of the fundus is delivered through the hiatus. The dotted line indicates the myotomy made with the knife. The myotomy is carried down just barely beyond the esophagogastric junction and up the esophagus for 6 to 10 cm.

B. The submucosa gapes widely, and dissection under the muscle edges with a Metzenbaum scissors (not shown) is often performed to increase the herniation of the submucosa. We have not seen the necessity for suturing the muscularis in its new position to the submucosa. With an incision of the length described, and the wide bulging of the submucosa, a regrowth of the musculature to recreate the original condition has seemed to us extremely unlikely. Not shown is a single suture tacking the fundus to the left border of the esophageal hiatus to recreate the angle of His (see pages 394–395, *Hill Procedure, B*). By the same token, we frequently place one or several sutures behind the esophagus to snug up the hiatus and further discourage the likelihood of reflux.

REFERENCES

1. Heller, E.: Extramuköse Cardioplastik beim chronischen Cardiospasmus mit Dilatation des Oesophagus. Mitt. Grenzgeb. Med. U. Chir. 27:141–149, 1914
   Heller's original paper.
2. Steichen, F.M., Heller, E., and Ravitch, M.M.: Achalasia of the esophagus. Surgery 47:846–876, 1960
   Investigation of the various operations for achalasia and of the reasons for the 30-year eclipse of Heller's procedure.
3. Ellis, F.H., Jr., Kiser, J.C., Schlegel, J.F., et al.: Esophagomyotomy for esophageal achalasia: Experimental, clinical, and manometric aspects. Ann. Surg. 166:640–656, 1967

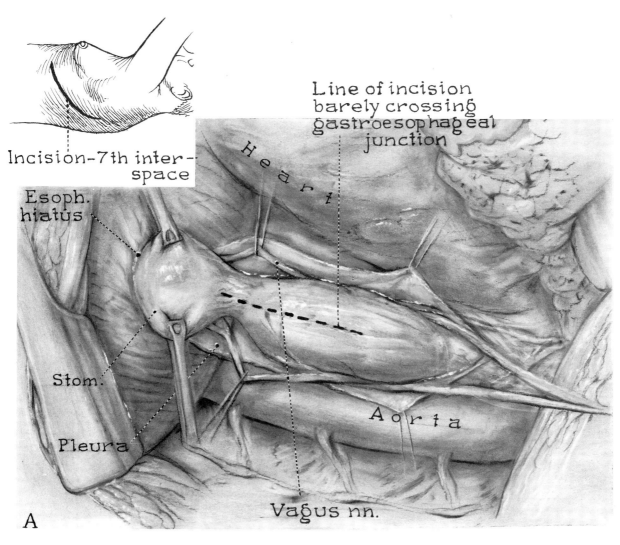

Incision–7th inter-space

Line of incision barely crossing gastroesophageal junction

Heart

Esoph. hiatus

Stom.

Pleura

Aorta

Vagus nn.

A

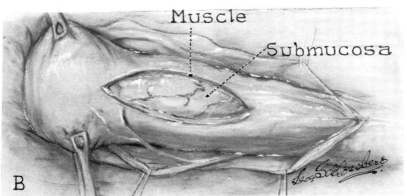

Muscle

Submucosa

B

Operations for Esophageal Atresia

TRACHEOESOPHAGEAL FISTULA—PRIMARY REPAIR—EXTRAPLEURAL APPROACH

A. The gastrostomy tube is shown, its insertion having been the initial procedure. This is routine in some clinics. We tend to reserve gastrostomy for sick infants—those with evidence of pneumonia or those in whom a large distal fistula has produced abdominal distention and respiratory distress, in which case gastrostomy is urgently required. In the absence of a specific need for gastrostomy, our own practice is to withhold gastrostomy unless the postoperative course indicates there will be a significant delay in establishing oral intake.

   Even more in infants than in older patients, it is important to avoid rib resection. The periosteum is reflected as shown and incision is carried through it posteriorly to the pleura, which is carefully stripped away from the underside of the ribs with blunt dissectors. With a little experience, it proves surprisingly easy to provide the wide mediastinal exposure shown, from the apex of the chest to the level of the carina or below, as required to expose the distal esophageal segment. The lung contained in its pleural sac is easily retracted without multiple abrasive gauze packs and trauma to the lung. From time to time, the retractor may be removed, the lung fully expanded for a few breaths, and exposure regained almost immediately by insertion of the retractor. The consequences of an anastomotic leak are minimized by the extrapleural approach. The controversy over the relative virtues of the transpleural and retropleural approach have been largely resolved with the general acceptance of the retropleural approach. If the dilated and hypertrophied proximal esophageal pouch does not present at once, its position is readily disclosed by the anesthetist's passing a catheter from above. The azygos vein is clearly shown.

B. The azygos vein has been ligated and divided, and the anatomical relationships are fully disclosed. The vagus, here shown with a tape around it, is best merely identified and left undisturbed. The lower ribbon retractor should be shown up over the bag of pleura and not pressing into it. Sharp dissection with small Metzenbaum scissors exposes the proximal segment. If the gap to be bridged is large, the proximal segment may be safely dissected into the cupola of the hemithorax. A second fistula, from the upper pouch, is not exquisitely rare and should be looked for. The circulation of the distal esophageal segment is less secure. Distal dissection should be held to the minimum required for anastomosis.

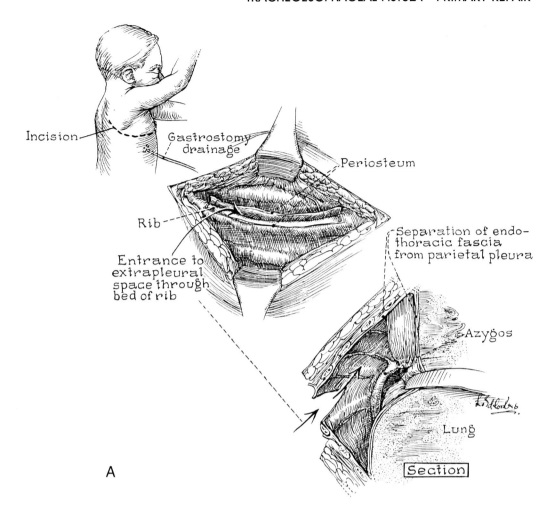

Incision

Gastrostomy drainage

Periosteum

Rib

Separation of endo-thoracic fascia from parietal pleura

Entrance to extrapleural space through bed of rib

Azygos

Lung

Section

A

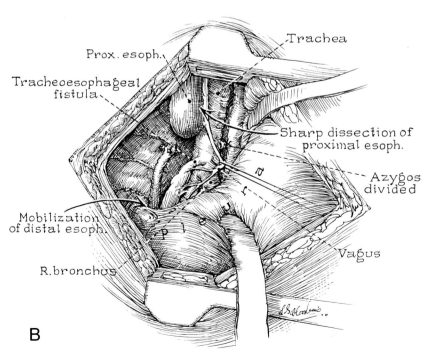

Prox. esoph.

Trachea

Tracheoesophageal fistula

Sharp dissection of proximal esoph.

Azygos divided

Mobilization of distal esoph.

Vagus

R. bronchus

B

C. The fistula is cut away from the trachea, leaving a millimeter or two of the fistulous tract attached to the trachea for closure by interrupted or continuous sutures of very fine nonabsorbable sutures. Cameron Haight's original technique of anastomosis is illustrated. Traction on the proximal pouch is made by a suture as shown. The submucosa is separated from the muscularis of the proximal segment. The anastomosis is made in two layers, the first with a series of interrupted, fine, nonabsorbable sutures through the submucosa and mucosa of the proximal segment and the full thickness of the distal segment. After the posterior closure has been completed, the muscularis of the proximal segment is brought down over the posterior anastomotic line and sutured to the distal segment. Advancing the esophageal catheter into the distal segment facilitates the identical insertion of the anterior sutures. This remains our preferred technique, although a good many surgeons are achieving equally good results with a single layer of through-and-through sutures. It is probable that the leakage rate is diminished by the Haight anastomosis, at the possible expense of an increased incidence of stricture. A suction catheter is placed posteriorly alongside, but not against, the anastomosis, held in place against the posterior wall by a fine catgut suture.

From Haller, J.A., Jr., and White, J.J.: Pediatric Surgery. In: *Operative Surgery—Principles and Techniques,* 2nd Edition, P.F. Nora (Ed.). Philadelphia, Lea & Febiger, 1980, with permission.

REFERENCES

1. Haight, C., and Towsley, H.A.: Congenital atresia of the esophagus with tracheoesophageal fistula. Extrapleural ligation of fistula and end-to-end anastomosis of esophageal segments. Surg. Gynecol. Obstet. 76:672–688, 1943
   Haight's classic "first" in which his approach was posterior, and extrapleural, but from the left side.
2. Holder, T.M., and Ashcraft, K.W.: Esophageal atresia and tracheo-esophageal fistula. Current Problems in Surgery, August 1966
   Comprehensive monograph.

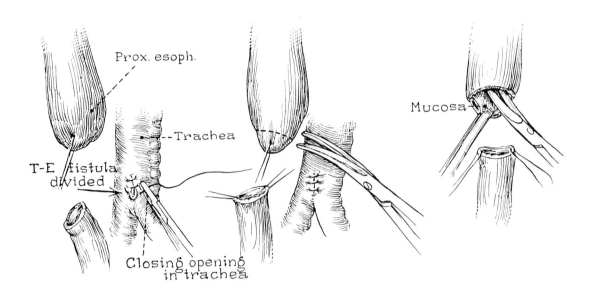

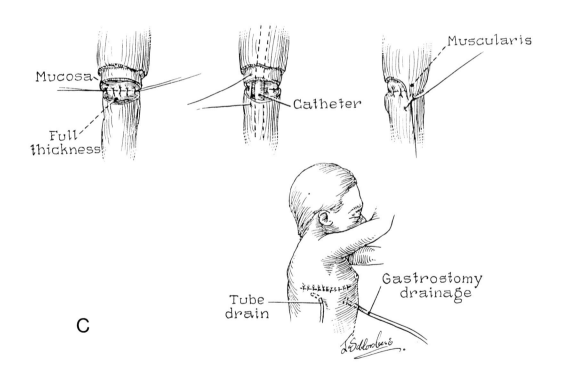

C

ESOPHAGEAL ATRESIA WITHOUT FISTULA—
TRANSTHORACIC COLON INTERPOSITION (WATERSTON PROCEDURE)

It has become increasingly possible to support some infants with isolated esophageal atresia by gastrostomy until, with growth, and with or without bougienage, the two ends of the esophagus approximate and direct anastomosis is feasible. Nevertheless, in many infants with a wide esophageal gap, with or without a fistula, and in some infants with failed repair, esophageal reconstruction is required. The two methods commonly employed are either the reverse greater curvature tube (see page 362, *Greater Curvature Gastric Tube for Replacement of the Esophagus*) or the colon interposition, usually by the technique of David Waterston, shown here.

A. The chest has been entered through the periosteal bed of the unresected 7th rib. Waterston gained access to the abdomen in the manner shown by peripheral incision in the diaphragm, leaving just enough of an edge attached to the wall for subsequent closure (see page 382, *Esophageal Replacement, Colon Interposition—Transthoracic, Transdiaphragmatic Approach*). Currently, often a separate incision is generally made in the abdominal midline, leaving the diaphragm undisturbed. The patient will in almost all cases already have a gastrostomy (not shown).

B. The stomach and colon are readily exposed through the long, curved peripheral diaphragmatic incision. The gastrocolic ligament is divided, freeing up the colon. We prefer merely to elevate the omentum from the colon.

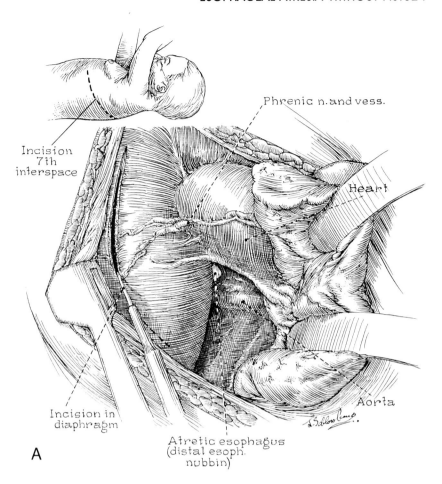

Phrenic n. and vess.

Heart

Incision 7th interspace

Aorta

Incision in diaphragm

Atretic esophagus (distal esoph. nubbin)

A

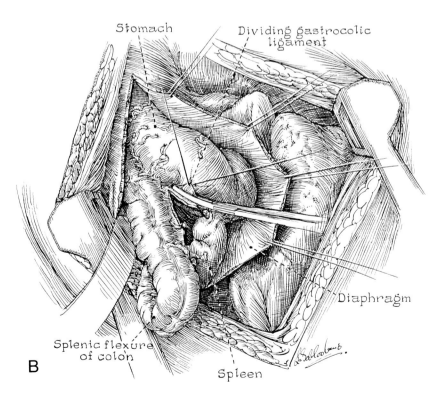

Stomach

Dividing gastrocolic ligament

Diaphragm

Splenic flexure of colon

Spleen

B

ESOPHAGEAL ATRESIA WITHOUT FISTULA *(Continued)*

C. The desired segment of colon has been isolated by proximal and distal division, and continuity of the colon is restored. Waterston's usual preference was for the use of the left colon. Our own preference is for the right colon. The drawings show the use of the left colon inserted isoperistaltically. The indifferent peristalsis in the colon permits successful use of the left colon antiperistaltically. Before dividing the colon, it is essential to measure the gap that must be bridged and to determine that the isolated colonic segment will be of sufficient length. In the illustration, the left transverse colon, splenic flexure, and proximal descending colon are shown being brought up in the chest; the circulation is entirely dependent upon the marginal vessels and the ascending branch of the left colic artery.

D. If there is a nubbin of distal esophagus sufficient for anastomosis, the colon is brought up as shown through a separate incision in the diaphragm. It is always brought up behind the stomach and may be brought up behind the pancreas as well, providing the shortest possible course. If the distal esophageal stump appears to be inadequate for anastomosis, it is ignored, the colon is brought up through the esophageal hiatus and the cologastrostomy is performed below the diaphragm.

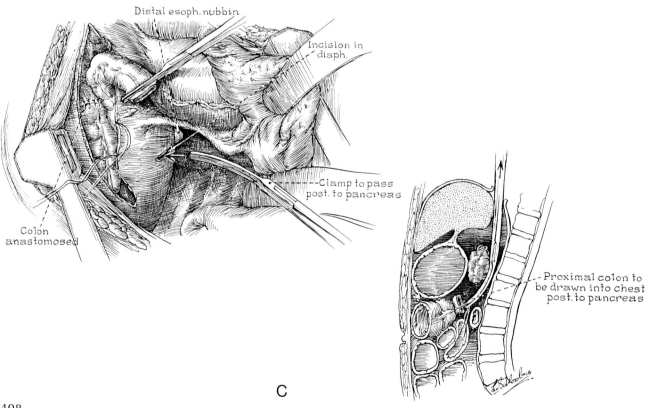

Distal esoph. nubbin

Incision in diaph.

Clamp to pass post. to pancreas

Colon anastomosed

Proximal colon to be drawn into chest post. to pancreas

C

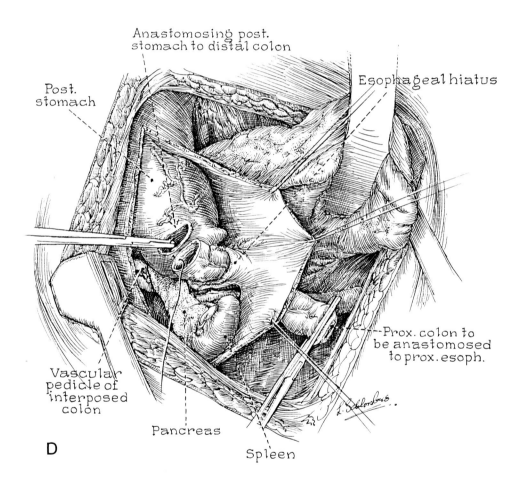

Post.
stomach

Anastomosing post.
stomach to distal colon

Esophageal hiatus

Vascular
pedicle of
interposed
colon

Prox. colon to
be anastomosed
to prox. esoph.

Pancreas

Spleen

D

E. Frequently a prior cervical esophagostomy requires making the anastomosis in the neck, which is, in any case, preferred by many. Here a satisfactory proximal pouch *in situ* is shown being directly anastomosed to the colon, end-to-end. The risk of this procedure is that if a leak occurs, it will be in the thorax. However, the need for the greater length of colon required to reach the neck and the tunneling into the neck through the cupola of the hemithorax are avoided.

The peripheral incision in the diaphragm is closed as in *Esophageal Replacement, Colon Interposition—Transthoracic, Transdiaphragmatic Approach.*

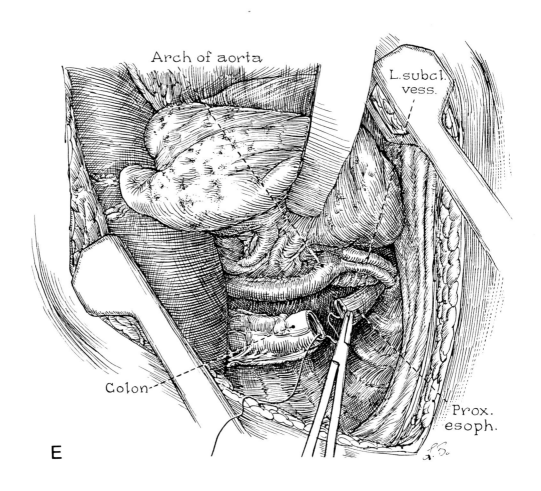

E

F. Final reconstruction. The top figure shows the colon that has been brought isoperistaltically through the stab wound in the diaphragm and anastomosed to the esophageal stump, below, and to the cervical esophagus, above. The lower figure shows the segment of colon brought up in the same manner through the small incision in the diaphragm, with the distal end then brought down through the hiatus for anastomosis to the stomach and the proximal end anastomosed end-to-end to the esophagus in the chest. If the colon is to be brought through the esophageal hiatus, we prefer to pass the colon with its vascular pedicle through the hiatus without the need for a counterincision in the diaphragm.

From Haller, J.A., Jr., and White, J.J.: Pediatric Surgery. In: *Operative Surgery—Principles and Techniques*, 2nd Edition, P.F. Nora (Ed.). Philadelphia, Lea & Febiger, 1980, with permission.

REFERENCES

1. Waterston, D.J.: Replacement of oesophagus with transverse colon. Thoraxchirurgie 11:73–74, 1963
2. Waterston, D.J.: Colonic replacement of esophagus (intrathoracic). Surg. Clin. North Am. 44:1441–1447, 1964

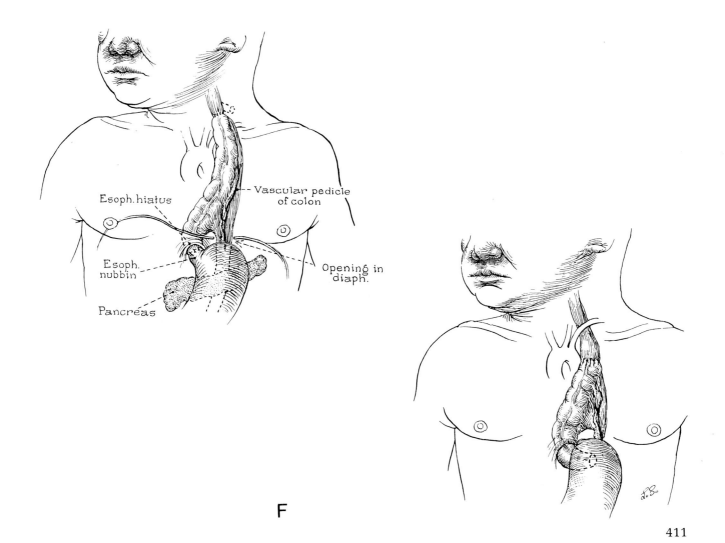

F

TRACHEOESOPHAGEAL "H" FISTULA

The "H" fistula, usually obliquely directed, is almost invariably best approached in the neck by the exposure shown. The difficulty is generally in the diagnosis and not in the operation if the fistula is low in the neck, as it usually is. The approach is medial to the sternocleidomastoid muscle, usually low enough so that the middle thyroid vein need not be divided. The two ends of the fistula are divided a millimeter or two outside the walls of the trachea and the esophagus, and the ends are oversewn.

From Haller, J.A., Jr., and White, J.J.: Pediatric Surgery. In: *Operative Surgery—Principles and Techniques,* 2nd Edition, P.F. Nora (Ed.). Philadelphia, Lea & Febiger, 1980, with permission.

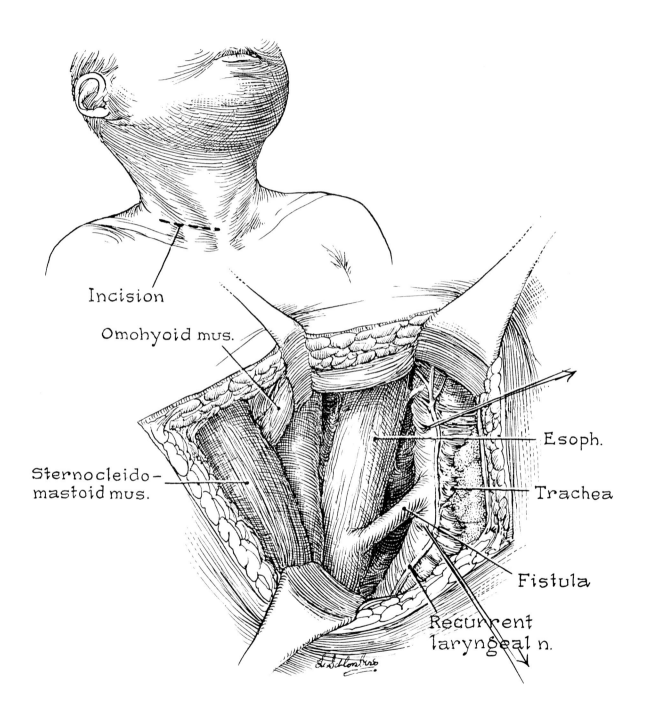

Incision

Omohyoid mus.

Sternocleido-
mastoid mus.

Esoph.

Trachea

Fistula

Recurrent
laryngeal n.

INDEX

Note: Page numbers in *italics* refer to illustrations.

415